Recent Advances in the Science of Cannabis

Recent Advances in the Science of Cannabis

Edited by
Robert M. Strongin, Jiries Meehan-Atrash, and Monica Vialpando

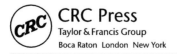

CRC Press
Taylor & Francis Group
Boca Raton London New York

CRC Press is an imprint of the
Taylor & Francis Group, an **informa** business

First edition published 2022
by CRC Press
6000 Broken Sound Parkway NW, Suite 300, Boca Raton, FL 33487-2742

and by CRC Press
2 Park Square, Milton Park, Abingdon, Oxon, OX14 4RN

© 2022 Taylor & Francis Group, LLC

CRC Press is an imprint of Taylor & Francis Group, LLC

ISBN: 978-0-367-22442-4 (hbk)
ISBN: 978-1-032-11959-5 (pbk)
ISBN: 978-0-429-27489-3 (ebk)

DOI: 10.1201/9780429274893

Typeset in Times
by Deanta Global Publishing Services, Chennai, India

Contents

Preface

On behalf of my two co-editors, Dr. Jiries Meehan-Atrash and Dr. Monica Vialpando, we hope you find this book to be a valuable resource, regardless of your level of expertise in the cannabis field. This volume was conceived during the 2019–2020 EVALI outbreak, and was completed during the Covid era. I first met Jiries several years earlier, when he inquired about earning his doctoral degree in organic chemistry in my research group. I already had an ongoing project focused on ENDS (electronic nicotine delivery systems) chemistry, and it was a logical transition for us to investigate cannabis extracts and vaping, which were becoming increasingly prevalent. Jiries and I soon published the first papers on the chemistry of vaping and dabbing terpenes, cannabinoids, and concentrated THC formulations. Apart from being a brilliant and dedicated scientist, it turns out that Jiries was also a talented and experienced science writer, and was thus an obvious choice to co-edit this book. After our first paper in the cannabis field was published in 2017, Nigam Arora (to whom I will always be indebted), invited me to give a talk at an upcoming American Chemical Society (ACS) meeting in the Cannabis Chemistry Subdivision (CANN) session. Soon after the meeting, Nigam introduced me to Monica Vialpando, another ACS CANN co-organizer. Monica turned out to be one of the most dynamic innovators and entrepreneurs that I have ever met. She is a leading expert in formulations for vaping, oral and topical products. We had much in common in that Monica also had extensive prior experience in the tobacco vaping field, but from the industry side. During the EVALI outbreak, there was a relatively high degree of misinformation and uncertainty surrounding the emerging cannabis field. We thus felt that a timely, new contribution highlighting evidence-based studies and ongoing scientific research was needed. This is what motivated the creation of this book.

The cannabis science field is currently too broad and too dynamic to allow for coverage of all significant and timely areas of interest in just one volume. However, the reader will find a diverse collection of important current topics herein, with contributions from leading experts from both academia and industry. The first five chapters cover cultivation toward optimizing the production of medicinally relevant secondary metabolites, the relationship between cannabis aroma, chemotypes, and pharmacology, an extensive overview of classical as well as new and unique cannabinoid structures, and cannabis analytical chemistry with a focus on mass spectrometry, chromatographic techniques, and sample processing. Chapters 6–10 cover issues in microbial testing, cannabis extract vaping and associated potential public health and regulatory issues, the science of transdermal delivery of cannabinoids, cannabis vaping chemistry, and cannabinoid pharmacokinetics and pharmacodynamics.

We would like to thank Carolyn Burek, who helped us greatly early on with editing. A very special thanks goes to Jessica Painter whose effort and dedication to this effort were invaluable, and at times, bordering on the heroic. Finally, we owe a great deal of gratitude to the contributing authors of each chapter. Writing a quality book chapter of course requires a non-trivial effort, and takes precious time away from one's busy career. We deeply appreciate all of you. Without your hard work and timely contributions this book would not have been possible.

Professor Robert M. Strongin
Portland, Oregon

Editors

Robert M. Strongin is a Professor of Organic Chemistry at Portland State University. He has studied the chemistry of vaping since 2013. He has been interested in determining how flavorings, including terpenes and other vape constituents, react and degrade when heated and aerosolized. In 2017 he began to investigate cannabis vaping and published the first peer-reviewed reports on the specific byproducts formed when dabbing terpenes, and, more recently, on the reactions and products that form upon vaping and dabbing concentrated cannabis oil mixtures. Dr. Strongin runs an internationally recognized research program, is a founder of two biotech startup companies, and is known for his contributions to STEM education. In addition to tobacco control and cannabis science, he is an expert in the field of biosensors and targeted molecular probes for imaging cancer tissue.

Jiries Meehan-Atrash graduated from the State University of New York at New Paltz with a Bachelor of Science in Chemistry in 2014 and in 2021 earned his PhD in Chemistry from Portland State University after studying e-cigarette aerosol chemistry and analytical methods under the mentorship of Dr. Robert M. Strongin. Jiries is currently a postdoctoral fellow at the University of Rochester Medical Center in the laboratory of Dr. Irfan Rahman.

Monica Vialpando is a pharmaceutically trained product development scientist, specializing in the formulation of poorly water-soluble drugs. As founder and CEO of Via Innovations, a bespoke product development company, she integrates this background with plant-based medicines to create fit-for-purpose designed products. In addition to her entrepreneurial endeavors, she is active in education and thought leadership and often focuses on cannabis-based strategies to support women's health, and is a scientific advisor to multiple organizations. With a passion for diversity and global connection, Dr. Vialpando's reach extends beyond typical barriers to collaborate with international experts and companies. She also leverages this throughout her company to design their differentiated products through the integration of plant-based medicines, science, technology, and art.

Contributors

John S. Abrams
The Clinical Endocannabinoid System
Consortium
San Diego, CA

Kyle Boyar
Skaggs School of Pharmacy and
Pharmaceutical Sciences
University of California
San Diego, CA

Carolyn Burek
Via Innovations
Desert Hot Springs, CA

David Dawson
CW Analytical
Oakland, CA

Brad Douglass
The Werc Shop
Seattle, WA
and
Portland State University
Portland, OR

William J. T. Ellyson
The Clinical Endocannabinoid System
Consortium
San Diego, CA

Victor J. Gomez
The Clinical Endocannabinoid System
Consortium
San Diego, CA

Zacariah L. Hildenbrand
University of Texas at El Paso
El Paso, TX

Allegra Leghissa
Shimadzu France

Roberto Mandrioli
University of Bologna
Bologna, Italy

Jiries Meehan-Atrash
Portland State University
Portland, OR

Laura Mercolini
University of Bologna
Bologna, Italy

Jessica Painter
Via Innovations
Desert Hot Springs, CA

Michele Protti
University of Bologna
Bologna, Italy

Markus Roggen
Delic Labs
Vancouver, BC

Callie Seaman
AquaLabs Ltd.
Sheffield, UK

Ted W. Simon
Ted Simon LLC
Winston, GA

Robert M. Strongin
Portland State University
Portland, OR

Jean L. Talleyrand
The Clinical Endocannabinoid System
Consortium
San Diego, CA

Monica Vialpando
Via Innovations
Desert Hot Springs, CA

1 Cultivation Stress Techniques and the Production of Secondary Metabolites in *Cannabis sativa*

Callie Seaman

CONTENTS

DOI: 10.1201/9780429274893-1

1.1   INTRODUCTION

Cannabis sativa could be described as one of the most chemically complex plants used in Western medicine today. It has been propagated and utilized by humankind for numerous purposes through thousands of years of our history as a source of nutrition for both animals and humans, as well as for fibers, building materials, fuel, and medicine (Romero et al. 2020). Differing levels of prohibition from the 14th century to today have undoubtedly slowed progress in our understanding of the full potential of the plant.

Cannabis sativa is dioecious, meaning male and female blossoms generally appear on separate plants. It is the resinous oil produced by the unpollinated mature female flowers that holds the greatest scientific and monetary value today. Although they can be found throughout the plant, this oil contains the highest concentration of hundreds of different secondary metabolites each with a potential array of medicinal properties (Andre, Hausman, and Guerriero 2016) (Flores-Sanchez and Verpoorte 2008b). While other secondary metabolites, including flavonoids, stilbenoids, lignans, and alkaloids all have important qualities, terpenoids, comprised of terpenes and cannabinoids, are the most widely acknowledged for their medical potential.

Before the 2012 legalization of its recreational use in Colorado and Washington, there was a particular and narrow focus on the major cannabinoids, cannabidiol (CBD) and tetrahydrocannabinol (THC), driven by the interests of the therapeutic sector. Since legalization, there has been a dramatic surge in academic publications on cannabis, with end-user demand fueling a wider understanding of properties and factors beyond the plants' psychoactive components such as flavor (de la Fuente et al. 2020). A more sophisticated understanding of cannabis has flourished as a result (Romero et al. 2020).

It has been well documented that the ratio of phytocannabinoids is important for the successful treatment of specific diseases (Lowe et al. 2018) (McPartland and Russo 2001) (Gordon 2020) (Nelson 2018) (Goldstein 2016) (Rosenburg et al. 2015). With increased research and understanding of the entourage effect, there is a greater demand from physicians for full plant extract alongside the isolate form of the compound (Romano and Hazekamp 2018) (Russo 2019) (Ben-Shabat et al. 1998) (Blasco-Benito, Seijo-Vila, et al. 2018). The ratios of phytocannabinoids and terpenes are now being further investigated to better understand their effects when used in conjunction with one another (de la Fuente et al. 2020) (Heblinski et al. 2020). In turn, this drives demand for strains to be bred to produce ratios of secondary metabolites that are disease-specific and will therefore require less processing, potentially reducing the cost of the end product (Thomas and Pollard 2016). Safeguarding patients is the top priority, but many factors must be considered when cultivating medicinal crops, with the consistency of production of both biomass and active ingredients of particular importance. In response to biotic and abiotic stress, plants produce phytoalexins, a large group of diverse secondary metabolites, which can cause a reduction in biomass. In this review, we will take a brief look at how stress to the plants affects the production of secondary metabolites such as phytocannabinoids, terpenes, and flavonoids.

1.2   WHAT ARE SECONDARY METABOLITES?

Secondary metabolites are compounds produced by the plant that are not essential for plant growth and are produced to enhance the chances of survival either through defense or increased attraction for reproduction.

1.2.1   Types of Secondary Metabolites

Approximately 565 secondary metabolites have been identified in cannabis (Romero et al. 2020), which can be split into six classes: cannabinoids, terpenes, flavonoids, stilbenoids, lignans, and alkaloids (Flores-Sanchez and Verpoorte 2008b). Here we will focus on the three most reported groups of active compounds of therapeutic interest. To date, these include over 140 cannabinoids (Gülck and Møller 2020), 110 terpenes (Hanuš and Hod 2020), and 20 flavonoids (Andre, Hausman, and Guerriero 2016). Table 1.1 summarizes the most documented secondary metabolites found in *Cannabis sativa* (Andre, Hausman, and Guerriero 2016).

1.2.1.1   Phytocannabinoids

Phytocannabinoids are primarily produced in nature by *Cannabis sativa*; however, research has shown that small quantities of cannabinoids have been found in hops and flaxseed (ElSohly 2017) (Andre, Hausman and Guerriero 2016). These compounds mimic our own endocannabinoids and interact with the endocannabinoid system (see also Chapter 10), enabling them to be used as a treatment for a variety of conditions, from epilepsy to pain (Gordon 2020) (Rosenburg et al. 2015). These are found in their highest concentration within the oils produced in the hair-like structures known as trichomes on the female flower and "sugar leaves" close to the flowers, though they have been detected in seeds, seedlings, roots, stems, leaves, and pollen (Aizpurua-Olaizola et al. 2016) (Frassinetti et al. 2018).

These compounds are the most studied group of secondary metabolites in cannabis research. To date, there are over 140 cannabinoids recorded that can be divided into ten main structural types (Table 1.1).

The major cannabinoids found in fresh plant material are tetrahydrocannabinolic acid (THCA) and cannabidiolic acid (CBDA), which decarboxylate to the more psychoactive neutral forms, THC and CBD (Hanuš, Meyer et al. 2016).

Cannabinoids are composed of 22 carbon atoms in their acid form, and after decarboxylation, 21 carbons in their neutral form. They are derived from diterpene structures and are terpenophenolic and are therefore much larger than the predominant terpenes found in cannabis (Hanuš and Hod 2020).

TABLE 1.1
The Three Major Groups of Secondary Metabolites Found in *Cannabis sativa*

	Phytocannabinoids	Terpenes		Flavonoids
		Monoterpenes	*Sesquiterpenes*	
Main production site	Bulbous trichomes on flowers and leaves	Bulbous trichomes on flowers and leaves	Sessile trichomes on flowers and leaves	Roots, leaves, seedlings, and stems
Precursors	Hexanoyl-CoA Olivetolic acid	Pyruvate G3P	Acetyl-CoA	Phenylalanine
Biosynthesis pathways	Polyketide pathway DOXP/MEP pathway	MEP pathway	MVA pathway	Phenylpropanoid pathway
Groups (number recorded) and examples	Δ^9-THC type (23) Δ^8-THC type (5) CBG type (16) CBD type (7) CBE type (5) CBN type (11) CBC type (9) CBT type (9) CBL type (3) CBND type (2) CBDV – cannabidivarin THCV – tetrahydrocannabivarin CBCV – cannabichromevarin CBGV – cannabigerovarin CBV – cannabivarin CBGM – cannabigerol monomethyl ether CBDHQ – cannabidiol hydroxyquinone THCP – tetrahydrocannabiphorol	β-pinene Myrcene Limonene Linalool α-pinene Terpinolene β-thujone Terpineol Cineole α-terpinene β-ocimene Borneol Geraniol Eucalyptol Isopulegol Pulegone Delta 3 Carene	α-humulene β-farnesene β-caryophyllene α-cubebene α-elemol β-farnesol Guaiol Bisabolol α-bergamotene δ-cadinene Valencene Eremophilene Nerolidol *Diterpenes* Camphorene	*Aglycones* Kaempferol Apigenin Luteolin Quercetin Vitexin Isovitexin Orientin Apigenin-7-O-Glu Cannaflavin A Cannaflavin B Cannaflavin C Anthocyanin Peonidin

Notes: The cannabinoids are split into the ten types of cannabinoids and the number identified in brackets. THC = tetrahydrocannabinol; CBG = cannabigerol; CBD = cannabidiol; CBE = cannabielsoin; CBN = cannabinol; CBC = cannabichromene; CBT = cannabicitran; CBL = cannabicyclol; CBND = cannabinodiol; MVA = mevalonate; MEP = methylerythritol phosphate (ElSohly 2017) (Flores-Sanchez and Verpoorte 2008a) (Booth and Bohlmann 2019).

1.2.1.2 Terpenes/Terpenoids

Terpenes are found within many plants and are volatile compounds that produce the distinctive aromas of cannabis. Their aromatic properties serve many purposes, including antimicrobial and antiherbivory defense, plant-to-plant interaction, and insect attraction for pollination (Hanuš and Hod 2020) (Booth and Bohlmann 2019). Terpenoids are the largest group of secondary metabolites and encompass some cannabinoids. A plant's age plays an important role in its yield and the degree of aroma from its flowers (Flores-Sanchez and Verpoorte 2008b).

Terpenes are grouped depending on the number of isoprene units and size. These include monoterpenes ($C_{10}H_{16}$, MW = 136), sesquiterpenes ($C_{15}H_{24}$, MW = 204), diterpenes ($C_{20}H_{32}$, MW = 272), and triterpenes ($C_{30}H_{50}$, MW = 410). Each of these groups can then be further divided into the structural arrangements of either acyclic (open chain), monocyclic (one fused ring), bicyclic (two fused rings), or tricyclic (three fused rings) (Hanuš and Hod 2020).

The two major groups found in cannabis with the largest diversity of terpenes are monoterpenes and sesquiterpenes. Table 1.1 lists some of the most common terpenes found in cannabis (Hanuš and Hod 2020) (Hillig 2004) (Booth and Bohlmann 2019).

Adverse reactions within humans are most often attributed to terpenes, and it is usually a particular allergy to a specific molecule (Nelson 2018). An increase in production of a particular terpene by the plant will result in the full plant extract and end product altering in composition between batches.

1.2.1.3 Flavonoids

Flavonoids are a highly diverse group of secondary metabolites and are found throughout the plant kingdom. They are responsible for the red, blue, and purple coloring in leaves produced by the anthocyanin pigment in cannabis. Some of the less well-known flavonoids are found in the roots of the plant and have been shown to play a role in resistance to aluminum toxicity in maize (Winkel-Shirley 2002).

Flavonoids provide nutritional and health benefits to humans and contribute to a well-balanced diet. Although a large body of research has been conducted into flavonoids within other plants, significantly less has been carried out on flavonoids within cannabis. Relative to the other major secondary metabolites in cannabis, flavonoids are much larger molecules, in the region of 430 g/mol. Their production can be genetically upregulated and downregulated. The more colorful flavonoids such as Peonidin have also been shown to play a role in absorbing harmful UV light that can cause cellular damage.

Unlike terpenoids, flavonoids have not been found in the glandular trichomes of the cannabis plant and are much more widespread throughout the plant kingdom than cannabinoids (Flores-Sanchez and Verpoorte 2008a). Within *Cannabis sativa*, flavonoids such as cannaflavins are found at high levels within seedlings (Flores-Sanchez and Verpoorte 2008a) (Werz et al. 2014) and the roots (Frassinetti et al. 2018). In contrast, another study found no flavonoids in the roots, and the flavonoid present varied from one tissue to another. It also demonstrated that the production was cultivar dependent (Flores-Sanchez and Verpoorte 2008b).

1.2.2   WHY SECONDARY METABOLITES ARE PRODUCED

Plants are robust and adaptable organisms, producing thousands of compounds that mimic many of those made by humans. But why do plants produce these metabolites? The answer is survival. They form a chemical arsenal against attack. This can be in the form of repelling insects (J. McPartland 1997); sunscreen (Hazekamp et al. 2005); defense against disease such as fungus; response to extreme temperatures; exposure to salts; response to drought; prevention of herbivore attack (Roy and Dutta 2003) (Rothschild, Rowan, and Fairbairn 1977); and overcrowding. In addition, survival is enhanced by secondary metabolites rendering them more attractive to insects for pollination. The compounds are part of the signaling system within the plant that allows homeostasis to be achieved. Stress causes interesting responses from the plant, including flavonoid expression (Winkel-Shirley 2002).

1.2.3   METABOLIC PATHWAYS FOR PRODUCTION

Phytocannabinoids and terpenes belong to the same class of compounds called terpenoids and share a biosynthesis pathway. Cannabinoid precursors are synthesized from two pathways: the deoxyxylulose phosphate/methylerythritol phosphate (DOXP/MEP) pathway and the polyketide pathway (Gülck and Møller 2020) (Flores-Sanchez and Verpoorte 2008b) (Romero et al. 2020) (Booth and Bohlmann 2019).

The synthesis of these terpenoids begins in the plastid of disk cells within the glandular trichome on the female flower (Romero et al. 2020). Smaller precursor molecules, such as isopentenyl diphosphate (IPP) and dimethylallyl diphosphate (DMAPP), are condensed to farnesyl diphosphate (FPP) and go on to become sesquiterpenes in the cytosol of the disk cells or geranyl diphosphate (GPP) within the plastid (Booth and Bohlmann 2019) (Gülck and Møller 2020) (Romero et al. 2020). GPP is further converted to either monoterpene via terpene synthase (monoterpene pathway) or cannabigerolic acid (CBGA) by condensing with olivetolic acid (cannabinoid pathway). CBGA then migrates through a currently unknown mechanism from the plastid of the disk cells to the apoplastic space where further cannabinoids are then produced via additional enzymes, such as cannabinoid synthase. These are then stored in a bubble-like structure with a cavity at the top of the trichome hair (Romero et al. 2020). It has been shown that the morphology of the trichome dictates the type of terpenoid present, with higher concentrations of monoterpenes within stalked bulbous trichomes, while sesquiterpenes are more prevalent in sessile trichomes (Livingston et al. 2020). Therefore, anything influencing the development of the morphology will shape the terpene profile of the plant. Figure 1.1 summarizes this process.

Flavonoids are unique compared with the terpenoids, stemming from the amino acid phenylalanine, which enters the phenylpropanoid pathway to produce p-coumaroyl-CoA, 3-malonyl-CoA, and feruloyl CoA, undergoing several enzymatic reactions to form vibrant red, blue, and purple leaves (Winkel-Shirley 2002) (Andre, Hausman and Guerriero 2016). Flavonoids act as scavengers and antioxidants toward the harmful reactive oxygen species produced as a response to abiotic stress from the

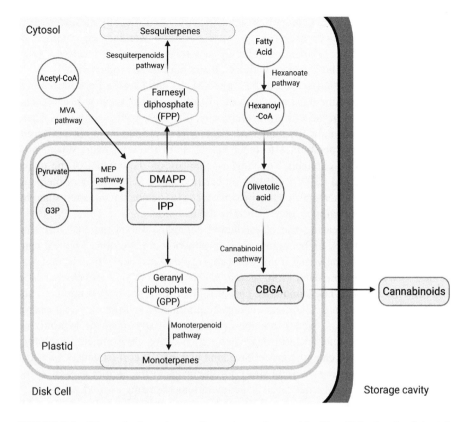

FIGURE 1.1 Biosynthetic pathway of terpenes and cannabinoids within the glandular trichome. CBGA = cannabigerolic acid; G3P = DMAPP = dimethylallyl diphosphate; IPP = isopentenyl diphosphate; MEP = methylerythritol phosphate; MVA = mevalonate. Modified from Romero 2020. Created with BioRender.com.

environment (Sharma et al. 2019). These reactive oxygen species are the elicitors for the phenylpropanoid pathway (Sharma et al. 2012). They are found in both male and female plants in equal concentrations within the leaves and roots. These are phenolic compounds also known as phenylpropanoids and are initially produced in the cytoplasm before being relocated to either the vacuole or the cell wall (Andre, Hausman, and Guerriero 2016). Many of these compounds display a pigment and thus color the cells. The production of flavonoids is regulated by several transcription factors (Davies and Schwinn 2006).

1.3 CULTIVATION

The cultivation of cannabis around the world has resulted in thousands of different strains, or chemovars, being bred from the original landrace strains that largely hail from India, Afghanistan, and Europe. Most strains are now hybrids with tendencies toward their origins.

Prohibition in the 20th century saw cannabis cultivated illegally in hidden grow rooms. Occupying spaces as varied as wardrobes and warehouses, commercial growing practices were adapted and entirely new techniques were developed, born out of the necessity to both remain undetected and maximize productivity.

The change of legislation within the United States and Canada for both medicinal and recreational cannabis has seen a multimillion-dollar industry develop. The demand for products in the form of flowers, oils, tinctures, edibles, balms, isolates, and cosmetics has dramatically increased. Each type of product requires a different profile of secondary metabolites to meet the needs of the consumer. Where previously the quality of cannabis was judged primarily on the content of the major cannabinoids THC and CBD, a greater appreciation and understanding of the plant among today's consumers has led to a broader focus to include flavor, determined by the terpenes, and appearance, determined by the flavonoids.

With the ever-increasing use of medicinal cannabis among patients suffering from severe conditions, higher standards of production are essential. Medical cannabis must be consistently free from pathogens, mycotoxins, heavy metals, and pesticides, as well as be traceable from seed to sale (Chandra et al. 2017) (McPartland and McKernan 2017). The cumulative cost of regular testing and prevention of contamination, in addition to significant energy requirements and the very real risk of crop failure, makes professional cannabis cultivation a costly endeavor. Minimizing potential risks is best achieved through automation of the environment, instituting and practicing regular cleaning procedures, and picking the correct genetics for disease resistance. Selecting the right strain for the needs of the facility as well as the patient/consumer is vital when large-scale operations are being created.

Many factors must be considered when choosing a strain, including high yield-potential, commercial viability, disease resistance, suitability for large-scale production, flowering time, and genetic stability. Plant genetics determine the chemical profile and cannabinoid content of plants, while biomass yield and crop consistency are largely determined by the growing environment (Jin, Jin, and Chen 2019).

There are three stages to the growth cycle of *Cannabis sativa*: (1) propagation, seeds are germinated or clones are produced. Root development takes place. (2) Vegetative stage, day length is longer (18 hours) and leaf growth is predominant. (3) Flowering stage, day length is shorter (12 hours) and flower production is initiated and becomes the focus of growth.

Every stage is heavily influenced by environmental factors: light, temperature, CO_2, humidity, and growing media all play a part in determining the rate of photosynthesis and therefore yield (Resh 2012).

Photosynthesis is the primary force that drives the production of biomass and secondary metabolites (Figure 1.2). *Cannabis sativa* utilizes C3 photosynthesis. Plants must perform a constant balancing act, allowing CO_2 assimilation via the stomata without losing too much water through transpiration. The interplay of the limiting factors means that simply increasing one factor will not automatically increase yield. For example, in response to an increase in the ambient CO_2 concentration in the growing environment, leaf temperature, relative humidity, and nutrient availability must also increase in order for the rate of photosynthesis to keep up with the rate at

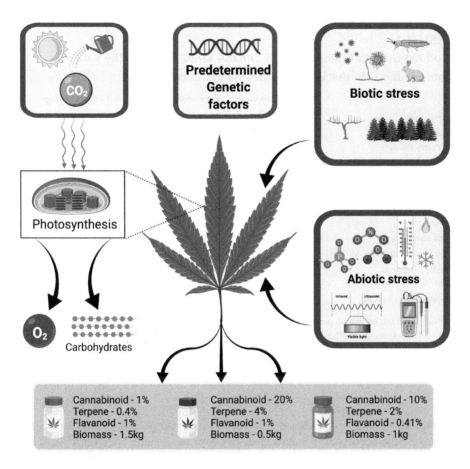

FIGURE 1.2 The influencing factors on secondary metabolite profile within *Cannabis sativa* oils. Created with BioRender.com.

which the CO_2 is assimilated. A balance must be found if productivity is to be maintained. Optimum conditions for the cultivation of *Cannabis sativa* have been studied extensively by many groups (ElSohly 2017) (Chandra et al. 2017) (Caplan, Dixon, and Zheng 2019) (De Backer et al. 2012) (Jin, Jin, and Chen 2019) (McPartland and Russo 2001) (Backer et al. 2019). A summary of the optimum growing conditions for cannabis is presented in Table 1.2.

1.3.1 GENETIC POTENTIAL

All plants have a genetic potential known as the genotype. This determines the potential chemotype or the chemical constitution of the plant. Phenotypes, or the characteristics of a particular plant, are the determining factor in choosing which plants to utilize for production. Environmental factors play a significant role in

TABLE 1.2

Optimal Growth Conditions for *Cannabis sativa* Based on the Rate of Photosynthesis Water Use Efficiency on the Leaves (WUE)

	Propagation stage	Vegetative stage	Flowering stage
Light			
Duration	18–24 hrs	18 hrs	12 hrs
Intensity (W m^{-2})	36–150	600	600
PPFD (μmol m^2/s)	–	1500	1500
Lamp	Fluorescent	Metal halide (MH)	High pressure sodium (HPS)
Predominate wavelength (nm)	420–620 nm	350–550 nm	540–650 nm
Relative humidity	75%	55–75%	55–60%
VPD	0.8 kPa	1.3–1.4 kPa	1.3–1.4 kPa
Leaf temperature	19–24°C	25–30°C	25–30°C
CO_2 concentration (μmol/mol)	–	–	750
Media conditions			
pH	5.5–6.5	5.5–6.5	5.5–6.5
Conductivity (mS/cm)	0.8–1.4	1.8–3.0	0.9–3.0

Notes: These are cultivar-dependent conditions. Plants utilize light between 400 and 700 nm, and this table demonstrates the typical types of artificial lamps used along with their predominating wavelength. VPD = vapor pressure deficit; PPFD = photosynthetic photon flux density; LED = light-emitting diode.

determining phenotype, although not beyond the base genetic potential as determined by the genotype. If a plant does not have the genetic code for a particular secondary metabolite, it will never be capable of producing it. Multiple studies have shown that the genetics of the plant is the biggest contributing factor to the yield and quality of secondary metabolite production (Vanhove, Van Damme, and Meert 2011) (Chandra et al. 2017). Commercialization and industrial production have for many years seen the breeding of cultivars that are more resistant to disease, drought, and frost in order to maintain a high standard of production.

Cannabis sativa can be categorized into three predominant chemotypes: drug-type, intermediate type, and fiber type. Those plants bred as hemp, for their fiber content and featuring a deficiency of cannabinoids, are known as fiber type. Those plants with a relatively equal ratio of THC and CBD fall into the intermediate type category. Plants with a high THC and low CBD content, generally bred illicitly for the recreational market, make up the drug type. Drug-type plants have been found to have THC concentrations as high as 26.4% (De Backer et al. 2012). As the connoisseur market has developed, breeding has shifted to focus on flavor from terpenes and coloring from flavonoids (de la Fuente et al. 2020). The development of the medicinal and wellness market has seen a shift in the chemovars being developed as there is a greater demand for CBD and other minor cannabinoids such as CBG. These three different ratio chemotypes are controlled by the expression genes for the enzymes

THCA synthase and CBDA synthase (Rodziewicz and Kayser 2020). Analytical techniques such as polymerase chain reaction (PCR) have allowed the identification of the genetic markers that indicate whether a young plant is of fiber type, intermediate THC type, or high THC.

1.3.2 INDOORS VS OUTDOORS

In the Northern Hemisphere, many growers have migrated to climate-controlled indoor facilities utilizing artificial lighting, optimized temperature, relative humidity, and a vapor pressure deficient (VPD) environment. While security concerns are evident, the prime instigator for the move to indoor environments allows for continuous year-round production. The vast majority of *Cannabis sativa* is photoperiod sensitive, requiring 12 hours of light to trigger flowering (short day). Therefore, indoor environments are not at the mercy of seasonal light cycles. There is a trend among some growers toward autoflowering plants, however, they do not yield as much biomass or resin as some of the other strains descending from India and Central Asia (McPartland 2018).

Through the end of the 20th century, Dutch growers led a technical revolution in indoor cultivation, perfecting hydroponic techniques such as nutrient film technique (NTF), Rockwool dripper systems, deep water culture (DWC), and flood and drain (Seaman 2017) (Bricklebank and Seaman 2011) (Resh 2012). These techniques became popular with the "closet cultivator" in the 1990s in the UK. Over time, these techniques have coalesced into a focus on coir-based systems due to the medium's forgiving nature and water buffering capacity. However, despite greater efficiency in terms of water and nutrient usage, most commercial facilities have chosen not to adopt pure hydroponics techniques for large-scale production, as the associated costs and time and maintenance requirements have been found to outweigh increases in yield (Jin, Jin and Chen 2019) (Potter 2014).

Cannabis cultivators face a number of disease and pest issues, including Fusarium (root disease), Pythium, botrytis (gray mold), powdery mildew, tobacco mosaic virus, russet mites, spider mites, and onion thrips (Rodziewicz and Kayser 2020). Air filtration is common practice in medicinal-grade growing facilities using HVAC purification systems to prevent infestations of molds, pathogens, and insects. Since the turn of the 21st century, there has been a move toward greater automation in pruning, repotting, moving plants, and harvesting, further reducing the risk of contamination.

Vertical growing systems and methods have been developed to maximize the efficient use of otherwise limited space in indoor growing environments (Seaman 2017). This can take on one of two forms, either with multiple layers of stacked platforms on which individual potted plants are grown, or as a wall in which plants are potted directly into media, such as Rockwool, and irrigated with a nutrient-enriched solution. The former method has been adopted by large-scale production facilities because the latter suffers from issues relating to crop density. Tightly packing plants reduces airflow between the plants and the media, creating the perfect microclimate for the proliferation of fungus.

Outdoor cultivation offers more space for root development and no restriction on the height to which plants can grow. While sunlight is free and offers plants the full spectrum of light necessary for healthy growth, seasonal and weather changes can be unpredictable and make it impossible to regulate light levels. Within glasshouses, supplementary lighting is often used to compensate for said changeability. Control over disease and infestation can become more difficult when operating outside as winds can carry spores and insects for miles. Weather damage is also a risk, coming in the form of frost, hail/rain, wind, and heat. The risk of contamination from pesticides is also increased outdoors, either as a result of leaching or drift from sprayers from neighboring fields or due to the persistent presence of now-banned pesticide residue, sometimes applied decades earlier. The lack of control over growing conditions outdoors in comparison to an indoor setting has been shown to result in a lack of consistent quality in the end product, with a significant disparity in THC:CBD ratios grown outdoors (Potter 2009).

1.3.3 REPRODUCTION AND PROPAGATION TECHNIQUES

Cannabis sativa, being diecious, has both male and female plants, with females producing the highest concentrations of oils rich in terpenoids. A sexing process must be undertaken when cultivating from seed. The traditional method is to germinate the seeds, place them into vegetative growth using a long-day light regime (18 hours) until large enough to take cuttings or clones, and then change the light regime to a short day (12 hours) so that flowers will be produced. Plants that display male flowers are then destroyed and females kept from which mother plants are selected. Multiple clones can be taken from these mother plants by simply cutting the end of a branch, treating the cut surface with auxins such as indole-butyric acid, placing it into the appropriate media, and then propagating the cutting at high humidity for 14 days until rooting occurs. Each plant is then guaranteed to be female and genetically identical to the other plants within that batch. This is the point at which the phenotype is chosen for its favorable characteristics. The process of cloning a plant reduces the time of propagation dramatically.

PCR has helped to speed up the sexing process through the amplification of genetic markers of male plants (Mandolino et al. 1999) (Medicinal Genomics 2020). Tissue from plants as young as five days old can be digested and the DNA extracted, amplified, and identified, saving valuable time (6–8 weeks) and space in the facility. D. J. Potter demonstrated the advantages of clones over seeds in his PhD thesis, concluding that cloning not only increased biomass and cannabinoid yield but also increased consistency of cannabinoid ratios (Potter 2009), which is also supported by other groups (De Backer et al. 2012) (Aizpurua-Olaizola et al. 2016).

Micropropagation, also known as "tissue culture," is a powerful new asexual propagation technique, similar to cloning (ElSohly 2017). It involves taking a small sample of leaf tissue and propagating it *in vitro* with a nutrient and hormone-rich broth. This technique allows for the large-scale production of genotypes from very little plant material (Lata et al. 2016). Disease-free plants can be created from this along with preserving the phenotype and genotype of the desired plant for long periods of time. As well as saving significantly on space, this method allows for rapid reproduction and helps to maintain consistency across the crop, as cannabinoid content is not affected by this technique (Chandra et al. 2010).

1.4 TYPES OF STRESSES

The definition of "stress" in this case is when pressure is applied to a system that prevents it from running at an optimal level, upsetting its balance and cellular homeostasis. Plants experience two types of stress that are inflicted by either living factors or non-living factors. Biotic stresses stem from living organisms and include insect attack, fungal disease, herbivore damage, and overcrowding (Figure 1.2).

Abiotic stress derives from non-living, environmental factors, such as levels of exposure to light, CO_2, drought, thermal stress, nutrition, salts, and heavy metals. These can be used to influence cannabinoid content and glandular density (Rodziewicz and Kayser 2020). From a scientific perspective, abiotic factors are easier to study, as variables can be kept constant and there is more data available about their effects.

Stress results in the increased production of reactive oxygen species (ROS) such as hydrogen peroxide, superoxide ions (O_2^-), and hydroxyl radicals (OH). This is a result of photosynthesis being an aerobic metabolic process. If one of the key factors (light, water, or CO_2) is limited or oversupplied, then a rapid build-up of ROS occurs. ROS can also be produced in response to an attack or metal toxicity. At low concentrations, ROS act as messengers for the release of a number of hormones that mediate a response in the plant (Sharma et al. 2012). They are the trigger pathways for the production of free radical scavengers, such as flavonoids. If the production of these scavengers does not keep up with ROS production, irreversible damage occurs to lipids, proteins, and DNA, leading to cell damage and even death (Sharma et al. 2019) (Sharma et al. 2012).

1.4.1 Biotic

1.4.1.1 Microbes, Arthropods, and Herbivores

Stress exerted by microbes, arthropods, and herbivores results in irreversible cell damage. Attack from microbes can come in various forms, with the main culprits being pathogenic fungi, in addition to threats from viruses, nematodes, bacteria, protozoa, and arthropods. When producing monocultures, there is always an increased risk of an infection affecting the whole crop. Cultivators should work to control the disease before it takes hold, damaging the plant, hindering its development, and reducing yield (J. M. McPartland 1996). One of the most common and problematic threats, thriving particularly in indoor growing conditions, is gray mold (*botrytis cinerea*), which manifests itself in the inflorescence and also on leaves and stems.

In response to microbial infections, plants produce phytoalexins, a large group of broad-spectrum antibiotics with low molecular weights that work as part of the defense system. These include terpenoids and flavonoids, along with other compounds such as stilbenes (Jeandet 2015). Plants also produce superoxide free radicals together with nitrogen monoxide as part of their defense mechanism (Heldt and Piechulla 2004). This release of chemicals needs to be triggered by an elicitor (cells from the pathogen) binding to the cell wall of the plant, triggering a cascade of signals that eventually stimulate the transcription of genes for the synthesis of the appropriate phytoalexins or other defense molecules (Heldt and Piechulla 2004). Many studies have shown that terpenes have antimicrobial properties (Kandi et al. 2015) (Andre, Hausman and Guerriero 2016) (ElSohly 2017) (Hanuš and Hod 2020), cannabinoids contain antibacterial and antifungal properties, and that cannabis whole plant extract is an effective repellent and pesticide (McPartland 1997).

Microbes are not entirely harmful, with research on symbiotic microbes showing a positive effect on biomass yield when applied to the roots (Conant et al. 2017). L. W. Robertson has hypothesized that the minor cannabinoid Δ^9-tetrahydrocannabutol (THCB) may be derived from microbial oxidation or decarboxylation of the precursor, as no enzymatic pathway has been found (Robertson, Lyle, and Billets 1975) (Citti et al. 2019). Endophytes, microbes that are most commonly fungus or bacteria, live between the cells of plants and have been proven to modulate and mimic secondary metabolites produced by the host plant (Taghinasab and Jabaji 2020).

Cannabis is not pollinated by insects, those present are only there to acquire food, be that from the plant itself or other insects (McPartland, Clarke, and Watson 2000). Some insects, such as thrip, whitefly, and spider mites, will feed on the sugar-rich sap in the leaf, destroying it from the inside out. Their effects can be devastating, and along with other insects, can be a source of further infection such as viruses.

Caterpillars eat the entire leaf and rabbits strip the bark from the base of the stem, while livestock and other mammals will demolish the entire plant. When plants are attacked or wounded, the glandular trichomes, full of cannabinoids and terpenes, are broken and release their contents. Many plant volatiles have been shown to be effective against herbivores. They are released to recruit parasitic wasps to repair wounded plants (Pare and James 1999) and produce a flavor that repels cattle in particular strains (McPartland, Clarke, and Watson 2000). Brushing past the plant can also cause itching and a rash in humans due to the terpenes.

Studies and reports to date have only mentioned the reduction in yield due to infestation, and the effectiveness of the extracts and compounds as antimicrobials. No data has been collected concerning effects on the precise secondary metabolite production in infected or attacked plants.

1.4.1.2 Space and Competing Plants

Cannabis is an allelopathic plant capable of secreting allelochemicals via its roots and leaves that exert a detrimental physiological effect on neighboring plants. The monoterpene limonene, pulegone, and the monoterpenoid 1,8-cineole are all produced by cannabis and serve to inhibit the growth of other plants. In heavy rain, trichomes rich with such compounds are washed from the leaves into the ground where they suppress the growth of competing plants. The herbicidal properties of hemp have seen it used as a smother crop in the practice of crop rotation (McPartland, Clarke, and Watson 2000). Extractions of varying concentrations from both cannabis leaves and flowers have been shown to inhibit the germination of monocots (Pudełko, Majchrzak, and Narożna 2014) and lettuce, however, the root extract had no effect (Mahmoodzadeh, Ghasemi, and Zanganeh 2015). This would suggest that it is the terpenes or cannabinoids that are stored in the glandular trichomes that serve this purpose. It has also been suggested that cannabinoids could play a role in this as THC levels have been found to be higher when competing with plants other than cannabis (McPartland, Clarke, and Watson 2000). Other studies have shown that this effect is plant-dependent, with inhibition of onions, carrots, and tomatoes all occurring at different concentrations of the same whole plant extract (Konstantinović et al. 2018). Assuming the nutrient needs of cannabis plants are met, this could be beneficial for increasing the production of particular terpenes.

It has been suggested the crop density of cannabis plants increases THC yields in overcrowded plants (Backer et al. 2019) (Latta and Eaton 1975). Although, as with the effects of many stress factors, this is cultivar dependent. Overall biomass yield per square meter is unaffected by plant density (Vanhove, Van Damme, and Meert 2011), though the data for optimum crop density has yet to be established based on cannabinoids or any other secondary metabolite.

It has been found that increasing the size of a plant pot has a negative effect on THC per square meter of growing space (Backer et al. 2019). Constricting roots into a tight ball helps to reduce the size of the plant as a whole, making the plant shorter and stockier; this is a similar method to bonsai practice.

1.4.1.3 Physical Damage

Physical damage can be caused by both biotic and abiotic factors. Being trampled upon, eaten, and enduring strong weather, particularly wind and rain, can result in deformed growth, although the stem and root structure are strengthened in response to regular vigorous movement. An interesting study showed that shaking Liquidambar trees for 30 seconds daily reduced growth by 70% creating much shorter and stumpier plants (Neel and Harris 1971).

During the initial stages of plant development, pruning is the normal practice within indoor facilities (Chandra et al. 2017) (Jin, Jin, and Chen 2019). Many lower branches are removed during the long-day light period, the most aggressive growth phase. Leaves are removed not only to increase light penetration into the canopy but also to increase air movement and reduce humidity to help combat and prevent disease. Some studies have shown that heavy pruning of certain cannabis varieties can reduce THC, CBG, and some terpene content (Fischedick et al. 2010).

Training plants with a frame, weaving the branches between a net, is a technique referred to as the ScrOG method ("Screen of Green") and has been employed with great success, increasing yield dramatically (Knight et al. 2010). This can be attributed to the increased light penetration into the canopy, and consequently, higher levels of photosynthesis. The effects on the secondary metabolite profile still need further investigation.

1.4.2 ABIOTIC

1.4.2.1 Light Stress

Light is the primary energy source that plants utilize in photosynthesis for the production of cells, sugars, oils, and secondary metabolites. The effects of light can be pleiotropic with three main parameters affecting plant growth: morphology, physiology, and secondary metabolite production (Gorelick and Bernstein 2017). Photoreceptors on the leaves are affected by the intensity, wavelength, and duration (photoperiod) of the light to which they are exposed.

Light intensity can be measured as photosynthetically active radiation (PAR). However, a more accurate method is to measure the photosynthetic photon flux density (PPFD), which is the number of photons that hit the plant per square meter per second. In the past, particularly within the illicit market, light intensity was measured in watts per meter ($W \cdot m^{-1}$), as the power consumption of the light is directly related to intensity. However, this does not give an accurate picture of what the plant is actually able to use. Light efficiency is better measured as the number of grams of biomass the plant produces per square meter (g W^{-1} m^2) based on the power input of the light. The rate of photosynthesis (P_n) is related to light intensity, with increased intensity leading to higher levels of photosynthesis. Photosynthesis decreases as the distance from the light source increases, following the inverse square law as applied to traditional artificial light sources, such as high pressure sodium (HPS) and metal halide (MH) lamps. Light intensity is also decreased beyond the canopy cover. Cannabis has been found to be able to tolerate high PPFD (+1500 μmol m^{-2} s^{-1}) without a significant reduction in yields (Chandra et al. 2015). However, when the light intensity is too great, biomass yield will decrease if the other limiting factors, such as water or CO_2 assimilation, are not increased proportionally. Eventually, there is a saturation point after which increased light intensity is no longer a benefit (Eichhorn Bilodeau et al. 2019). Often with increased intensity, particularly with high-pressure sodium (HPS) and metal halide (MH) lamps, there is an increase in temperature that can have an adverse effect on photosynthesis. However, research has demonstrated that both CBD and THC content increases with amplified light intensity, which supports the theory that these cannabinoids are produced as a defense mechanism against photo-radiation damage, limiting the harmful effects of light stress (Backer et al. 2019). The same study demonstrated that there was a decrease in mass per watt biomass yield as a result of increased light intensity, further supported by the work of Potter and Duncombe (2012). However, these studies were performed with MH and HPS lamps, which have low PPFD, energy efficiency issues, and limited wavelength bands. In contrast to Backer's 2019 paper, the 2012 Potter study found that THC concentration is not affected by the irradiance of light, and an increase in flower number boosted THC yield as opposed to an increase in THC accumulation by the leaf (Potter and Duncombe 2012). It is not yet clear if higher photosynthesis rates are related to higher cannabinoid yields (Jin, Jin, and Chen 2019).

With the advancement of light-emitting diodes (LEDs), precise control of the light spectrum is easier to achieve, along with greater efficiency of energy use. LED lights can be created that better mimic the full spectrum of sunlight and can be finely tuned to the growth phase.

Plants consume light between the wavelengths of 400 and 700 nm and the intensity of a particular wavelength can alter plant development, morphology, and physiology. Ultraviolet (UV) light (100–400 nm), particularly UVB (280–315 nm), has been shown to have dramatic pleiotropic effects. It is well documented that plants produce phenolic compounds such as flavonoids, anthocyanins, and other secondary metabolites as a protection mechanism against UV radiation (Zhang and Björn 2009). UVB in particular harms DNA and causes deep tissue damage, resulting in the production of ROS (Sharma et al. 2012) (Sharma et al. 2019) (Heldt and Piechulla 2004). Numerous studies have shown THC levels in plants rise in response to UVB exposure, suggesting THC protects against its harmful effects (Pate, Chemical Ecology of Cannabis 1994) (Pate 1983) (Lydon, Teramura, and Coffman 1987). Lydon also found that vegetative and flora material were stimulated to produce more THC when exposed to UVB for 40 days. However, this effect was not seen with any of the other cannabinoids. Further evidence to support THC as a protector against UVB can be found in research comparing HID and two LEDs, each with differing light spectrums (Magagnini, Grassi, and Kotiranta 2018). The results demonstrated that not only can the morphology of the plant be altered by changes in the spectrum but that there is also an increase in all of the cannabinoids. Interestingly, the light with the highest levels of UVA in its spectrum induced CBG accumulation in addition to THC. This is a very promising area of research and more needs to be done for conclusive data to be produced.

UVC (100–280 nm) has been shown to induce the production of cinnamic acid amide derivatives, which are precursors to flavonoids. However, no significant effect on cannabinoid content was found (Marti et al. 2014).

A review by Eichhorn Bilodeau et al. (2019) concluded that green light (520–560 nm) inhibited THC production, whereas red light had been shown to stimulate monoterpene production, and far red-light treatment and UV blue increased flavonoid content.

The production of THC has been found to be higher in plants descended from landrace strains from India (Indica) and Central Asia (Afghanica) than in sativas originating in Europe, where the light intensity is not as great, and result in a higher CBD content instead (McPartland 2018). This supports the notion that THC is produced as a photo-radiation protector.

As a photoperiod plant, *Cannabis sativa* is stimulated to flower via a complex set of pathways when the day length falls to 12 hours. Interrupting the dark period with light can cause morphological change and regenerative growth within the flowers. The plant can then revert to its vegetative growth phase. This method can be employed to regrow a plant once it has had its flowers harvested. As the root network is established, the plant will focus on reproducing leaves and flowers.

Light duration is shown to have some interesting effects on the lesser-known cannabinoids such as tetrahydrocannabivarin (THCV) and CBG (Potter 2009). Potter found that by extending the day length to 13 hours, the CBG content was increased, whereas THC and THCV were reduced. Another study demonstrated that by increasing the duration of the flowering phase (short day) and reducing the number of weeks for the vegetative phase, THC yields increased per meter (Backer et al. 2019).

1.4.2.2   Carbon Dioxide

Carbon dioxide (CO_2) from the atmosphere is the primary source of carbon utilized by plants through photosynthesis. *Cannabis sativa* is a C_3 plant relying heavily on CO_2 for photosynthesis. The biggest limiting factor to the rate of P_n is the ambient CO_2 concentration with the Earth's current atmospheric concentration standing at 372–450 µmol mol^{-1}. S. Chandra demonstrated that a concentration of CO_2 at 750 µmol mol^{-1}, a temperature of 30°C, and a PPFD of 1500 µmol m^{-2} s^{-1} is the optimal growing condition for *Cannabis sativa*. This figure is based on the net photosynthesis, transpiration, stomatal conductance, internal CO_2 concentration, the ratio of internal to external CO_2 concentration, and water use efficiency on the leaf (WUE) (Chandra et al. 2008). A higher concentration of 1500 µmol mol^{-1} is a common recommendation for indoor growing, as anything above this level is toxic to humans (Haupt 2018). This concentration can be used successfully, however, in larger growing facilities that can cover hundreds of thousands of meters, where it is no longer cost-effective to further raise the concentration, factors such as leaf temperature must also be raised to keep up with the rate of photosynthesis. S. Chandra et al. went on to find that the effect of increasing CO_2 was significant and cultivar dependent. They concluded that cannabis was still productive in drier conditions as long as CO_2 concentrations were elevated (Chandra et al. 2011).

At present, further data pertaining to the effects of CO_2 on secondary metabolites have yet to be reported.

1.4.2.3   Drought

Drought is one of the major stimulators of secondary metabolite production. Water, a key component of photosynthesis, makes up over 80% of the plant. It is drawn up through the plants' roots and lost through the leaves, via the stomata, through the process of transpiration. The rate of transpiration is driven by temperature and the relative humidity of the surrounding air. The vapor pressure deficit (VPD) is the maximum amount of water the air can hold at a given temperature and is what ultimately controls the opening and closing of the stomata on the leaves, and therefore the rate of photosynthesis and water vapor exchange. A high VPD is an indication of a drier/warmer environment, which increases transpiration and causes leaf wilt and ultimately leading to necrosis and loss of yield. Whereas a low VPD, an indication of relative high humidity, encourages fungi, such as botrytis, to flourish in the flowers. Elevated CO_2 levels allow cannabis to maintain productivity in drier conditions with a high VPD (Chandra et al. 2008) (Chandra et al. 2015).

As with other plants, drought stress can decrease yield in cannabis, however, it can have a positive effect on the production of both the major cannabinoids and specific terpenes (Caplan 2018) (Caplan, Dixon, and Zheng 2019). This is time dependent and relative to the stage of the growth cycle. By allowing the media to dry over an 11-day period on the seventh week of the flowering stage, without reducing the photosynthetic rate, cannabinoid and terpene content were increased by 50% compared with the control. Elevated concentrations of THCA, CBDA, THC, and CBD were observed without loss of inflorescence biomass, while CBG was unaffected (Caplan, Dixon, and Zheng 2019). Other studies have shown elevated THC levels in plants found in drier climates (Pate, Chemical Ecology of Cannabis 1994).

The Caplan 2018 study also revealed the importance of the timing of drought on secondary metabolite production, as drought stress at an early stage increases the terpenes cis-ocimene and linalool, whereas drought stress at a later stage increases trans-ocimene and alpha-bisabolol.

1.4.2.4   Thermal Stress

Plants can experience stress through both extremes of temperature, cold stress and heat stress, leading to reduced growth and even senescence. Cold stress reduces the rate of photosynthesis, increases ROS, and the expression of cold response genes (COR). Frosts can even cause crystals of ice to form between the cells, piercing them and causing them to burst (Miura and Furumoto 2013). Heat stress causes photosynthesis to stop, increases ROS, and triggers a cascade of complex responses. The optimum temperature for growing *Cannabis sativa* in controlled environments has been found to be 25–30°C, although this is cultivar dependent (Chandra et al. 2008). This data was based on the maximum rate of photosynthesis and water use efficiency (WUE) on the leaves.

Secondary metabolite production in many plants has been shown to increase with both types of thermal stress (Gorelick and Bernstein 2017). *Cannabis sativa* that has derived from hotter climates such as India and Afghanistan before hybridization, produces higher concentrations of cannabinoids (McPartland 2018). It is still not fully clear if temperature has an effect on the biosynthesis of cannabinoids, as much of the work that seemingly proved the effect was not performed under controlled conditions, and results have been contradictory.

LED lights have been shown to reduce the temperature of the leaf as they emit less radiant heat compared with traditional grow lamps, and in some cases, have been shown to increase the cannabinoid content (Magagnini, Grassi, and Kotiranta 2018). This could be attributed to the spectrum of light being broader, including more UV light. Similarly, cooler conditions, for example, 23°C as opposed to 32°C, have been shown to yield higher THC content (Bazzaz et al. 1975). In contrast, Boucher et al. (1974) observed an increase in cannabinoid content in warmer climates. Work needs to be done on a molecular level to better understand the precise effect of thermal stress on secondary metabolite production in cannabis.

1.4.2.5   Nutrition, Salts, and Heavy Metal Stress

Cannabis is a bioaccumulator of a variety of metals, salts, and hydrocarbons, and has been used to clean contaminated land (Linger et al. 2002). These elements are then stored in the plant and can become concentrated to a level that is toxic to humans when oils are extracted from the flowers. Routine testing of products for heavy metal stress is performed in both the pharmaceutical and recreational sectors, particularly as customers have become better educated on these matters (de la Fuente et al. 2020). Cannabis has been reported to have become tolerant to Cd, Ni, and Cr without displaying any signs of stunted growth (Linger et al. 2002). Accumulation of these heavy metals within the plant must first be addressed before consideration for use in triggering a response in the plant (Gorelick and Bernstein 2017).

Cannabis requires a great deal of calcium for growth. Many studies have been carried out on the nutritional needs of cannabis, in terms of accumulation, distribution, effects on biomass, and photosynthesis; particularly with regards to hemp for industrial use (Landi 1997) (Kalinowski et al. 2020) (Ivanyi and Izsaki 2009) (Tang et al. 2017) (Maļceva, Vikmane, and Stramkale 2011) (Da Cunha Leme Filho et al. 2020). Nutrition is crucial for the healthy development of the plant. Calcium, magnesium, iron, and molybdenum all accumulate in the leaves, whereas copper, manganese, and zinc accumulate within the flowers (Landi 1997).

Caplan, Dixon, and Zheng ran trials to establish the benefits of nitrogen application on cannabinoid production during the vegetative and flowering phases (Caplan, Dixon, and Zheng 2017a) (Caplan, Dixon, and Zheng 2017b). It was concluded that supplying high concentrations (389 mg/L) of nitrogen from an organic fertilizer during the vegetative phase increases THC yields. However, excessive application of organic fertilizers in the flowering stage should be avoided to keep cannabinoid content high (Caplan, Dixon, and Zheng 2017b). A Hungarian study on hemp confirmed that increasing nitrogen application during the flowering phase decreased overall THC concentration (Bócsa, Máthé, and Hangyel 1997).

A metadata analysis of over ten datasets concluded that slow-release fertilizers affected THC content of the plants, but only stated the yield increase not THC compared with liquid mineral fertilizer (Backer et al. 2019), further supporting the need for specific feed regimes and application times to optimize consumption and stimulation of secondary metabolites.

Early work by Hanuš and Dostálová (1994) demonstrated that fertilization had an effect on cannabinoid content, particularly THC. Five treatments of fertilizers were applied to hemp fields: (1) nitrogen and potassium (NK); (2) phosphorus and potassium (PK); (3) nitrogen and phosphorus (NP); (4) nitrogen, phosphorus, and potassium (NPK); and 5) a control. Plants treated with PK yielded the highest THC, whereas the plants treated with NK yielded the highest CBD content. The group treated with NP yielded the lowest THC, suggesting that potassium is important for the production of THC. This study supports the need for growth-phase-specific fertilization (Hanuš and Dostálová 1994).

It has been suggested that magnesium, manganese, and iron play a role in the regulation of THC synthase and other cannabinoid enzyme pathways. After observing an increase in these bivalent ions in the leaf tissue, there was a corresponding increase in THC production (Latta and Eaton 1975). In the same study, it was found that magnesium also had a positive effect on the production of the degradation product CBN. Microelements were also found to affect THC production, with some evidence concluding that iron is essential for THC production while copper acts as an inhibitor (Honma et al. 1971).

The most cannabinoid-diverse study ever carried out on plant nutrition examined the effects of NPK and humic acid on THC, CBD, CBG, CBN, THCV, CBCT, CBC, and CBL. It demonstrated that cannabinoid metabolism is affected by mineral nutrition. It also found this to have an organ-specific effect, altering the cannabinoid content between the leaves and the inflorescence. The study concluded that the exact relationship was not clear; however, the use of nutritional supplements helped to increase the homogeneity of cannabinoids through the plant (Bernstein et al. 2019).

The technique of flushing a plant two weeks before harvest with water alone is common practice among home growers that want to improve flavor. However, there is no scientific evidence that supports the belief that this enhances terpene or cannabinoid content. One study confirmed that this method of flushing does nothing to the nutrient content of the flower. It also found that nitrogen depletion is a signal for the plant to mature, while an increase in sulfur is a death signal to the plant (Stemeroff 2017). During the final phases of flowering, the plants stop taking up nutrients, so the reduction of feed makes sense.

The application of silver nitrate is well-documented to cause the production of male flowers in the localized area of application (Mohan Ram and Sett 1982). This in turn will reduce the production of cannabinoids. Further investigation is required into the effects of other metals on secondary metabolite production.

The media conditions have also been shown to affect cannabis. Plants grown in peat, coco coir, and a 30% green fiber substitute were compared, and no difference in the CBDA content between them was found. However, the peat-based product did yield higher biomass, and therefore proportionally more oil (Burgel, Hartung, and Graeff-Hönninger 2020).

1.5 OTHER FACTORS

1.5.1 TIME OF HARVEST

The point in the life cycle of the plant when harvest occurs is crucial for the concentration of secondary metabolites. CBGA concentrations are at their highest during propagation and then drop rapidly before remaining mostly constant throughout the rest of the life cycle of the plant. CBGA is the predominant cannabinoid produced within seedlings, with only trace concentrations of THCA and CBDA (<0.2%) (Aizpurua-Olaizola et al. 2016). Studies have shown that THCA and CBDA are present in cuttings, or clones, at the same concentration as the mother plant they were originally taken from. However, this drops significantly as the cutting grows (De Backer et al. 2012).

The change in cannabinoid profile starts early in the growth cycle of the plant, with CBC synthase being most efficient at converting CBG when it is in low concentrations in young plants. With the increase in growth and CBG concentration, THC and CBD synthase become more efficient and take over in overall yield (Potter 2014). The highest concentrations of THCA and CBDA are found in fresh plant material at full maturity when the pistils change to a ginger color and the glandular trichomes turn from transparent to a milky color (Livingston et al. 2020). CBDA concentration peaks before THCA concentration in flower sets (Aizpurua-Olaizola et al. 2016).

Within the European industrial hemp sector, legislation states that the flowers must be below 0.2% THCA/THC for cultivation under a hemp license. This is also true of any CBD product legally sold on the high street or internet. To comply with these regulations, farmers and cultivators will harvest their crop a couple of weeks before full maturation. Terpenes follow a similar pattern, in that their yield is increased with the maturation of the female flowers (Aizpurua-Olaizola et al. 2016).

1.5.2   DRYING AND CURING PROCESS

A change in flower composition occurs over time, with the loss of volatile compounds such as terpenes and the degradation of cannabinoids. Due to the nature of many of the secondary metabolites, they often further metabolize/degrade either through decarboxylation or oxidation. CBN, CBV, Δ^8-THC, and CBEV are all degradation products due to the oxidation of the neutral forms of the pre-existing cannabinoids.

These processes occur naturally over time, however, they are often accelerated with heat or UV light to produce the psychoactive neutral forms of the compounds (Wang et al. 2016).

Due to the volatile nature of terpenes, these are lost over time and can be easily destroyed if the curing process is rushed or performed at very high temperatures. Drying for 24 hours over 37°C decarboxylates all of the acid forms of cannabinoids, which is desirable for products that are taken orally. The optimum time for, and temperature of, decarboxylation was investigated by Wang et al. (2016) and there were found to be differences between THCA and CBDA, standing at 20 minutes at 110°C for the former and 20 minutes at 130°C for the latter. The acid forms of THC have been found to remain stable for up to 30 weeks below 4°C, but longer if stored at −18°C (Jin, Jin, and Chen 2019).

One of the major issues with the production of medicinal cannabis is the potential for the contamination of the flower by pathogenic microbes such as *Escherichia coli*, *Aspergillus niger*, and *Salmonella* (McPartland and McKernan 2017). All of these can be introduced into the growing facility via personnel or the media in which the plants are grown, the environment being perfect for the proliferation of microbes. This remains the primary challenge in the control and prevention of contamination, with treatment usually involving pesticides that are prohibited from use on medicinal crops. As many of the patients receiving cannabis-based medicine (CBM) are often seriously ill and severely immunocompromised, exposure to such pathogens or pesticides could be life-threatening. Gamma-irradiation can be used after harvest for decontamination purposes. Studies have shown that CBD and THC concentrations are not affected by this type of treatment, but volatile monoterpenes such as myrcene and linalool are negatively impacted. The same study concluded that this was also plant-variety dependent, as the reduction in myrcene was not consistent between cultivars. This may have been due to other secondary metabolite differences between the cultivars that offer protective properties (Hazekamp 2016).

1.6   SUMMARY

Due to its international origins and widespread hybridization through the 20th century, the chemical constitution of cannabis is exceptionally diverse across its many cultivars or "strains." The environment in which plants are cultivated can greatly influence their phenotypes and biomass yield, however, plant genotype remains the primary determinant of which metabolites they are capable of expressing.

Careful climate control, optimization, and disease prevention measures can result in consistently reproducible high biomass yields. However, many secondary metabolites are produced by plants as a defense mechanism in response to stress. Terpenoid expression tends to occur in response to biotic stress, while flavonoid expression is a result of abiotic stress. By intentionally stressing the plant in controlled measures, a greater diversity of secondary metabolites form across the crop, though these measures often reduce biomass yield. A balance must be perfected to maintain biomass yield while still producing the rarer, more medicinally interesting secondary metabolites.

Stress promotes evolution, helping to naturally breed resistance into strains. It is only through exposure to stress factors that plants are able to evolve. Secondary metabolites in *Cannabis sativa* are already utilized in the revolutionary treatment of severely debilitating conditions in humans. Through a greater understanding of the mechanisms and the elicitors of the stress response, more can be harvested and conscripted into the development of life-saving plant-based medicines.

BIBLIOGRAPHY

Aizpurua-Olaizola, Pier, Umut Soydaner, Ekin Öztürk, Daniele Schibano, Yilmaz Simsir, Patricia Navarro, Nestor Etxebarria, and Aresatz Usobiaga. 2016. "Evolution of the Cannabinoid and Terpene Content During the Growth of Cannabis sativa Plants from Different Chemotypes." *Journal of Natural Products* 49: 324–331.

Andre, Christelle M., Jean-Francois Hausman, and Gea Guerriero. 2016. "Cannabis sativa: The Plant of the Thousand and One Molecules." *Frontiers in Plant Science* 7: 19.

Backer, Rachel, Timothy Schwinghamer, Phillip Rosenbaum, Vincent McCarty, Samuel Eichhorn Bilodeau, Dongmei Lyu, and Md Bulbul Ahmed, et al. 2019. "Closing the Yield Gap for Cannabis: A Meta-Analysis of Factors Determining Cannabis Yield." *Frontiers in Plant Science* 10: 495.

Bazzaz, F. A., D. Dusek, D. S Seigler, and A. W. Haney. 1975. "Photosynthesis and Cannabinoid Content of Temperate and Tropical Populations of Cannabis sativa." *Biochemical Systematics and Ecology* 3 (1): 15–18.

Ben-Shabat, Shimon, Ester Fride, Tzviel Sheskin, Tsippy Tamiri, Man-Hee Rhee, Zvi Vogel, Tiziana Bisogno, Luciano De Petrocellis, Vincenzo Di Marzo, and Raphael Mechoulam. 1998. "An Entourage Effect: Inactive Endogenous Fatty Acid Glycerol Esters Enhance 2-Arachidonoyl-Glycerol Cannabinoid Activity." *European Journal of Pharmacology* 365 (1): 23–31.

Bernstein, Nirit, Gorelick Jonathan, Zerahia Roei, and Koch Sraya. 2019. "Impact of N, P, K, and Humic Acid Supplementation on the Chemical Profile of Medical Cannabis (Cannabis sativa L.)." *Frontiers in Plant Science* 10: 736.

Blasco-Benito, S., M. Seijo-Vila, M. Caro-Villalobos, I. Tundidor, C. Andradas, E. García-Taboada, J. Wade, et al. 2018. "Appraising the "Entourage Effect": Antitumor Action of a Pure Cannabinoid Versus a Botanical Drug Preparation in Preclinical Models of Breast Cancer." *Biochemical Pharmacology* 157: 285–293.

Bócsa, I., P. Máthé, and L. Hangyel. 1997. "Effect of Nitrogen on Tetrahydrocannabinol (THC) Content in Hemp (Cannabis sativa L.) Leaves at Different Positions." *Journal of the International Hemp Association* 4 (2): 78–79.

Booth, Judith K., and Jörg Bohlmann. 2019. "Terpenes in Cannabis sativa – From Plant Genome to Humans." *Plant Science* 284: 67–72.

Boucher, F., L. Cosson, J. Unger, and M. R. Paris. 1974. "Cannabis sativa L. Chemical Races or Varieties." *Plantes Médicinales et Phytothérapie* 8 (1): 20–31.

Bricklebank, Neil, and Callie Seaman. 2011. "Soil-free Farming." *Chemistry and Industry Magazine* 6, 19–21. www.soci.org/Chemistry-and-Industry/CnI-Data/2011/6/Soil-free -farming.

Burgel, Lisa, Jens Hartung, and Simone Graeff-Hönninger. 2020. "Impact of Different Growing Substrates on Growth, Yield and Cannabinoid Content of Two Cannabis sativa L. Genotypes in a Pot Culture." *Horticulturae* 4 (6): 62.

Caplan, Deron. 2018. "Propagation and Root Zone Management for Controlled Environment Cannabis Production." PhD Thesis. University of Guelph, Canada.

Caplan, Deron, Mike Dixon, and Youbin Zheng. 2017a. "Optimal Rate of Organic Fertilizer During the Flowering Stage for Cannabis Grown in Two Coir-based Substrates." *HortScience* 52 (9): 1307–1312.

Caplan, Deron, Mike Dixon, and Youbin Zheng. 2017b. "Optimal Rate of Organic Fertilizer During the Flowering Stage for Cannabis Grown in Two Coir-based Substrates." *HortScience* 52 (12): 1796–1803.

Caplan, Deron, Mike Dixon, and Youbin Zheng. 2019. "Increasing Inflorescence Dry Weight and Cannabinoid Content in Medical Cannabis Using Controlled Drought Stress." *HortScience* 54 (5): 964–969.

Chandra, Suman, Hemant Lata, Ikhlas A. Khan, and Mahmoud A. Elsohly. 2008. "Photosynthetic Response of Cannabis sativa L. to Variations in Photosynthetic Photon Flux Densities, Temperature and CO_2 Conditions." *Physiology and Molecular Biology of Plants* 14 (4): 299–306.

Chandra, Suman, Hemant Lata, Ikhlas A. Khan, and Mahmoud A. Elsohly. 2011. "Photosynthetic Response of Cannabis sativa L., an Important Medicinal Plant, to Elevated Levels of CO2." *Physiology and Molecular Biology of Plants* 17 (3): 291–295.

Chandra, Suman, Hemant Lata, Mahmoud A. ElSohly, Larry A. Walker, and David Potter. 2017. "Cannabis Cultivation: Methodological issues for Obtaining Medical-grade Product." *Epilepsy & Behavior* 70: 302–312.

Chandra, Suman, Hemant Lata, Zlatko Mehmedic, Ikhlas A. Khan, and Mahmoud A. ElSohly. 2010. "Assessment of Cannabinoids Content in Micropropagated Plants of Cannabis sativa and Their Comparison with Conventionally Propagated Plants and Mother Plant During Developmental Stages of Growth." *Biochemistry, Molecular Biology and Biotechnology* 76 (7): 743–750.

Chandra, Suman, Hemant Lata, Zlatko Mehmedic, Ikhlas A. Khan, and Mahmoud A. ElSohly. 2015. "Light Dependence of Photosynthesis and Water Vapor Exchange Characteristics in Different High Δ^9-THC Yielding Varieties of Cannabis sativa L." *Journal of Applied Research on Medicinal and Aromatic Plants* 2 (2): 39–47.

Citti, Cinzia, Pasquale Linciano, Fabiana Russo, Livio Luongo, Monica Iannotta, Sabatino Maione, Aldo Laganà, et al. 2019. "A Novel Phytocannabinoid Isolated from Cannabis sativa L. with an In Vivo Cannabimimetic Activity Higher than Δ^9-Tetrahydrocannabinol: Δ^9-Tetrahydrocannabiphorol." *Scientific Reports* 1 (9): 1–13.

Conant, Richard T., Robert P. Walsh, Michael Walsh, Colin W. Bell, and Matthew D. Wallenstein. 2017. "Effects of a Microbial Biostimulant, Mammoth™, on Cannabis sativa Bud Yield." *Journal of Horticulture* 4 (191). doi: 10.4172/2376-0354.1000191.

Da Cunha Leme Filho, Jose F., Wade Thomason, Gregory K. Evanylo, Xunzhong Zhang, Michael S. Strickland, Bee K. Chim, and Andre A. Diatta. 2020. "Biochemical and Physiological Responses of Cannabis sativa to an Integrated Plant Nutrition System." *Agronomy Journal* 112: 5237–5248.

Davies, K. M., and K. E. Schwinn. 2006. "Molecular Biology and Biotechnology of Flavonoid Biosynthesis." In Anderson, O. M. and K. R. Markham (eds), *Flavonoids: Chemistry, Biochemistry and Applications*, 143–218. Boca Raton, FL: CRC Press-Taylor & Francis Group.

De Backer, Benjamin, Kevin Maebe, Alain G. Verstraete, and Corinne Charlier. 2012. "Evolution of the Content of THC and Other Major Cannabinoids in Drug-Type Cannabis Cuttings and Seedlings During Growth of Plants." *Journal of Forensic Sciences* 57 (4): 918–922.

de la Fuente, Alethia, Federico Zamberlan, Andrés Sánchez Ferrán, Facundo Carrillo, Enzo Tagliazucchi, and Carla Pallavicini. 2020. "Relationship Among Subjective Responses, Flavor, and Chemical Composition Across More than 800 Commercial Cannabis Varieties." *Journal of Cannabis Research* 1 (2): 1–18.

Eichhorn Bilodeau, S., B. S. Wu, A. S. Rufyikiri, S. MacPherson, and M Lefsrud. 2019. "An Update on Plant Photobiology and Implications for Cannabis Production." *Frontiers in Plant Science* 10: 296.

ElSohly, Mahmoud A. 2017. "Phytochemistry of Cannabis sativa L." In Kinghorn, A. Douglas, Heinz Falk, Simon Gibbons, and Jun'ichi Kobayashi (eds), *Phytocannabinoids Unraveling the Complex Chemistry and Pharmacology of Cannabis sativa*, 1–36. Cham: Springer International Publishing.

Fischedick, Justin Thomas, Arno Hazekamp, Tjalling Erkelens, Young Hae Choi, and Rob Verpoorte. 2010. "Metabolic Fingerprinting of Cannabis sativa L., Cannabinoids and Terpenoids for Chemotaxonomic and Drug Standardization Purposes." *Phytochemistry* 71 (17–18): 2058–2073.

Flores-Sanchez, Isvett Josefina, and Robert Verpoorte. 2008a. "PKS Activities and Biosynthesis of Cannabinoids and Flavonoids in Cannabis sativa L. Plants." *Plant Cell Physiology* 49 (12): 1767–1782.

Flores-Sanchez, Isvett Josefina, and Robert Verpoorte. 2008b. "Secondary Metabolism in Cannabis." *Phytochemistry Reviews* 7: 615–639.

Frassinetti, Stefania, Eleonora Moccia, Leonardo Caltavuturo, Morena Gabriele, Vincenzo Longo, Lorenza Bellani, Gianluca Giorgi, and Lucia Giorgetti. 2018. "Nutraceutical Potential of Hemp (Cannabis sativa L.) Seeds and Sprouts." *Food Chemistry* 262: 56–66.

Gülck, Thies, and Birger Lindberg Møller. 2020. "Phytocannabinoids: Origins and Biosynthesis." *Trends in Plant Science* 25 (10): 985–1004.

Goldstein, Bonni. 2016. *Cannabis Revealed*. United States of America.

Gordon, Dani. 2020. *The CBD Bible*. London: Orion Spring.

Gorelick, Johnathan, and Nirit Bernstein. 2017. "Chemical and Physical Elicitation for Enhanced Cannabinoid Production in Cannabis." In Chandra, S. (ed), Cannabis sativa L. – Botany and Biotechnology, 439–456. Cham: Springer International Publishing.

Hanuš, Lumír Ondřej, and Marie Dostálová. 1994. "The Effect of Soil Fertilization on the Formation and the Amount of Cannabinoid Substances in Cannabis sativa L. in the Course of One Vegetation Period." *Acta Universitatis Palackianae Olomucensis Facultatis Medicae* 138: 11–15.

Hanuš, Lumír Ondřej, Stefan Martin Meyer, Eduardo Muñoz, Orazio Taglialatela-Scafati, and Giovanni Appendino. 2016. "Phytocannabinoids: A Unified Critical Inventory." *Natural Product Reports* 33 (12): 1357–1392.

Hanuš, Lumír Ondřej, and Yotam Hod. 2020. "Terpenes/Terpenoids in Cannabis: Are They Important?" *Medical Cannabis and Cannabinoids* 3: 20–60.

Haupt, Joshua. 2018. *Three a Light*. Colorado: Pono Publications Ltd.

Hazekamp, A., R. Peltenburg, R. Verpoorte, and C. Giroud. 2005. "Chromatographic and Spectroscopic Data of Cannabinoids from Cannabis sativa." *Journal of Liquid Chromatography & Related Technologies* 28 (15): 2361–2382.

Hazekamp, Arno. 2016. "Evaluating the Effects of Gamma-irradiation for Decontamination of Medicinal Cannabis." *Frontiers in Pharmacology* 7: 108.

Heblinski, Marika, Marina Santiago, Charlotte Fletcher, Jordyn Stuart, Mark Connor, Iain S. McGregor, and Jonathon C. Arnold. 2020. "Terpenoids Commonly Found in Cannabis sativa Do Not Modulate the Actions of Phytocannabinoids or Endocannabinoids on TRPA1 and TRPV1 Channels." *Cannabis and Cannabinoid Research* 5 (4): 305–317.

Heldt, Hans-Walter, and Brigit Piechulla. 2004. "Secondary Metabolites Fulfil Specific Ecological Functions in Plants." In *Plant Biochemistry*, 403–411. Heidelberg: Elsevier Academic Press.

Hillig, Karl W. 2004. "A Chemotaxonomic Analysis of Terpenoid Variation in Cannabis." *Biochemical Systematics and Ecology* 32 (10): 875–891.

Honma, S, H. Kaneshima, M. Mori, and T. Kitsutaka. 1971. "Cannabis Grown in Hokkaido 2. Contents of Cannabinol, Tetrahydrocannabinol and Cannabidiol in Wild Cannabis." *Hokkaido Ritsu Eisei Kenkyusho* 21: 180–185.

Ivanyi, Ildiko, and Zoltan Izsaki. 2009. "Effect of Nitrogen, Phosphorus, and Potassium Fertilization on Nutritional Status of Fiber Hemp." *Communications in Soil Science and Plant Analysis* 40 (1–6): 974–986.

Jeandet, Philippe. 2015. "Phytoalexins: Current Progress and Future Prospects." *Molecules* 2 (20): 2770–2774.

Jin, Dan, Shengxi Jin, and Jie Chen. 2019. "Cannabis Indoor Growing Conditions, Management Practices and Post-Harvest Treatment: A Review." *American Journal of Plant Sciences* 10 (6): 925–946.

Kalinowski, Jennifer, Keith Edmisten, Jeanine Davis, Michelle McGinnis, Kristin Hicks, Paul Cockson, Patrick Veazie, and Brian E. Whipker. 2020. "Augmenting Nutrient Acquisition Ranges of Greenhouse Grown CBD (Cannabidiol) Hemp (Cannabis sativa) Cultivars." *Horticulturae* 6: 98.

Kandi, Sabitha, Vikram Godishala, Pragna Rao, and K. V. Ramana. 2015. "Biomedical Significance of Terpenes: An Insight." *Biomedicine* 1 (3): 8–10.

Knight, Glenys, Sean Hansen, Mark Connor, Helen Poulsen, Catherine McGovern, and Janet Stacey. 2010. "The Results of an Experimental Indoor Hydroponic Cannabis Growing Study, Using the 'Screen of Green' (ScrOG) Method – Yield, Tetrahydrocannabinol (THC) and DNA Analysis." *Forensic Science International* 202: 36–44.

Konstantinović, B., S. Vidović, A. Stojanović, M. Kojić, N. Samardžić, M. Popov, A. Gavarić, and B. Pavlić. 2018. "Allelopathic Effect of Essential Oil of Cannabis sativa L. on Selected Vegetable Species." *In* IX *International Scientific Agriculture Symposium "AGROSYM 2018,"* Jahorina, Bosnia and Herzegovina, 4–7 October 2018. Book of Proceedings, pp. 1212–1215. University of East Sarajevo, Faculty of Agriculture, Republic of Srpska, Bosnia.

Landi, S. 1997. "Mineral Nutrition of Cannabis sativa L." *Journal of Plant Nutrition* 20 (2–3): 311–326.

Lata, Hemant, Suman Chandra, Ikhlas Khan, and Mahmoud ElSohly. 2016. "In Vitro Propagation of Cannabis sativa L. and Evaluation of Regenerated Plants for Genetic Fidelity and Cannabinoids Content for Quality Assurance." *Methods in Molecular Biology* 1391: 275–88. Springer Science+Business Media.

Latta, R. P., and B. J. Eaton. 1975. "Seasonal Fluctuations in Cannabinoid Content of Kansas Marijuana." *Economic Botany* 29: 153–163.

Linger, P., J. Müssig, H. Fischer, and J. Kobert. 2002. "Industrial Hemp (Cannabis sativa L.) Growing on Heavy Metal Contaminated Soil: Fibre Quality and Phytoremediation Potential." *Industrial Crops and Products* 16 (1): 33–42.

Livingston, Samuel J., Teagen D. Quilichini, Judith K. Booth, Darren C. J. Wong, Kim H. Rensing, Jessica Laflamme-Yonkman, Simone D. Castellarin, Joerg Bohlmann,

Jonathan E. Page, and A. Lacey Samuels. 2020. "Cannabis Glandular Trichomes Alter Morphology and Metabolite Content During Flower Maturation." *The Plant Journal* 101: 37–56.

Lowe, Henry, Lorenzo Gordon, Tony Vendryes, Archibald McDonald, and Deborah Miran. 2018. *Medical Cannabis: The Way Forward for Health Care Practitioners.* Kingston: Pelican Publishers.

Lydon, John, Alan H. Teramura, and C. Benjamin Coffman. 1987. "UV-B Radiation Effects on Photosynthesis, Growth and Cannabinoid Production of Two Cannabis sativa Chemotypes." *Phytochemistry and Photobiology* 46 (2): 201–206.

Maļceva, Marija, Māra Vikmane, and Veneranda Stramkale. 2011. "Changes of Photosynthesis-related Parameters and Productivity of Cannabis sativa Under Different Nitrogen Supply." *Environmental and Experimental Biology* 9: 61–69.

Magagnini, Gianmaria, Gianpaolo Grassi, and Stiina Kotiranta. 2018. "The Effect of Light Spectrum on the Morphology and Cannabinoid Content of Cannabis sativa L." *Medical Cannabis and Cannabinoids* 1: 19–27.

Mahmoodzadeh, Homa, Mohsen Ghasemi, and Hasan Zanganeh. 2015. "Allelopathic Effect of Medicinal Plant Cannabis sativa L. on Lactuca sativa L. Seed Germination." *Acta Agriculturae Slovenica* 105: 233–239.

Mandolino, G., A. Carboni, S. Forapani, V. Faeti, and P. Ranalli. 1999. "Identification of DNA Markers Linked to the Male Sex in Dioecious Hemp (Cannabis sativa L.)." *Theoretical and Applied Genetics* 98: 86–92.

Marti, Guillaume, Sylvain Schnee, Yannis Andrey, Claudia Simoes-Pires, Pierre-Alain Carrupt, Jean-Luc Wolfender, and Katia Gindro. 2014. "Study of Leaf Metabolome Modifications Induced by UV-C Radiations in Representative Vitis, Cissus and Cannabis Species by LC-MS Based Metabolomics and Antioxidant Assays." *Molecules* 19 (9): 14004–14021.

McPartland, J. M., R. C. Clarke, and D. P. Watson. 2000. "Section 2 Disease and Pests of Cannabis." In *Hemp Disease and Pests*, 25–167. Wallingford: CABI Publishing.

McPartland, John. 1997. "Cannabis as Repellent and Pesticide." *Journal of the International Hemp Association* 2 (4): 87–92.

McPartland, John. 2018. "Cannabis Systematics at the Levels of Family, Genus and Species." *Cannabis and Cannabinoid Research* 144: 203–212.

McPartland, John M. 1996. "Cannabis Pests." *Journal of International Hemp Association* 3 (2): 49, 52–55.

McPartland, John M., and Ethan B. Russo. 2001. "Cannabis and Cannabis Extracts: Greater than the Sum of their Parts?" *Journal of Cannabis Therapeutics* 1 (3–4): 103–132.

McPartland, John, and Kevin McKernan. 2017. "Contaminants of Concern in Cannabis: Microbes, Heavy Metals and Pesticides." In Suman Chandra, Hemant Lata, and Mahmoud A. ElSohly (eds), Cannabis sativa L. – *Botany and Biotechnology*, 457–474. Cham: Springer.

Medicinal Genomics. 2020. *Medicinal Genomics.* Accessed January 10, 2021. https://www.medicinalgenomics.com/youpcr-platform/.

Miura, Kenji, and Tsuyoshi Furumoto. 2013. "Cold Signaling and Cold Response in Plants." *International Journal of Molecular Sciences* 14: 5312–5337.

Mohan Ram, H.Y., and R. Sett. 1982. "Induction of Fertile Male Flowers in Genetically Female Cannabis sativa Plants by Silver Nitrate and Silver Thiosulphate Anionic Complex." *Theoretical and Applied Genetics* 62 (4): 369–375.

Neel, P.L., and R.W. Harris. 1971. "Motion-induced Inhibition of Elongation and Induction of Dormancy in Liquidambar." *Science* 173: 58–59.

Nelson, Regina. 2018. *The Survivor's Guide to Medical Cannabis.* Columbia: Integral Education & Consulting.

Pare, Paul W., and Tumlinson H. James. 1999. "Plant Volatiles as a Defense Against Insect Herbivores." *Plant Physiology* 121: 325–331.

Pate, David W. 1983. "Possible Role of Ultraviolet Radiation in Evolution of Cannabis Chemotypes." *Economic Botany* 37: 396.

Pate, David W. 1994. "Chemical Ecology of Cannabis." *Journal of International Hemp Association* 2: 32–37.

Potter, David J. 2009. "The Propagation, Characterisation and Optimisation of Cannabis Sativa L as a Phytopharmaceutical." PhD Thesis. London: Kings College London, March.

Potter, David J. 2014. "A Review of Cultivation and Processing of Cannabis (Cannabis sativa L) for Production of Prescription Medicines in the UK." *Drug Testing and Analysis* 6: 31–38.

Potter, David J., and Paul Duncombe. 2012. "The Effect of Electrical Lighting Power and Irradiance on Indoor-Grown Cannabis Potency and Yield." *Journal of Forensic Sciences* 57 (3): 618–622.

Pudełko, Krzysztof, Leszek Majchrzak, and Dorota Narożna. 2014. "Allelopathic Effect of Fibre Hemp (Cannabis sativa L.) on Monocot and Dicot Plant Species." *Industrial Crops and Products* 56: 191–199.

Ramakrishna, Akula, and Gokare Aswathanarayana Ravishankar. 2011. "Influence of Abiotic Stress Signals on Secondary Metabolites in Plants." *Plant Signaling & Behavior* 6 (11): 1720–1731.

Resh, Howard. 2012. *Hydroponic Food Production: A Definitive Guidebook for the Advanced Home Gardener and the Commercial Hydroponic Grower.* New York: CRC Press.

Robertson, Larry W., Michael A. Lyle, and Stephen Billets. 1975. "Biotransformation of Cannabinoids by Syncephalastrum Racemosum." *Biomedical Mass Spectrometry* 2 (5): 266–271.

Rodziewicz, Paweł, and Oliver Kayser. 2020. "Cannabis sativa L. – Cannabis." In Novak, J., and W. D. Blüthner (eds), *Medicinal, Aromatic and Stimulant Plants*, 233–264. Cham: Springer.

Romano, Luigi, and Arno Hazekamp. 2018. "An Overview of Galenic Preparation Methods for Medical Cannabis." *Current Bioactive Compounds* 15 (2): 174–195.

Romero, P., A. Peris, K. Vergara, and J. T. Matus. 2020. "Comprehending and Improving Cannabis Specialized Metabolism in the Systems Biology Era." *Plant Science* 298: 110571. doi: 10.1016/j.plantsci.2020.110571.

Rosenburg, Evan, Richard Tsien, Benjamin Whalley, and Orrin Devinsky. 2015. "Cannabinoids and Epilepsy." *Neurotherapeutics* 12: 747–768.

Rothschild, M., M. G. Rowan, and J. W. Fairbairn. 1977. "Storage of Cannabinoids by Arctia Caja and Zonocerus Elegans Fed on Chemically Distinct Strains of Cannabis sativa." *Nature* 266: 650–651.

Roy, B. K., and B. Dutta. 2003. "In Vitro Lethal Efficacy of Leaf Extract of Cannabis sativa Linn on the Larvae of Chironomous Samoensis Edward: An Insect of Public Health Concern." *Indian Journal of Experimental Biology* 41: 1338–1341.

Russo, Ethan B. 2019. "The Case for the Entourage Effect and Conventional Breeding of Clinical Cannabis: "No Strain" No Gain." *Frontiers in Plant Science* 9: 1969.

Seaman, Callie. 2017. "Investigation of Nutrient Solutions for the Hydroponic Growth of Plants." PhD Dissertation. Sheffield Hallam University. Sheffield, UK.

Sharma, Anket, Babar Shahzad, Abdul Rehman, Renu Bhardwaj, Marco Landi, and Bingsong Zheng. 2019. "Response of Phenylpropanoid Pathway and the Role of Polyphenols in Plants under Abiotic Stress." *Molecules* 24 (13): 2452.

Sharma, Pallavi, Ambuj Bhushan Jha, Rama Shanker Dubey, and Mohammad Pessarakli. 2012. "Reactive Oxygen Species, Oxidative Damage, and Antioxidative Defense

Mechanism in Plants Under Stressful Conditions." *Journal of Botany* 2012, Article ID 217037,26 pages, 2012. https://doi.org/10.1155/2012/217037 .

Stemeroff, Jonathan. 2017. "Irrigation Management Strategies for Medical Cannabis in Controlled Environments." PhD Thesis. Ontario: University of Guelph, November.

Taghinasab, Meysam, and Suha Jabaji. 2020. "Cannabis Microbiome and the Role of Endophytes in Modulating the Production of Secondary Metabolites: An Overview." *Microorganisms* 8 (3): 855.

Tang, K., P. C. Struik, X. Yin, D. Calzolari, S. Musio, C. Thouminot, M. Bjelková, V. Stramkale, G. Magagnini, and S. Amaducci. 2017. "A Comprehensive Study of Planting Density and Nitrogen Fertilization Effect on Dual-purpose Hemp (Cannabis sativa L.) Cultivation." *Industrial Crops & Products* 107: 427–438.

Thomas, Brian, and Gerald Pollard. 2016. "Preparation and Distribution of Cannabis and Cannabis-Derived Dosage Formulations for Investigational and Therapeutic Use in the United States." *Frontiers in Pharmacology* 7: 385.

Vanhove, Wouter, Patrick Van Damme, and Natalie Meert. 2011. "Factors Determining Yield and Quality of Illicit Indoor Cannabis (Cannabis spp.) Production." *Forensic Science International* 212: 158–163.

Wang, Mei, Yan-Hong Wang, Bharathi Avula, Mohamed M. Radwan, Amira S. Wanas, John van Antwerp, Jon F. Parcher, Mahmoud A. ElSohly, and Ikhlas A. Khan. 2016. "Decarboxylation Study of Acidic Cannabinoids: A Novel Approach Using Ultra-high-performance Supercritical Fluid Chromatography/Photodiode Array-Mass Spectrometry." *Cannabis and Cannabinoid Research* 1 (1): 262–271.

Werz, Oliver, Julia Seegers, Anja Maria Schaible, Christina Weinigel, Dagmar Barz, Andreas Koeberle, Gianna Allegrone, et al. 2014. "Cannflavins from Hemp Sprouts: A Novel Cannabinoid-Free Hemp Food Product, Target Microsomal Prostaglandin E2 Synthase-1 and 5-Lipoxygenase." *PharmaNutrition* 2 (3): 53–60.

Winkel-Shirley, Brenda. 2002. "Biosynthesis of Flavonoids and Effects of Stress." *Current Opinion in Plant Biology* 5 (3): 218–223.

Zhang, Wen Jing, and Lars Olof Björn. 2009. "The Effect of Ultraviolet Radiation on the Accumulation of Medicinal Compounds in Plants." *Fitoterapia* 80 (4): 207–218.

2 Aroma in Cannabis
A Foundation for Chemotype Classification

John S. Abrams, William J. T. Ellyson,
Victor J. Gomez, and Jean L. Talleyrand

CONTENTS

2.1 INTRODUCTION

It is not far-fetched to hypothesize that the mutualistic coevolution of plants and humans has resulted in a broad range of interactions between cannabis and the human endocannabinoid system (ECS). Like other botanicals, cannabis contains many biologically active ingredients. Phytocannabinoids, a major chemical class in cannabis, interact with the constituents of the ECS, which are located on nerve and immune cells in every human organ. The effects of this interaction are broad and involve the mediation of pain, mood, sleep, and appetite.

DOI: 10.1201/9780429274893-2

The Clinical Endocannabinoid System Consortium (CESC) is composed of a multi-disciplinary group of scientists engaged in understanding the many interactions between cannabis active ingredients and the ECS. Our initial goal is to categorize cannabis active ingredients based on clinical effects. The key to this approach relies on the validation of historical use categories in a cannabis-prevalent population. The CESC is located in California where cannabis users have prevailed through nearly a century of prohibition. Lacking access to mainstream science, our cannabis community developed an organoleptic approach to assessing cannabis value and effect.

This chapter exhibits the CESC's analysis of cannabis aroma, its use in drug categorization, and its predicted effects. Our work includes an analysis of the terpenoid content of proposed aroma groups. Next, relying on our crowd-sourced web-based Dosing Project™ work for validation, we note the influence of harvest and storage practices on aroma. We also demonstrate gender preference for a particular aroma group. Finally, we identify a terpene ratio discriminant feature that may be predictive of two commonly described cannabis effects.

Statistical analysis of crowd-sourced responses allows us to understand the known and discover the unknown. Our investigations initially described terpenoid content, as terpenes are a significant class of aromatic compounds found in cannabis. In this approach, we also reveal a second class of aromatic compounds that have yet to be fully explored, esters. This perspective fulfills an unmet need for accessible chemotype descriptive features for cannabis beyond major phytocannabinoids, Δ^9-tetrahydrocannabinol (THC), and cannabidiol (CBD). Our observational study and analyses expedite the understanding of active cannabis ingredients, including a preliminary understanding of dose-effect relationships and interactions.

2.1.1 THE LINGUISTICS OF AROMA

It has been recognized that English speakers appear to have only two to three dedicated smell words in their active vocabulary ("stinky", "fragrant", "musty"). This is a significant contrast to the 15 smell terms in Maniq (Majid 2015). Moreover, English speakers utilize nouns to describe odors, while speakers of Jahai and Maniq rely on verbs. The striking mechanistic similarities between human and rodent data with respect to vision, audition, and olfaction lead us to believe that odors are universally encoded as objects (Olofsson and Gottfried 2015).

Aromatic designations are language and culture specific. In the English language, many words are used to describe aroma. Jason Castro at the Bates College Program in Neuroscience uses non-negative matrix factorization to compare 144 monomolecular odors with 146 semantic labels in order to determine if there is hierarchical clustering in the language of aroma that correlates with neurological pathways (Castro, Ramanathan, and Chennubhotla 2013). They identified a set of ten near orthogonal aromatic axes that each represents a single odor quality. The descriptors involve words such as fragrant/floral, woody/resinous, citrus/lemon, sickening/putrid, fruity/sweet, chemical, minty, popcorn/earthy, sharp/pungent, and aromatic/almond.

Evidence suggests that perfumers and enologists in Western countries learn designated odor terms and categories well beyond those present in everyday language. However, "The lack of cultural and art discourse pertaining to the sense of smell is simply the lack of vocabulary to describe scent phenomena" (Raspet 2016). In a study with speakers of Jahai, abstract terminology was used to identify different scents. However, there was a consistent and very high response rate of agreement of these terms. In English, we tend to refer to scents based on visual aspects, these terms are limited to their referent, and abstract terminology allows for greater flexibility and accuracy. Utilizing terms such as earth, floral, and fuel are excellent examples of how we can use specific terminology from a categorical standpoint. We can go even further and produce descriptors that identify a single odor quality categorizing them as descriptive features of these aroma categories. By establishing a nomenclature in the cannabis industry, we can obtain a very similar result as speakers of Jahai. Compiling an abstract terminology to represent terpene and other odorant profiles would result in a stronger foundation for understanding cannabis pharmacology, including organoleptic responses and characteristic anticipated effects.

2.1.2 TERPENOIDS

Terpenes are an important active component of *Cannabis sativa L*. These aromatic compounds make up approximately 10% of cannabis trichome content by weight (Potter 2009). Terpenes have been studied for the reduction of pain (Guimarães, Serafini, and Quintans-Júnior 2014). They contribute to the anxiolytic effect of cannabis (Pamplona et al. 2018). In addition, certain terpenes may paradoxically contribute to a stimulating effect of cannabis (Gulluni et al. 2018). Terpenes also contribute to aroma, which may correlate with distinct effects of cannabis cultivars.

Terpene content ratio can be used to validate the cannabis plant. To the inexperienced consumer, members of the Cannabaceae family may have a similar appearance and aroma. It is noted that *Cannabis sativa L*. and *Humulus lupulus L*. (Hops) produce similar terpenes. However, an analysis of the β-caryophyllene and α-humulene content demonstrates that terpenes develop in ratios. *Cannabis sativa L*. contains a 3:1 ratio of β-caryophyllene to α-humulene and *Humulus lupulus* has a 1:3 β-caryophyllene to α-humulene ratio (Abrams et al. 2016; Miller and Abrams 2016). We believe terpene content ratio analysis to be useful in the chemotaxonomy of cannabis cultivars.

Cannabis sativa L. produces over 100 distinct terpene compounds (Brenneisen 2007). Terpene clusters represent the link of multiple biosynthetic pathways in the plant (Booth, Page, and Bohlmann 2017). By sampling multiple cannabis cultivars, multivariate analysis can expose dominant terpene clusters. In a study of multiple high THC cultivars, the use of principal component analysis (PCA) reduced an extensive list of terpenes to a limited number of terpene clusters (Fischedick 2017). Further evaluation of these clusters of terpenes may readily correlate with the effects described by cannabis consumers.

2.2   IDENTIFYING CANNABIS AROMA CATEGORIES BASED ON TERPENOID CONTENT

2.2.1   THE 2015 GOLDEN TARP AWARDS COMPETITION

Cannabis aroma can be used to assess the quality attributes of the product. California cannabis farmers propose an organoleptic approach to plant categorization and effect. It has yet to be proven whether the aroma of cannabis influences its effect. Cannabis aroma likely attracts or repels insects and other consumers. As a result of market forces, aroma is an important consideration in cannabis agronomy and formulation development. Our analysis of aroma begins with terpene profiles from a set of cannabis flower samples submitted to a northern California cannabis competition. The event reflects a population that has cultivated cannabis for a substantive number of years. We took advantage of this event in order to develop a cannabis chemotaxonomy based on aroma. The Golden Tarp Award (GTA) competition (Figure 2.1) carried out late in the summer of 2015 is foundational to our work.

The GTA required that contestants submit their dried cannabis flowers into "Earth", "Floral", "Fruity", or "Fuel" aroma groups. The underlying cannabinoid and terpenoid content for each sample was determined, producing a rich dataset for analyses. A distribution of submitted samples in each aroma group is depicted in Figure 2.1. It can be seen that the dominant aroma was "Fuel", with roughly equal proportions of samples in the other categories. This is not unexpected for a sample set derived from summer light deprivation cultivation in the Emerald Triangle region of California in 2015. We applied both univariate and multivariate analysis to the GTA terpene content dataset and examined how specific terpenes corresponded to these aroma groups. The results are summarized in the following section.

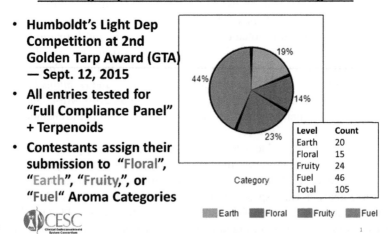

FIGURE 2.1   Details of the 2015 Golden Tarp Awards Cannabis competition in California.

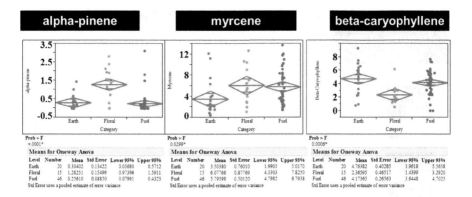

FIGURE 2.2   Univariate terpenoid analyses of the "Earth", "Floral", and "Fuel" aroma categories.

Our analysis begins from a somewhat empirical departure point. We uncovered through trial and error that a small set of terpenes were significantly different between aroma groups. These results are depicted in Figure 2.2. We utilized JMP v10 software (SAS Institute, Cary, NC) for statistical and graphical analyses throughout this work. Using simple univariate analysis ANOVA, we determined that the terpene α-pinene was significantly elevated in the "Floral" aroma group, with a mean value that was roughly four-fold greater than that observed in the "Earth" or "Fuel" categories. The terpene myrcene was found to be present in the "Earth" category at roughly half the levels found in the "Floral" and "Fuel" categories. The sesquiterpene beta-caryophyllene (BCP) was observed in this study to be decreased by half, on average, in the "Floral" category.

Prior studies have shown that these terpenes, which appear to correlate with the olfactory classification of cultivars into "Earth", "Floral", or "Fuel", are also responsible for modulating the endocannabinoid system (ECS). Indeed, β-caryophyllene is shown to have direct activity on the cannabinoid$_2$ receptor (CnR2/CB$_2$) in mouse models of neuropathic pain (Klauke et al. 2014). α-Pinene has been implicated as an acetylcholine esterase inhibitor, thereby believed to promote memory and cognition (Miyazawa and Yamafuji 2005). Yet, it displays zolpidem-like (Ambien) activity in mice at the GABA$_A$ receptor (Yang et al. 2016). Myrcene has demonstrated sedative properties in mice (Do Vale et al. 2002). We postulate that these aromatic compounds are important in correlating chemotypic categorizations to the effect of cannabis.

2.2.2   Multivariate Analyses of Terpenoids and Aroma Groups

The two-way hierarchical clustering dendrogram and heat map for the GTA dataset (Figure 2.3) is a multivariate analysis approach that identifies which samples are most similar based on their overall terpenoid content (i.e., data vector). It is carried out computationally as an iterative process, starting with joining individual samples and expanding each cluster until all samples are connected successively into clusters

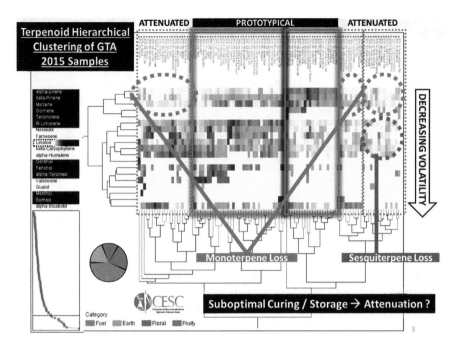

FIGURE 2.3 Dendrogram from two-way hierarchical clustering analysis (HCA) of the Golden Tarp Award (GTA) samples by terpenoid and color-coded for aroma category.

of increasing sample counts, resulting in one large cluster. The dendrogram lengths represent relative (Euclidean) distances of clusters from each other. The sample labels are color-coded by GTA aroma category. The terpenoids in this two-way clustering are also labeled on the left as monoterpenes (black background) or sesquiterpenes (white background). The heat map colors represent terpenoid content depicted as a gradient from low (pale) to high (dark).

We identify two main clusters visually from the dendrogram and heat map: one labeled "Prototypical" and one "Attenuated". Within the "Prototypical" clusters, there are two subsets. One is trending "Floral", and another trending "Fuel". There are distinct patterns of monoterpene or sesquiterpene content across each aroma group. Furthermore, the two-way clustering of the terpenoids themselves appears to follow both a trend to cluster mono- or sesquiterpenoid classes. A notable exception is linalool, which is made along with nerolidol by the same terpene synthase in snapdragons (Nagegowda et al. 2008), suggesting similarity in cannabis. There is also a trend to align from most to least volatile, and we note that α-bisabolol is consistently present. We further note that in the clusters labeled "Attenuated", large swaths of terpenoid content appear to be diminished. We interpret this as the loss of terpenes resulting from suboptimal handling and storage post-harvest. Furthermore, the lower myrcene content in the "Earth" category (Figure 2.2) may be reflective of a general terpenoid loss. Overall, this figure suggests that both terpenoid content patterns and patches of loss may contribute to aroma category assignments.

A second form of multivariate analysis is employed to determine how well a categorical value can be predicted by a set of continuous variables. We employ discriminant analysis to evaluate how well the set of continuous terpenoid content values for each sample can predict the various aroma groups of the samples submitted in the 2015 GTA competition. In contrast to logistic regression, which is employed later in the chapter (*vide infra*), discriminant analysis classifications are fixed, and a multivariate set of Y variables are considered to be the random variables. We are utilizing this discriminant analysis approach to predict the categorical value based on the continuous ones.

We present a linear discriminant analysis canonical bi-plot in Figure 2.4. The observations and the multivariate means of each group are points on the bi-plot. They are expressed in terms of the first two canonical variables, which are represented by the bi-plot axes Canonical1 and Canonical2 respectively. These define two dimensions that provide maximum separation among the aroma category groups. Linear discriminant analysis assumes that the Y variables are normally distributed with the same variances and co-variances. We also display a hybrid type of discriminant analysis result in the Figure 2.4 insert. Here, the co-variances are assumed to be different across aroma groups. The analyses present the aroma group means as a series of plus ("+") markers within each group centroid. Each sample is a symbol representing a contestant-submitted aroma category. Its position is the Mahalanobis distance based on its distance to the aroma group mean. This takes into account the variances and co-variances between the variables. An ellipse denoting a 50% contour is plotted for each group, which depicts a region in the space of the first two canonical variables that contains approximately 50% of the observations, assuming

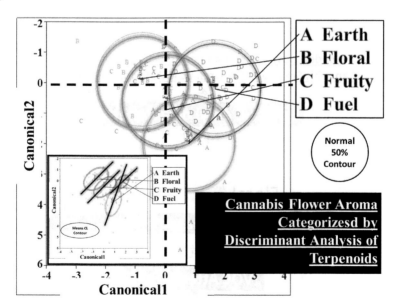

FIGURE 2.4 Canonical score plot from discriminant analysis of the Golden Tarp Award (GTA) samples predicting aroma category based on individual terpenoid content.

normality. The point (0,0) represents the grand mean of the data in terms of the canonical variables and is shown as the intersection of the two bold dotted lines in the figure. Overall, the relative degree of overlap indicates how well these aroma categories can be discriminated.

Our analysis reveals a clear distinction between the "Floral" and "Fuel" categories in the horizontal (Canonical1) dimension of Figure 2.4, indicating a primary distinctive feature across the cannabis flower samples tested. These two categories are moved rightward and leftward of the overall canonical center. In contrast, the "Earth" category moved downward from the canonical center, indicating that it is influenced by a different set of underlying terpenoid content values. The "Fruity" category lies at the canonical center and overlaps with the other categories, indicating that it is not well defined by any of the terpenoid content values. The means CL contours depicted in the Figure 2.4 insert were determined using a hybrid discriminant analysis method. Here, we observe that the long axes of the contours are basically parallel for the "Floral", "Fuel", and "Fruity" categories, and differ from that of the "Earth" category. This is consistent with the hypothesis that the underlying factors driving these three categories are largely similar, whereas that of "Earth" differs. The simplest unifying explanation for this is that "Floral" and "Fuel" are influenced by different terpenoid content and that "Fruity" is independent of terpenoid content and is likely a function of a different class of natural products. We currently attribute this feature to the ester category. "Earth" represents attenuation, as described previously, and would likely have a different set of co-variances, reflecting differences in relative volatility across the set of terpenoids. This is the explanation for its different contour position and dimension in the hybrid discriminant analysis canonical space.

Taken together, we propose a model as depicted in Figure 2.5. The model illustrates how aroma categories may correlate with cannabis small volatile organic

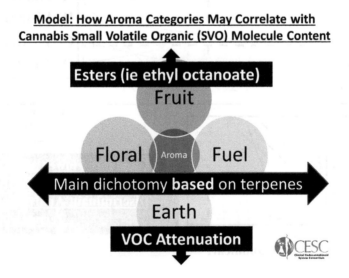

FIGURE 2.5 Modeling aroma category correlations with cannabis small volatile organic (SVO) molecule content.

(SVO) compound content. Elements of the canonical plot (Figure 2.4) have been incorporated into this model, which is seen as a collection of non-overlapping Venn diagram circles. The principal (horizontal) dimension is defined by the terpenoid content and underlies the "Floral" and "Fuel" categories. The vertical dimension reflects overall attenuation as described for "Earth". In this two-dimensional scheme, "Fruity" is not yet well defined based on the current state of cannabis chemotype knowledge. Advances in this area (such as for the ester category of natural products) will become another principal discriminant feature and provide a crucial third axis to the aroma-based chemotype scheme underlying the cannabis commodity.

2.3 VALIDATING CANNABIS AROMA CATEGORIES USING THE DOSING PROJECT™

In a proof of concept (POC) version of its flagship study called the Dosing Project™, the CESC takes an observational study approach to the use of smoked or vaporized cannabis for the improvement of pain and disordered sleep. Initial results identify a predictable dosage (in milligrams per kilograms body weight) from smoked high THC flowers with a significant probability of completely improving pain and sleep. The analyses of independent and dependent variables inform more than dosage. They provide pertinent information on user preferences and habits. Most importantly, our results demonstrate a valid, novel approach to investigating dose, effect, and adverse events.

The Dosing Project™ captured both categorical and continuous responses in a short series of query screens of a crowd-sourced, web-based format. Summaries of this work have been previously presented, and additional manuscripts detailing analyses of CBD effects and interactions with adverse events and aroma groups are available. The clinical data described herein validates certain aroma categories detailed previously using an observational study approach. Based on the conclusions obtained from our initial aroma group analyses detailed previously, we elected to query respondents for the three categories comprising: "Floral", "Earth", and "Fuel". The absence of any discriminant power in the "Fruity" group influenced us to omit it from the early version of the survey. The query screen for aroma group is shown in Figure 2.6. In addition, we included text descriptive queues as a modal help screen, which is shown in the lower left.

The aim of including these aroma prompts is to investigate whether a respondent's assessment of aroma adds validity as a significant factor affecting therapeutic response to smoking or vaping cannabis. The fraction of responses in each of the three aroma groups is shown in Figure 2.6. About half of the respondents identified "Earth", which we attribute to a category of attenuated cannabis botanical material likely processed or stored under suboptimal conditions. These conditions likely lead to a loss of volatile organic compounds, many of which contribute to Cannabis aroma. The remaining half of the responses are split into roughly two-thirds "Floral" and one-third "Fuel".

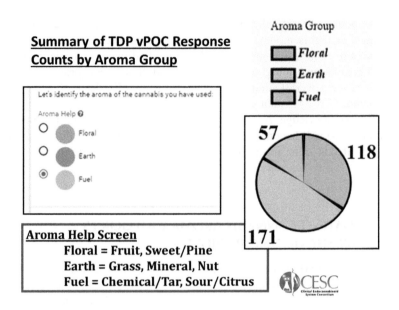

FIGURE 2.6 Details of the Dosing Project™ vPOC response counts by aroma category including modal help lexical definitions.

2.3.1 CANNABIS AROMA CATEGORY RESPONSE RATES CORRELATE WITH THE ANNUAL COMMODITY PRODUCTION CYCLE

We present a time series analysis by aroma group in Figure 2.7. These results reflect the availability of cannabis flowers. The trend in harvest release by farmers may help explain a seasonal pattern of available aroma groups reflected in the Dosing Project™ responses. The aroma group, in turn, may reflect package and storage stability and the content of volatile terpene content. We illustrate this using cannabis grown in the Emerald Triangle as an example. The "Floral" group best represents this trend. Cannabis produced in this region is predominantly grown in both greenhouses and full sun. The Emerald Triangle is believed to produce a significant portion of the cannabis likely to have been reported in the Dosing Project™. The seasonality of sun-grown cannabis in California results in a glut of available product in the fall and winter months. This glut lowers the price point for a pound of processed flowers significantly and has driven two strategies by farmers to maximize their profits. First, by using light deprivation techniques, crops can be forced into early flowering, which provides a mid-summer harvest when product levels are low, and second, by storing a portion of fall harvest carefully to release in spring and summer when prices are back up. In this scenario, the rising "Earth" group of Figure 2.7 represents the market release of stored cannabis flowers where the content of volatile terpenes is attenuated. Furthermore, we note that a study of consumer perceptions of strain differences in cannabis aroma (Gilbert and DiVerdi 2018) observed that the most frequently reported aroma descriptor was "earthy".

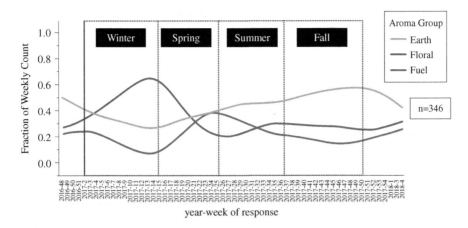

year-week of response

FIGURE 2.7   Time series: Fraction of weekly response counts in the Dosing Project™ by aroma category.

2.3.2 CANNABIS AROMA CATEGORY PREFERENCES BY HEIGHT: A SURROGATE FOR GENDER

The Dosing Project™ did not ask specifically about the gender of responders. Nonetheless, we wanted to see if we could establish any preliminary indication for gender skewing in cannabis botanical products. We did collect responder height information, and after outlier removal for inappropriate height responses (caused by a coding oversight in the application), we observed distribution for responder height as shown in Figure 2.8. The distribution was fitted by a normal two-mixture continuous fit and we obtained a result showing around 40% in the lower height class and 60% in the higher height class. We are attributing female gender to the shorter height class, and male gender to the taller height class. This two-fifths female/three-fifths male assignment is consistent with previously reported gender use patterns for cannabis and supports our using height as a surrogate for gender in this case.

We therefore carried out a series of ordinal logistic regressions against height as the continuous variable and obtained the series of results shown in Figure 2.9. These plots reflect the probability of falling into a Y-axis category level graphed against the continuous variable of height on the X-axis. Significant regression models are framed in gray and demonstrate probabilities that change (curves) as height increases. We observed that taller responders skewed toward "No CBD", which is the cohort of responses not using High CBD or THC EQUIV CBD cannabis flowers (a) high THC (b) cannabis botanical product, as well as showing a preference for the "Fuel" aroma category (c). There was no height effect on either mode of administration (d) or indication (e). These results are therefore consistent with a hypothesis that men prefer high THC, "Fuel" categories in comparison with women. The results support "Floral", "Earth", and "Fuel" as valid organoleptic descriptors that produce a consistent narrative. Our future initiatives are aimed at extending these initial findings.

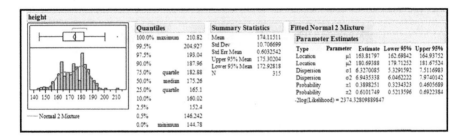

FIGURE 2.8 Distribution and moments for responder height in the Dosing Project™.

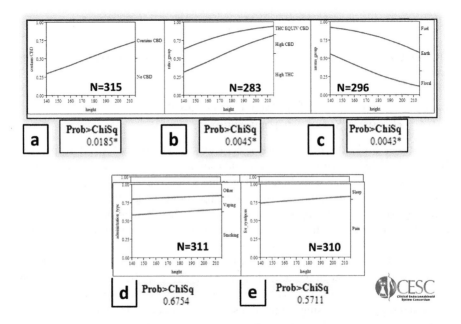

FIGURE 2.9 Ordinal logistic regression series against height for a set of categorical Dosing Project™ variables including cannabinoid ratio group (a), contains cannabidiol (CBD) (b), aroma category (c), mode of administration (d), and indication (e).

2.4 IDENTIFYING BIOCHEMICAL MARKERS THAT DEFINE CANNABIS AROMA CATEGORIES

We have investigated whether any biochemical markers may correlate with our perceived aroma groups. In Figure 2.10, we show that "Floral" and "Fuel" demonstrate differences when two monoterpenes, β-pinene and limonene, are plotted for each sample. The main figure shows a contour plot, color-coded by aroma category, and the inset shows the actual individual sample data. We observe good distinction and discrimination between the two aroma categories using β-pinene and limonene as surrogate markers. It can be observed that the "Fuel" category shows roughly a 10:1

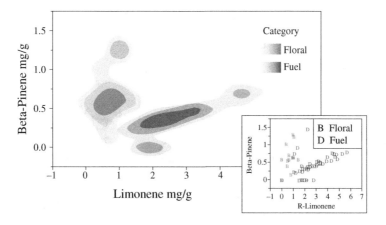

FIGURE 2.10 "Floral" and "Fuel" aroma categories demonstrate differences in a β-pinene vs limonene scatterplot.

difference in limonene content compared with β-pinene, whereas the "Floral" category is closer to 1:1. This observation is correlative and not necessarily causative. It does, nonetheless, provide a useful biochemical index for assigning cannabis flowers to either of these two classes. Furthermore, it is our hypothesis that the two aroma categories, "Floral" and "Fuel", correspond well with the popular "Sativa" and "Indica" effect class distinguishing attributes currently in widespread use. Sativa and Indica are misnomers for effect. They are traditionally terms used by botanists to describe phenotypic qualities of cannabis. However, popular nomenclature applies the term "Sativa" to an energetic or stimulating effect of cannabis, whereas "Indica" is used to describe a sedative or hypnotic effect of cannabis.

Pinenes, as a class, have demonstrated multiple clinical effects (Salehi et al. 2019). β-Pinene is one of two isomers normally found in cannabis; α-pinene is the other. β-Pinene is ubiquitous in cannabis, likely because of co-production by several of its different (promiscuous) monoterpene synthases, whereas α-pinene is observed to be more strain-restricted. Limonene, also commonly found in the essential oil of citrus, is proposed to have an uplifting mood effect and contributes to a pleasant aroma. It has also been suggested that pleasant aromas can be uplifting (Hoenen et al. 2016). We point out, however, that the β-pinene:limonene ratio groupings are best considered to be good surrogate markers for an uplifting "Sativa" and sedating "Indica" effects classification. We emphasize, though, that we consider their presence to be correlative and not causative of the perceived "Sativa" and "Indica" effects. Moreover, it is currently unclear to what extent such effect differences pertain to ingested cannabis as compared with inhaled cannabis.

We evaluated the general applicability of a discriminant categorization based on the relative content of limonene to β-pinene. In our process, we examined multiple cannabis flower terpenoid content databases obtained over the last five years. We present this as a series of scatterplots. Figure 2.11 summarizes the per sample limonene to β-pinene results for four different datasets, which together comprise greater than 790 samples. A clear discriminant pattern is evident in all cases.

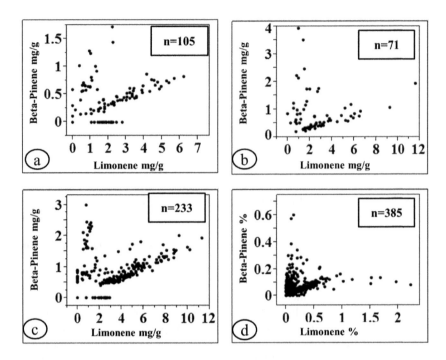

FIGURE 2.11 β-Pinene vs limonene scatterplots from different cannabis flower terpenoid analysis datasets.

Each of the databases was an independent analysis employing different sets of samples and standards, as well as analysis methodologies. A different contract lab produced the data for each analysis. The dataset in panel (a) is the complete GTA dataset. The dataset in panel (b) consists of samples included in the sampling analysis plan report derived from 2016 Humboldt Test plot studies. Panel (c) illustrates data derived from a cannabis flower strain terpenoid multivariate analysis dataset (kindly provided by J. Fishedick). Panel (d) represents a large dataset accrued for the Humboldt Sun Growers Guild (HSGG), using yet another contract analysis lab.

Overall, the pattern is largely similar, with two discernible groups corresponding to an approximate 1:1 and 10:1 β-pinene to limonene ratio groupings. Because ratios are without units, the analysis can compare across the terpenoid content units (either mg/g or %) currently in use within the industry. We suggest that this global class assignment based on biochemical parameters can predict organoleptic responses and characteristic anticipated effects of cannabis products.

2.5   SUMMARY AND FUTURE DIRECTIONS

2.5.1   SUMMARY

Our work employed a multi-disciplinary approach aimed at understanding the many-to-many interactions between cannabis active ingredients and the ECS. Our initial effort categorizes cannabis active ingredients based on their anticipated clinical effects.

We start by taking an organoleptic approach to assessing cannabis value. We relied on observation of cannabis aroma, its use in drug categorization, and its potential to predict effect as a foundation. Our work includes an analysis of the terpenoid content of proposed aroma categories. We have identified a biochemical foundation for key cannabis aroma categories through multivariate analysis approaches including hierarchical clustering analysis and discriminant analysis. Our hypothesis is described by a simple Venn diagram model of four cannabis aroma categories comprising: "Earth", "Floral", "Fruit", and "Fuel" and their relationships. We propose that the "Floral" and "Fuel" groups are distinguishable based on terpene group differences. These may underlie the major popular cannabis dichotomy of an uplifting "Sativa" effect and a sedative "Indica" effect. Furthermore, the "Earth" aroma group reflects attenuated cannabis, and the "Fruit" aroma group may result from another class of odorants such as esters.

Guided by the results such as those obtained by discriminant analysis, we elected to query respondents about the three aroma categories comprising "Floral", "Earth", and "Fuel". We believe that an aroma category "lexicon" should help tell a consistent and informative "narrative". We proceeded to validate aroma categories through the crowd-sourced responses from our Dosing Project™ survey and determined that they support coherent conclusions. The key to this approach relies on validation through historical use in a cannabis-prevalent population. We found that we were able to uncover the influence of harvest and storage practices on aroma categories and that this interpretation supported our overall model. Moreover, we demonstrated what appeared to be a gender preference among men for "Fuel" strains.

Finally, we identify a terpene ratio distinctive feature that appears predictive of the "Floral" and "Fuel" aroma categories that may actually facilitate assignment to two main cannabis effect categories of "Sativa" and "Indica", respectively. Our future work is aimed at clarifying this further through quantitative electro-encephalography (qEEG) studies with smoked flowers in cannabis-experienced volunteers (manuscript in preparation). We show that the β-pinene:limonene ratio dichotomy is generally applicable across multiple datasets obtained from analysts using different approaches and standards. In conclusion, the concept of assessing terpene ratio types is useful for defining cannabis distinctive features. This approach provides a robust, coherent, accessible, and evidence-based classification framework for the cannabis commodity.

2.5.2 FUTURE DIRECTIONS

Our set of aroma categories is foundational for further elucidating and predicting cannabis effects. The concept of elaborating a series of distinctive features is fundamental to the study of linguistics and was originally codified for phonological descriptive features (Chomsky and Halle 1968). It can be considered broadly applicable. This approach provides a framework for future work identifying other cannabis product chemical classes pertinent to aroma (esters, aldehydes, thiols). We present a working model for this framework in Figure 2.12 as a distinctive features matrix pertinent to cannabis aromatics. Interestingly, Gilbert and DiVerdi (2018) reported that the number of odorant descriptors most frequently reported for a given cannabis sample was around four. Our work opens the door to advances in analytical technologies applicable to this field. Similar to how this is understood in a linguistics context, we consider this a critical link to underlying physiology. Our current view is that top-level aroma

Aroma Category	Flos	Earth			Fuel		Fruit		
Distinctive Feature	Sweet/pine	Grass	Mineral	Nut	Chemical/Tar	Sour/Citrus	$Fruit_1$	$Fruit_2$	$Fruit_n$
$Cultivar_1$	+	-	-	-	-	-	-	-	-
$Cultivar_2$	-	+	-	-	-	-	-	-	-
$Cultivar_3$	-	-	+	-	-	-	-	-	-
$Cultivar_4$	-	-	-	+	-	-	-	-	-
$Cultivar_5$	-	-	-	-	+	-	-	-	-
$Cultivar_6$	-	-	-	-	+	+	-	-	-
...					...				
$Cultivar_n$	+	-	-	-	-	-	-	-	+

FIGURE 2.12 A preliminary model for an aroma-based distinctive features matrix for cannabis.

distinctive features may reflect multiple receptor class activations (GPCRs, TRPs) by the same aromatic (odorant). We anticipate that multiple features will be present in any given cultivar (strain). Our approach provides the framework for understanding universal concepts underlying the pharmacology of cannabis.

2.6 ACKNOWLEDGMENTS

We appreciate Kevin Jodrey for his helpful discussions about the 2015 Golden Tarp Awards Cannabis competition, as well as his introducing us to the world of cannabis aroma categories. Particular gratitude is extended to Emanuele Tozzato and Erik Wahlstrom for coding the initial POC version of the Dosing Project™. We acknowledge in memory of Jerry Chaney of North Coast Laboratories, Arcata, CA (DBA HQAL), their kind provision of the dataset included in Figure 2.11b. We are grateful to Justin Fischedick for kindly providing the dataset included in Figure 2.11c (Fischedick 2017). We relied on Joseph Casey for critical reading of the manuscript.

The GTA dataset discussed in this chapter was embedded in a digital token recorded on a public blockchain ledger. Scan the QR code to access this dataset which includes cannabinoid and terpenoid content for each sample along with its cultivator-submitted aroma category designation. We would like to acknowledge the help of Christian Saucier of The Ethical Data Alliance (EDA) in getting this set up.

ABBREVIATIONS

ANOVA:	Analysis of Variance
BCP:	Beta-caryophyllene
CBD:	Cannabidiol
CnR2 (CB2):	Cannabinoid$_2$ receptor$_2$
ECS:	Endocannabinoid System
GPCR:	G-Protein Coupled Receptor
GTA:	Golden Tarp Award, northern California cannabis competition
HCA:	Hierarchical Clustering Analysis
PCA:	Principal Component Analysis
POC:	Proof of Concept
qEEG:	Quantitative Electro-Encephalography
SVO:	Small volatile organics
TDP:	The Dosing Project™
THC:	Δ^9-tetrahydrocannabinol
TRP:	Transient receptor potential

BIBLIOGRAPHY

Abrams, J. S. et al. 2016. "The Clinical Endocannabinoid System Consortium (CESC) Responds to: Request for Information: Increasing the Varieties of Marijuana and Marijuana Products for Research Notice Number: NOT-DA-16-034." https://ced5782 d-48ef-4276-a15c-7799d0314977.filesusr.com/ugd/4c83e8_3f735f08964547e7b0837 c4f6a7c495e.pdf.

Booth, Judith K., Jonathan E. Page, and Jörg Bohlmann. 2017. "Terpene Synthases from Cannabis Sativa." *PLoS ONE* 12 (3): e0173911. https://doi.org/10.1371/journal.pone.0173911.

Brenneisen, R. 2007. "Chemistry and Analysis of Phytocannabinoids and Other Cannabis Constituents." In Mahmoud A. ElSohly (ed), *Marijuana and the Cannabinoids*, 17–49. Totowa, NJ: Humana Press. https://www.medicinalgenomics.com/wp-content/uploads/2011/12/Chemical-constituents-of-cannabis.pdf.

Castro, Jason B., Arvind Ramanathan, and Chakra S. Chennubhotla. 2013. "Categorical Dimensions of Human Odor Descriptor Space Revealed by Non-Negative Matrix Factorization." *PLoS ONE* 8 (9): e0073289. https://doi.org/10.1371/journal.pone.0073289.

Chomsky, Noam, and Morris Halle. 1968. *The Sound Patterns of English*. New York: Harper Row.

Fischedick, Justin T. 2017. " Identification of Terpenoid Chemotypes Among High (–)- Trans −Δ^9-Tetrahydrocannabinol-Producing Cannabis Sativa L. Cultivars ." *Cannabis and Cannabinoid Research* 2 (1): 34–47. https://doi.org/10.1089/can.2016.0040.

Gilbert, Avery N., and Joseph A. DiVerdi. 2018. "Consumer Perceptions of Strain Differences in Cannabis Aroma." Edited by John I. Glendinning. *PLoS ONE* 13 (2): e0192247. https://doi.org/10.1371/journal.pone.0192247.

Guimarães, Adriana G., Mairim R. Serafini, and Lucindo J. Quintans-Júnior. 2014. "Terpenes and Derivatives as a New Perspective for Pain Treatment: A Patent Review." In *Expert Opinion on Therapeutic Patents*. Abingdon: Taylor & Francis. https://doi.org/10.1517/1 3543776.2014.870154.

Gulluni, Nadia, Tania Re, Idalba Loiacono, Giovanni Lanzo, Luigi Gori, Claudio MacChi, Francesco Epifani, Nicola Bragazzi, and Fabio Firenzuoli. 2018. "Cannabis Essential Oil: A Preliminary Study for the Evaluation of the Brain Effects." *Evidence-Based Complementary and Alternative Medicine* 2018 24: 243–65. https://doi.org/10.1155/2018/1709182.

Hoenen, Matthias, Katharina Müller, Bettina M. Pause, and Katrin T. Lübke. 2016. "Fancy Citrus, Feel Good: Positive Judgment of Citrus Odor, but not the Odor Itself, Is Associated with Elevated Mood during Experienced Helplessness." *Frontiers in Psychology* 7 (February): 74. https://doi.org/10.3389/fpsyg.2016.00074.

Klauke, A. L., I. Racz, B. Pradier, A. Markert, A. M. Zimmer, J. Gertsch, and A. Zimmer. 2014. "The Cannabinoid CB2 Receptor-Selective Phytocannabinoid Beta-Caryophyllene Exerts Analgesic Effects in Mouse Models of Inflammatory and Neuropathic Pain." *European Neuropsychopharmacology* 24 (4): 608–20. https://doi.org/10.1016/j.euroneuro.2013.10.008.

Majid, Asifa. 2015. "Cultural Factors Shape Olfactory Language." *Trends in Cognitive Sciences.* Elsevier Ltd. https://doi.org/10.1016/j.tics.2015.06.009.

Miller, E. P., and J. S. Abrams. 2016. "Levels of the Sesquiterpenes β-Caryophyllene and α-Humulene Are Highly Correlated in Cannabis Varietals." In *AOCS 2016 Annual Meeting,* Salt Lake City. https://ced5782d-48ef-4276-a15c-7799d0314977.filesusr.com/ugd/4c83e8_c9df3392019f4a1c8f06c9507aa3c57c.pdf.

Miyazawa, Mitsuo, and Chikako Yamafuji. 2005. "Inhibition of Acetylcholinesterase Activity by Bicyclic Monoterpenoids." *Journal of Agricultural and Food Chemistry* 53 (5): 1765–8. https://doi.org/10.1021/jf040019b.

Nagegowda, Dinesh A., Michael Gutensohn, Curtis G. Wilkerson, and Natalia Dudareva. 2008. "Two Nearly Identical Terpene Synthases Catalyze the Formation of Nerolidol and Linalool in Snapdragon Flowers." *Plant Journal* 55 (2): 224–39. https://doi.org/10.1111/j.1365-313X.2008.03496.x.

Olofsson, Jonas K., and Jay A. Gottfried. 2015. "Response to Majid: Neurocognitive and Cultural Approaches to Odor Naming Are Complementary." *Trends in Cognitive Sciences* 19: 629–30. Elsevier Ltd. https://doi.org/10.1016/j.tics.2015.06.010.

Pamplona, Fabricio A, Entourage Phytolab, Sachin Patel, Daniel E Lantela, Brishna S Kamal, and Fatima Kamal. 2018. "Cannabis and the Anxiety of Fragmentation-A Systems Approach for Finding an Anxiolytic Cannabis Chemotype." *Frontiers in Neuroscience* | Www.Frontiersin.Org 12: 730. https://doi.org/10.3389/fnins.2018.00730.

Potter, David J. 2009. "The Propagation, Characterisation and Optimisation of Cannabis Sativa L as a Phytopharmaceutical." Available Online. https://extractionmagazine.com/wp-content/uploads/2018/06/THE-PROPAGATION-CHARACTERISATION-AND-OPTIMISATION-OF-CANNABIS-SATIVA-L-AS-A-PHYTOPHARMACEUTICAL.pdf.

Raspet, Sean. 2016. "Toward an Olfactory Language System." *Future Anterior: Journal of Historic Preservation, History, Theory, and Criticism,* 13 (2): 139–53.

Salehi, Bahare, Shashi Upadhyay, Ilkay Erdogan Orhan, Arun Kumar Jugran, Sumali L.D. Jayaweera, Daniel A. Dias, Farukh Sharopov, et al. 2019. "Therapeutic Potential of α- and β-Pinene: A Miracle Gift of Nature." *Biomolecules. MDPI AG* 9: 738. https://doi.org/10.3390/biom9110738.

Vale, T. Gurgel Do, E. Couto Furtado, J. G. Santos, and G. S.B. Viana. 2002. "Central Effects of Citral, Myrcene and Limonene, Constituents of Essential Oil Chemotypes from Lippia Alba (Mill.) N.E. Brown." *Phytomedicine* 9 (8): 709–14. https://doi.org/10.1078/094471102321621304.

Yang, Hyejin, Junsung Woo, Ae Nim Pae, Min Young Um, Nam Chul Cho, Ki Duk Park, Minseok Yoon, Jiyoung Kim, C. Justin Lee, and Suengmok Cho. 2016. "α-Pinene, a Major Constituent of Pine Tree Oils, Enhances Non-Rapid Eye Movement Sleep in Mice through GABAA-Benzodiazepine Receptors." *Molecular Pharmacology* 90 (5): 530–9. https://doi.org/10.1124/mol.116.105080.

3 Cannabinoid Chemistry of Cannabis

David Dawson and Markus Roggen

CONTENTS

3.1 INTRODUCTION

For over five millennia, the cannabis plant has been used by people around the world for medical, recreational, and industrial purposes. It is believed to have been first cultivated in central and northeastern Asia, where it was used to produce both strong

DOI: 10.1201/9780429274893-3

hemp-derived fibers as well as medicinal formulations, such as tinctures and teas made from extracts of cannabis (Russo 2001; ElSohly 2002). Therapeutic use of the plant was ubiquitous in Ancient Egypt, and evidence of cannabis usage is widespread across the varied cultures of continental Asia (Russo 2007). A transitional moment in the history of cannabis came in 1840 when an Irish physician studying in India named William O'Shaughnessy introduced cannabis to the European and North American pharmacopeia. Nearly 200 years later, cannabis has become one of the most studied plants in the world, with well over 10,000 papers describing the biology and chemistry of this ancient plant (Hazekamp et al. 2010).

Despite this intense focus from the scientific community, the cannabis plant and its metabolites (see also Chapter 1) are still considered a "neglected pharmacological treasure trove" (Mechoulam 2005). This is in part due to the rich and varied metab-olome of cannabis—the plant produces numerous sugars, hydrocarbons, steroids, mono- and sesquiterpenes, flavonoids, nitrogenous compounds, glycoproteins, and more. The biological profile of the cannabis plant is not only vast but ever-expand-ing. In an early survey of the cannabis metabolome, Turner et al. (1980) reported 423 distinct compounds; 15 years later, that number had increased to 483 (Ross and ElSohly, 1995). As of this writing, the most recent comprehensive review places the number of cannabis metabolites at 565 (ElSohly et al. 2017). As legalization efforts progress and the barriers to scientific research continue to fall, the number of known metabolites is sure to increase.

One of the most studied categories of cannabis metabolites is cannabinoids, a class of terpenophenolic compounds that are considered the main bioactive compo-nent of the plant, and almost exclusively found in cannabis (Hazekamp et al. 2010). New cannabinoids are being identified at a stunning rate. In 2005, 72 cannabinoids had been reported in the literature; the subsequent ten years saw the identification of 48 additional cannabinoids (ElSohly et al. 2017). As the number of known cannabi-noids increases, so too does the degree of structural variation. Thus, it is increasingly difficult to compare cannabinoids with disparate structures with one another. In this chapter, cannabinoids will be discussed in depth, first introducing their origins through biosynthesis and chemical transformation, then individual cannabinoids are described, primarily organized by a molecular skeleton (*vide infra*), and subdivided by their proposed chemical origin (e.g., decarboxylation, oxidation, isomerization). In this way, subtle differences in substituents, oxidation patterns, and positions of unsaturation will be highlighted.

3.2   THE CHEMISTRY BEHIND CANNABINOIDS

3.2.1   Biosynthesis

The fundamental biosynthetic transformations that form all cannabinoid types are shown in Figure 3.1. The first biogenic step involves the condensation of hex-anoyl-CoA and three malonyl-CoA molecules. Incorporation of the six-carbon hexanoyl-CoA affords cannabinoids with a five-carbon alkyl side chain, which is the most common alkyl chain length for cannabinoids. The biosynthetic importance

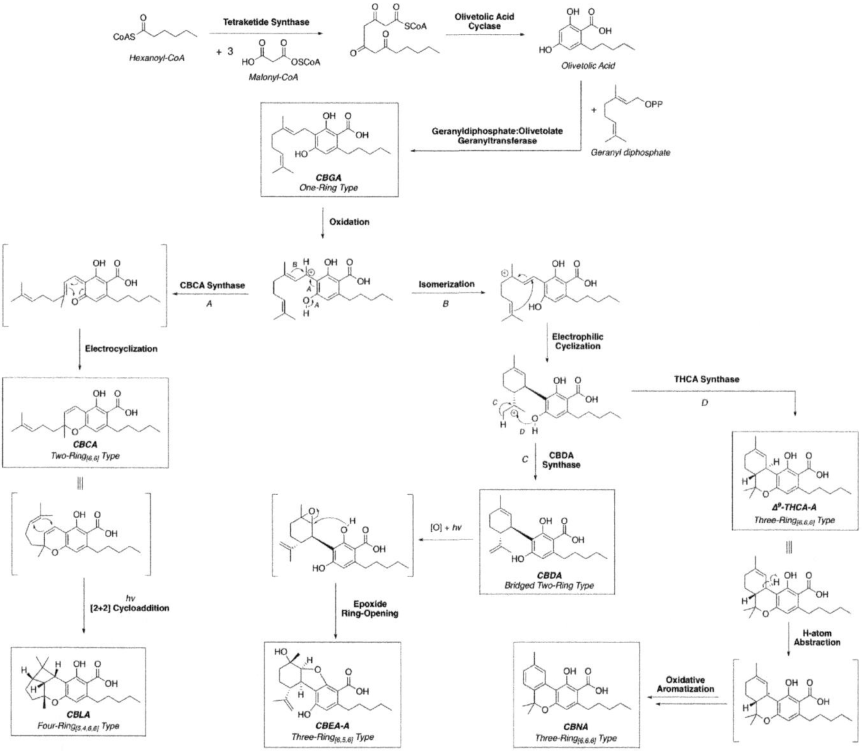

FIGURE 3.1 Biosynthetic pathway of cannabinoids.

of hexanoyl-CoA is supported by the reported correlation between levels of hexanoyl-CoA in the cannabis plant and the *in vivo* concentration of cannabidiolic acid (CBDA) (Hanus et al. 2016a). The enzymes involved with this biosynthetic pathway are not selective for the chain length of this initial synthon; depending on the number of carbons, cannabinoids with various alkyl chain lengths can be created. For example, biosynthesis that starts with ethyl-CoA affords orcinoids, cannabinoids with C1-length chains, and incorporation of butyl-CoA yields varinoids, which feature C3-length chains. Other cannabinoids with shortened or elongated carbon chains (C4-, C6-, and C7-length analogs) have been isolated from the cannabis plant. Although it was originally proposed that shortened alkyl chain lengths could arise from fungal-induced oxidation (Robertson et al. 1975), isotopic labeling experiments performed by Kajima and Piraux (1982) provided evidence that varinoid compounds were not formed by chain shortening of common C5-length cannabinoids.

The product of this first biosynthetic step is an activated polyketide, which then undergoes cyclization by the action of olivetolic acid cyclase (OAC) (Gagne et al. 2012). This step involves a formal intramolecular aldol condensation and is notable for its retention of the carboxylic acid group, which is rare in plant polyketides. The resulting cyclized product is olivetolic acid (OA), which, in the presence of geranyl diphosphate (GPP), undergoes an isoprenylation reaction mediated by the enzyme geranyl diphosphate:olivetolate geranyltransferase (Mechoulam and Gaoni 1967; Shoyama et al. 1975a; Fellermeier and Zenk 1998). This reaction forms a carbon–carbon bond between GPP and OA without further cyclization, which affords cannabigerolic acid (CBGA) and other one-ring type cannabinoids. All naturally occurring cannabinoids are derived from CBGA (see compound **3.1**), or related one-ring type analogs, as various enzymatic transformations convert the long, linear isoprenyl moiety into the varied molecular skeletons seen across the cannabinoid family. The biosynthetic importance of CBGA was first proposed by Gaoni and Mechoulam (1964a), who cited the low oxidation level along with the isoprenyl moiety as evidence that CBGA was formed early in the biosynthetic pathway.

All downstream biosynthetic transformations begin with formal hydride abstraction from the benzylic isoprenyl carbon of CBGA. The enzyme CBCA synthase (Morimoto et al. 1998) allows for rearrangement of this resonance stabilized carbocation to an ortho quinone methide (Path A), which can then undergo an electrocyclic reaction to form CBCA and other two-ring$_{[6,6]}$ type cannabinoids. Subsequent exposure of two-ring$_{[6,6]}$ type cannabinoids to light causes a photoinduced stereoselective [2+2] cycloaddition, which yields four-ring$_{[5,4,6,6]}$ type cannabinoids such as CBLA. If the oxidized CBGA species instead undergoes double-bond isomerization to form a tertiary carbocation (Path B), a cyclohexene ring can be formed via electrophilic cyclization. CBDA synthase (Taura et al. 1996) terminates this electrophilic cyclization by formal deprotonation that forms the exocyclic double bond of CBDA and analogous bridged two-ring type cannabinoids (Path C). Alternatively, THCA Synthase (Taura et al. 1995a) can affect a ring closure via attack of the carbocation by the resorcinol hydroxyl group at C1 to form Δ^9-THCA-A and other three-ring$_{[6,6,6]}$ type cannabinoids (Path D). Both CBDA and Δ^9-THCA-A undergo distinct oxidative degradation pathways when exposed to air. When subjected to both oxygen and photoirradiation, CBDA forms CBEA-A and analogous three-ring$_{[6,5,6]}$ type cannabinoids. This reaction is proposed to proceed via an epoxide intermediate (Shani and Mechoulam 1974). Oxygen-induced abstraction of the benzylic hydrogen atom from Δ^9-THCA-A and other three-ring$_{[6,6,6]}$ type cannabinoids form a stabilized radical and can initiate an oxidative aromatization reaction to afford CBNA.

3.2.2 DECARBOXYLATION

The decarboxylation reaction is a key step in the production or consumption of cannabis products. In this reaction, a thermally unstable acidic cannabinoid loses its carbonyl group to produce its neutral counterpart and one molecule of CO_2. For example, the decarboxylation reaction of Δ^9-THCA-A to form Δ^9-THC can be seen in Figure 3.2. Decarboxylation is generally desirable, as cannabinoid acids have minimal bioactivity (Brenneisen 2007). To this point, only the neutral form of Δ^9-THC is intoxicating (Mechoulam and Gaoni 1967). To better understand the underlying mechanism (Figure 3.2), a few reported studies have used computational models of decarboxylation for Δ^9-THCA-A or simplified structural analogs. This work has shown that an intermolecular proton donor lowers the activation energy of the

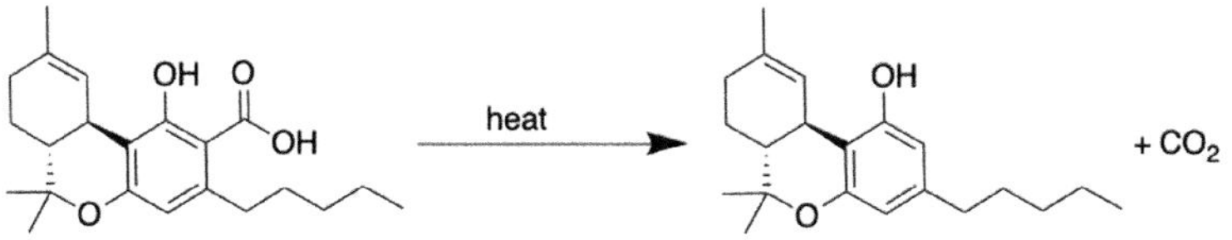

FIGURE 3.2 Decarboxylation reaction of THCA to THC.

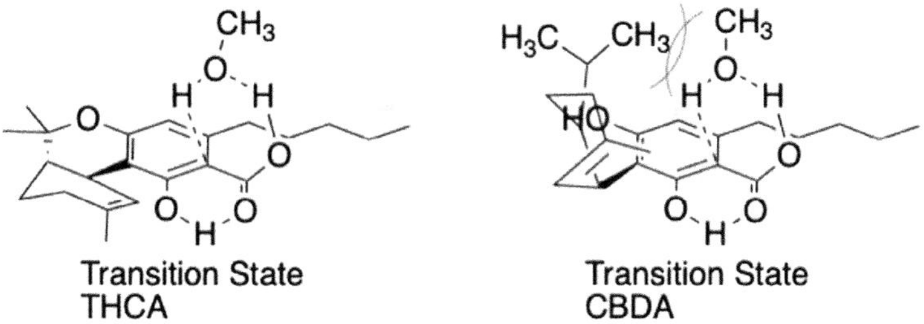

FIGURE 3.3 Transition states of rate-limiting step for THCA and CBDA decarboxylation.

decarboxylation reaction, ortho hydroxyl groups crucially influence the transition state of the reaction, and the reaction proceeds via a keto-type intermediate (Ruelle 1986; Li and Brill 2003; Chuchev and BelBruno 2007).

Perrotin-Brunel et al. (2011) further refined such mechanistic proposals and provided further evidence that direct keto-enol tautomerism was a key step in the HCOOH-catalyzed decarboxylation of Δ^9-THCA-A. These studies have provided a foundation for understanding the mechanistic pathway of benzoic acid derivatives and even Δ^9-THCA-A decarboxylation. He et al. (2020) further expanded on this model to explain rate differences observed between Δ^9-THCA-A and CBDA decarboxylation (Wang et al. 2016). The authors identified the tautomerization step as the critical step in defining decarboxylation rates. The observed differences in reactivity hinge on the greater rigidity of the Δ^9-THCA-A framework when compared with CBDA (Figure 3.3). The study demonstrated that the relative conformational flexibility of CBDA hindered the intermolecular proton donor (methanol) from accessing the ipso position on the aromatic ring, thus slowing the decarboxylation reaction.

3.2.3 OXIDATION

Cannabinoids are prone to oxidation, which makes them desirable antioxidant targets with potential medical applications (Pellati et al. 2018). Oxidation reactions of cannabinoids are common in cannabis production, and the resulting products can be desired or undesired. The most notorious oxidation plaguing cannabis production is the oxidation of Δ^9-THC to CBN (Figure 3.4), a reaction that occurs naturally in dried cannabis when stored over long periods (Turner et al. 1973a). The ratio of Δ^9-THC to CBN can even be used to determine the age of stored cannabis samples (Ross and ElSohly 1999). The reaction pathway of this oxidation was first proposed by Turner and ElSohly (1979), who invoked epoxy and hydroxylated intermediates.

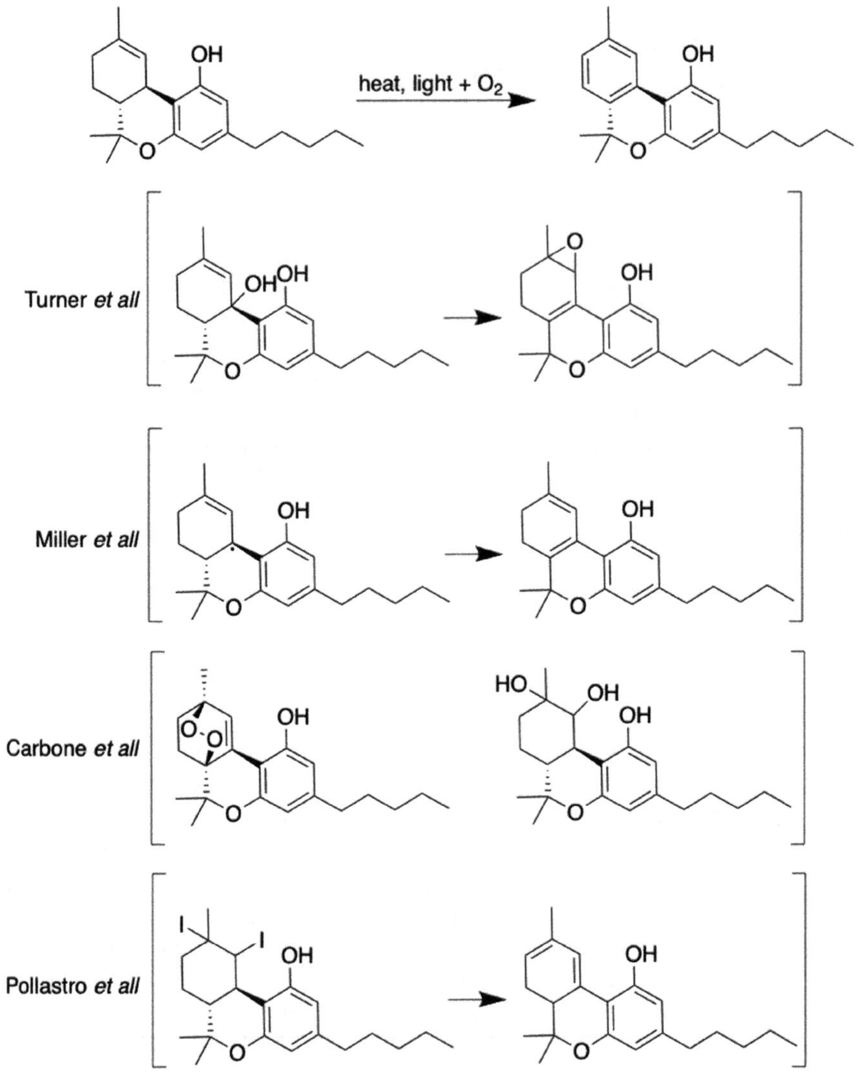

FIGURE 3.4 THC to CBN oxidation with proposed intermediates.

Miller et al. (1982) proposed a free radical oxidation pathway that hinged on the abstraction of the labile proton at C-10a (*vide infra*). Carbone et al. (2010) isolated potential reaction intermediates from an ethanol/propylene glycol solution that was stored for five years. Recently, Pollastro et al. (2017) disclosed a one-step synthetic method involving iodine in refluxing toluene to obtain CBD in larger quantities for pharmacologic studies.

Another category of cannabinoid oxidation products is cannabinoquinoids (Figure 3.5). The first hydroquinone, HU331, was isolated by Mechoulam et al.

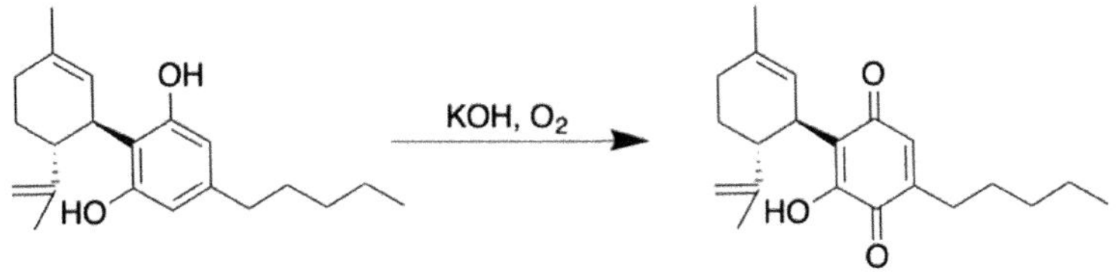

FIGURE 3.5   Beam Test of CBD resulting in cannabinoquinoid HU331.

(1968) and identified as the molecule giving color to the Beam Test (Grlic 1962). The Beam Test relies on basic aerobic conditions but is beset by side reactions, including oxidative dimerization. Therefore, Caprioglio et al. (2020) developed cleaner oxidation to cannabinoquinoids by $\lambda 5$-periodinanes, such as Dess–Martin periodinane or 2-iodoxybenzoic acid.

3.2.4   ISOMERIZATION

Double-bond isomerization is an important chemical transformation that is responsible for the formation of several three-ring$_{[6,6,6]}$ type cannabinoids. A detailed analysis of double-bond isomerization trends in a controlled laboratory setting was undertaken by Srebnik et al. (1984). Naturally occurring and synthetically modified cannabinoids were subjected to high-temperature reflux in the presence of a base, reaction conditions that affect isomerization in the given substrates. By comparing cannabinoids with different double bond positions and substitution patterns, a clearer picture of the mechanism behind isomerization begins to emerge.

The authors found that Δ^9-THC readily isomerizes into Δ^8-THC. This rapid isomerization is due in part to the labile proton at C10a, where deprotonation forms an anion with both allylic and benzylic stabilization. When Srebnik et al. subjected Δ^8-THC to reflux conditions, no reaction occurred. The desired isomerization to Δ^{10}-THC only occurred at 0°C in the presence of a strong alkyl lithium base. This finding strongly suggests that Δ^8-THC is the thermodynamic product, as isomerization only occurred when reaction conditions favored the kinetic product (low temperature, strong base). This is further supported by the lack of a reaction when conditions favor the formation of the thermodynamic product (high temperature, weaker base).

Similar follow-up experiments with CBD suggested that free unsubstituted phenolic –OH groups and the presence of the exocyclic double bond were important factors for double-bond isomerization. Recent studies have shown that double-bond isomerization is promoted by the presence of an acid, which suggests an intermolecular proton transfer is a key mechanistic step (Webster et al. 2008).

3.3   CANNABINOIDS

In this chapter, cannabinoids are organized by molecular structure and classified according to both the number and size of rings. The molecular skeleton of a

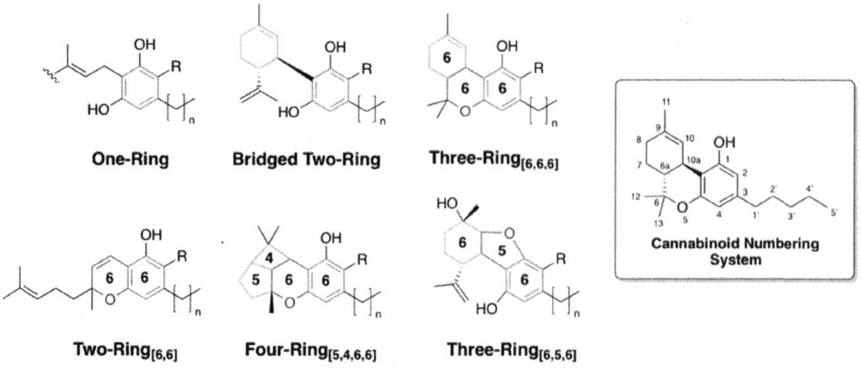

FIGURE 3.6 Left: Basic nomenclature used to classify cannabinoids in this work. Right: Formal numbering system for cannabinoids, with Δ^9-THC as an example.

cannabinoid provides insight into if the compound was formed via enzymatic or chemical processes and where it is located along the biosynthetic pathway. In grouping cannabinoids by the overall structure of the ring systems, differences concerning degrees of unsaturation, alkyl chain lengths, and positions of oxidation are highlighted, which, in turn, helps the reader focus on the subtle variations between cannabinoids. The nomenclature used in this chapter is shown in Figure 3.6. Cannabinoid types are referred to by the number of rings present with a subscript listing the size of the rings. Additionally, on the right of Figure 3.6 is the formal carbon numbering conventions for cannabinoids that will be referred to throughout this chapter. Of note, several cannabinoids mentioned in the text have the distinct nomenclature prefix "Δ^x-" where x is a number between six and ten. This number corresponds to the location of a double bond in the molecular structure. For example, Δ^9-THC refers to tetrahydrocannabinol with a double bond starting at the C9 position, as seen in Figure 3.6.

3.3.1 ONE-RING TYPE

3.3.1.1 Biogenic Compounds

One-ring type cannabinoids are among the least structurally complex cannabinoids and are defined by a unique molecular skeleton containing a single ring, such as in CBGA (**3.1**) (Figure 3.7). The relative structural simplicity of one-ring type cannabinoids is in part due to their role as the first cannabinoid created by the biosynthetic pathway of the cannabis plant (Shoyama et al. 1975a). The proposed one-ring type cannabinoids with shortened chain lengths ([C1-length] cannabigerorcolic acid (CBGOA, **3.2**); [C3-length] cannabigerovarinic acid (CBGVA, **3.3**); [C4-length] cannabigerobutolic acid (CBGBA, **3.4**) and elongated chain lengths ([C6-length] cannabigerohexolic acid (CBGHA, **3.5**); and [C7-length] cannabigerophorolic acid (CBGPA, **3.6**)) are formed via the same biosynthetic pathway as the most common C5-length cannabinoid, CBGA. Of these alkyl chain analogs, only CBGVA has been

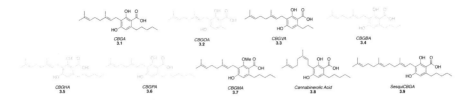

FIGURE 3.7 Biogenic one-ring type cannabinoid structures. Grayed-out structures indicate cannabinoids that have not yet been isolated but are assumed to exist due to the existence of related downstream cannabinoids.

isolated in its acidic form from the cannabis plant (Shoyama et al. 1977). Despite this fact, it can be assumed that the other alkyl chain analogs must exist in the acidic form *in vivo*, as the isolation of downstream biosynthetic products implies their existence. In this work, the structures of cannabinoids that are reasonably assumed to exist are illustrated in gray.

Another source of structural variation is present in cannabinoids with *O*-alkylated substituents on the resorcinol ring. Only one such type of cannabinoid has been isolated from cannabis: cannabigerolic acid monomethylether (CBGMA, **3.7**) features a single methyl alkylation of one of the resorcinol –OH groups and was first found in an Asian hemp varietal (Shoyama et al. 1970). This monomethyl ether analog of CBGA is the parent compound of all monomethyl ether cannabinoid derivatives found in the other cannabinoid types.

Structural variation along the isoprenyl chain affords another two distinct one-ring type cannabinoids. Cannabinerolic acid (**3.8**) is a CBGA analog that contains a double bond in a Z-configuration at the proximal side of the isoprenyl chain (Taura et al. 1995b). It is unclear if this Z-isomer of CBGA is compatible with cannabinoid synthases and thus participates in the biosynthetic pathway. Farnesyl prenylogue Sesqui cannabigerolic acid (SesquiCBGA, **3.9**), first found in its neutral form, has recently been identified by detailed ESI-LC/MS analysis (Berman et al. 2018). There is no evidence that any cannabinoids are biosynthetically derived from this unique isoprenyl variant.

3.3.1.2 Compounds Formed by Heat

One commonality shared between all cannabinoid types is the decarboxylation of acidic cannabinoids upon treatment with heat. Subjecting the naturally occurring acidic forms of cannabinoids to sustained heat will expel CO_2 and yield the neutral cannabinoid, which lacks substitution at the C-2 position (Thomas and ElSohly 2016) (Figure 3.8). Decarboxylation of CBGA-type compounds CBGA, CBGVA, and CBGMA affords cannabigerol (CBG, **3.10**), cannabigerovarin (CBGV, **3.11**), and cannabigerol monomethyl ether (CBGM, **3.12**), respectively (Gaoni and Mechoulam 1964a; Shoyama et al. 1977; Yamauchi et al. 1968).

In addition to the decarboxylated cannabinoids mentioned previously, there have been a few one-ring type compounds isolated from the cannabis plant in their neutral form. It is likely that these cannabinoids were originally biosynthesized in their acidic

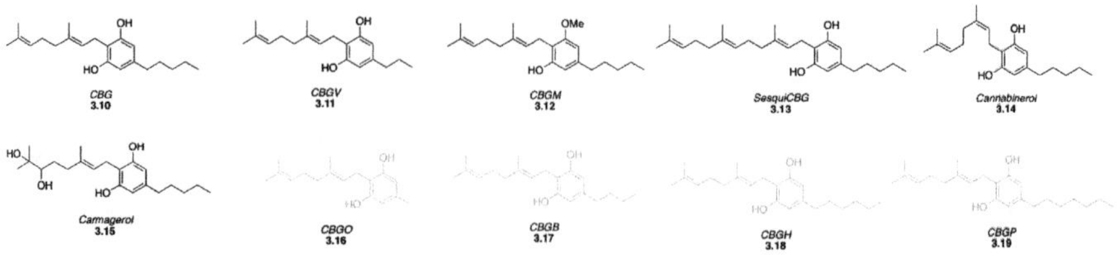

FIGURE 3.8 Neutral one-ring type cannabinoid structures. Grayed-out structures indicate cannabinoids that have not yet been isolated but are assumed to exist due to the existence of related downstream cannabinoids.

forms and underwent decarboxylation upon isolation. A farnesyl prenylogue of CBG, SesquiCBG (**3.13**), was isolated as a minor constituent (~100 mg/kg dry weight) from Carmagnola derived hemp, a northern Italian fiber hemp varietal (Pollastro et al. 2011). Cannabinerol (**3.14**), a neutral form of CBG with a Z-configuration at the isoprenyl double bond has recently been isolated (Hanus et al. 2016b). A dihydroxylated form of CBG, carmagerol (**3.15**), was isolated from the aerial portions of the *Carma* hemp varietal (Appendino et al. 2008). The acidic form of this dihydroxylated CBG analog has not been reported in the literature. Compounds **3.16–3.19** have not yet been isolated in their neutral forms but are presumed to exist due to the isolation of downstream biosynthetic products.

3.3.2 BRIDGED TWO-RING TYPE

3.3.2.1 Biogenic Compounds

Bridged two-ring type cannabinoids are more structurally complex than one-ring type cannabinoids and are typified by an aromatized resorcinol ring connected to a *p*-menthyl ring by a single C–C bond (Figure 3.9). The long, linear isoprenyl chain found in one-ring type cannabinoids has undergone oxido-cyclization to form the *para*-menthyl ring, a transformation mediated by CBDA synthase. The oxido-cyclization affected by CBDA synthase does not require coenzymes, oxidants, or metal ion cofactors to proceed (Taura et al. 1996) and is not selective for alkyl chain length. Therefore, the one-ring type cannabinoids with varying alkyl chain lengths seen in Figure 3.7 are transformed to their corresponding bridged two-ring type analogs via a single enzymatic pathway.

The predominant bridged two-ring type cannabinoid found in both *Cannabis sativa* L. and fiber hemp is CBDA (**3.20**). CBDA is the major cannabinoid formed in fiber hemp and was the first acidic cannabinoid to be isolated and characterized (Krejci and Santavy 1955). Decades later, the varinoid analog cannabidivarinic acid (CBDVA, **3.21**) was found in cannabis from the Meao village in Thailand (Shoyama et al. 1977). In addition to CBDA and CBDVA, several other acidic bridged two-ring type cannabinoids with varying alkyl chain lengths and structural features are presumed to naturally exist but have yet to be officially documented due to the difficulties associated with isolating and purifying the trace quantities found in the plant.

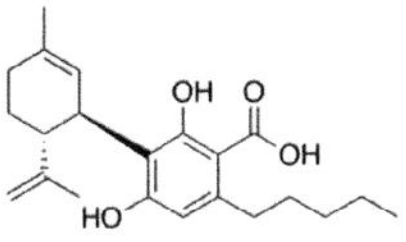

CBDA
3.20

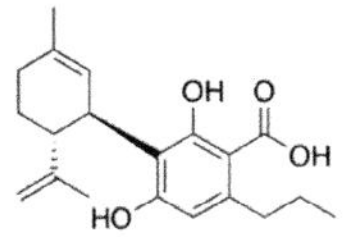

CBDVA
3.21

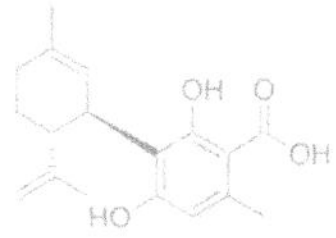

CBDOA
3.22

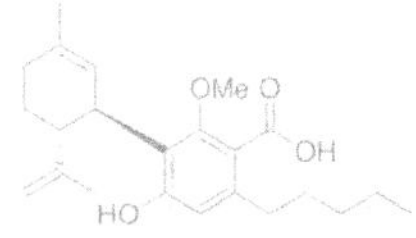

CBDMA
3.23

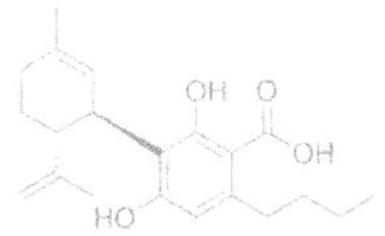

CBDBA
3.24

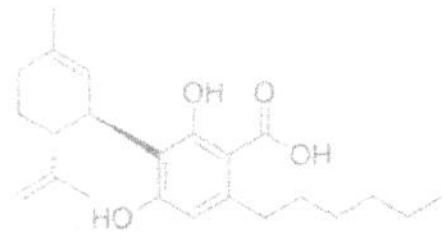

CBDHA
3.25

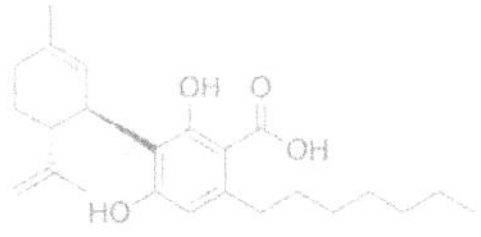

CBDPA
3.26

FIGURE 3.9 Biogenic bridged two-ring type cannabinoid structures. Grayed-out structures indicate cannabinoids that have not yet been isolated but are assumed to exist due to the existence of related downstream cannabinoids.

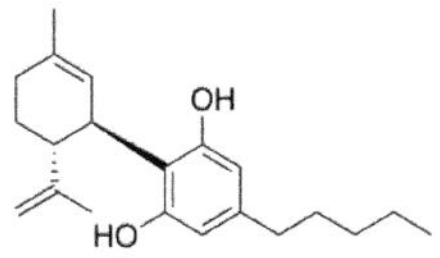

CBD
3.27

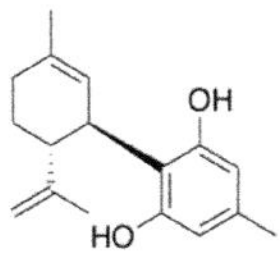

CBDO
3.28

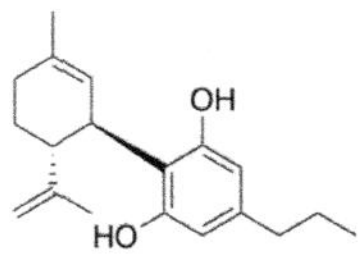

CBDV
3.29

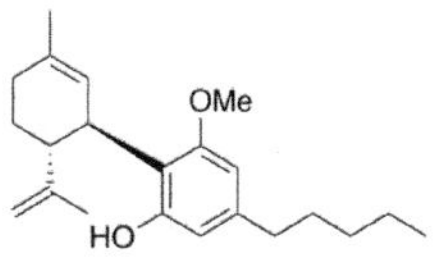

CBDM
3.30

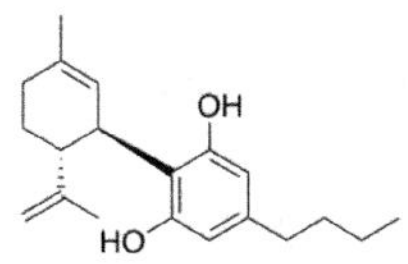

CBDB
3.31

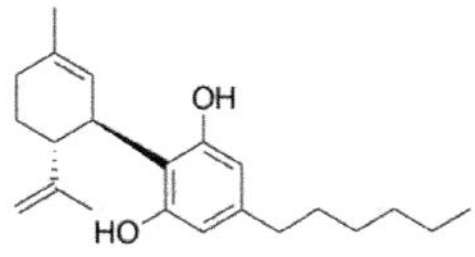

CBDH
3.32

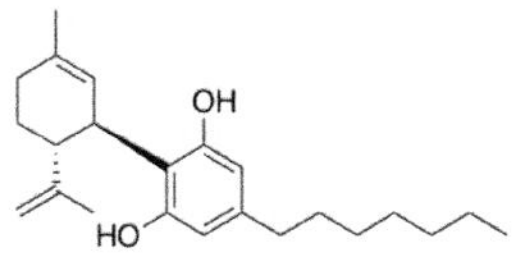

CBDP
3.33

FIGURE 3.10 Neutral bridged two-ring type cannabinoid structures.

These compounds, including the orcinoid and monomethyl ether analogs, as well as newly discovered C4-, C6-, and C7-chain length analogs, can be seen in gray in Figure 3.9.

3.3.2.2 Compounds Formed by Heat

Unlike the acidic bridged two-ring type cannabinoids, the majority of decarboxylated, neutral bridged two-ring type cannabinoids have been isolated and characterized (Figure 3.10). Cannabidiol (CBD, **3.27**) was the first naturally occurring cannabinoid to be isolated (Jacob and Todd 1940; Adams et al. 1940), although it would take over two decades and the emergence of NMR spectroscopy to deduce the correct chemical structure (Mechoulam and Shvo 1963). In the subsequent years, the orcinoid analog of CBD, cannabidiorcol (CBDO, **3.28**) was found in a Lebanese cannabis strain, but not in a similar Brazilian strain (Vree et al. 1972a). Varinoid analog cannabidivarin (CBDV, **3.29**) was isolated and characterized by Vollner et al. (1969). The presence of CBDV in cannabis strains has chemotaxonomic significance, as higher levels of varinoid compounds are more common in cannabis indica strains when compared with cannabis sativa (Hillig and Mahlberg 2004; Welling et al. 2016). The monomethyl ether analog of CBD was isolated in its neutral form (CBDM, **3.30**) from a northern Asian hemp varietal, and is proposed to exist as the acidified form *in vivo* (Shoyama et al. 1972a).

In recent years, three new alkyl chain length variants of CBD have been isolated and characterized by the Cannazza group. Cannabidibutol (CBDB, **3.31**), a CBD analog with a four-carbon alkyl chain, was first identified by mass spectrometric profile by Harvey (1976). Over 40 years later, Citti et al. (2019a) characterized an impurity in a hemp extract and unambiguously confirmed the presence of CBDB. Furthermore, cannabidihexol (CBDH, **3.32**) and cannabidiphorol (CBDP, **3.33**), two bridged two-ring type cannabinoids with elongated alkyl chain lengths have been isolated from hemp extracts (Linciano et al. 2020; Citti et al. 2019b). Although these novel alkyl analogs have only been reported for CBD- and THC-type cannabinoids, it suggests that there is substantially more structural variation in the cannabis pharmacopeia than previously thought.

3.3.2.3 Thymyl-Type Compounds

The final class of bridged two-ring cannabinoids involves CBD analogs with a fully aromatized *p*-menthyl fragment. This aromatization forms a thymyl-type moiety, which results in extensive pi-conjugation throughout the molecule (Figure 3.11). Not much is known about this class of cannabinoids, and early scientific accounts of the class are questionable. The first isolation of an aromatized form of CBD, termed cannabinodiol (CBND, **3.34**), was reported by Van Ginneken (1972). After subsequent investigations from other researchers (Friedrich-Fiechtl and Spiteller 1975), it is now widely considered that Van Ginneken et al. isolated the oxidatively cyclized analog cannabifuran (see Section 3.3.6). Thus, it is suggested that references to Van Ginneken's isolation reports of CBND and propyl analog cannabinodivarin (CBNDV) be treated with skepticism (Van Ginneken et al. 1972; Vree et al. 1972b).

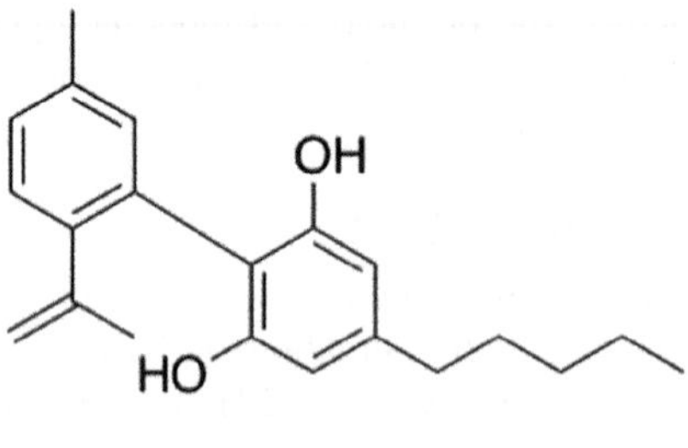

CBND
3.34

FIGURE 3.11   Thymyl-type bridged two-ring cannabinoid structures.

Subsequently, the conclusive isolation of CBND was published by Lousberg et al. (1977), who isolated and characterized CBND in a strain of Lebanese cannabis.

Little is known of the chemical origins of thymyl-type bridged two-ring cannabinoids. Unlike other aromatized cannabinoids, such as cannabinol (CBN, see Section 3.3.3.3), thymyl-type cannabinoids are believed to have a biogenic origin, despite the lack of a known synthase (Hanus et al. 2016a). This hypothesis is rooted in the differences in both the molecular structure and oxidative stability between Δ^9-THC and CBD. Because Δ^9-THC has an additional ring in its molecular skeleton (see Section 3.3.3), the molecule is nearly planar. Removal of a benzallylic proton from the C10a position of Δ^9-THC results in a conjugated radical, which is relatively stable and lowers the barrier for p-menthyl aromatization. Conversely, the two rings of CBD lie in different planes (Jones et al. 1977), as free rotation about the internal C–C bond allows for minimization of steric forces between the two substituted rings. Thus, the formation of a benzallylic radical at C10a has little to no stabilization from conjugation, which, in turn, disfavors oxidation and subsequent aromatization. It is therefore presumed that the formation of thymyl-type bridged two-ring cannabinoids occurs *in vivo*, and not from post-harvest oxidation.

3.3.3 THREE-RING$_{[6,6,6]}$ TYPE

3.3.3.1 Biogenic Compounds

Three-ring$_{[6,6,6]}$ type cannabinoids are similar to bridged two-ring type cannabinoids but feature an additional dihydropyran ring, formed by condensation of an –OH group on the resorcinol ring with the pendant allylic group on the p-methyl moiety (Figure 3.12). This class of cannabinoids are downstream biosynthetic products formed from CBGA (and its derivatives) by the action of THCA synthase (Taura et al. 1995a). The most common three-ring$_{[6,6,6]}$ type cannabinoid found in the cannabis plant is Δ^9-tetrahydrocannabinolic acid A (Δ^9-THCA-A, **3.35**), which was first

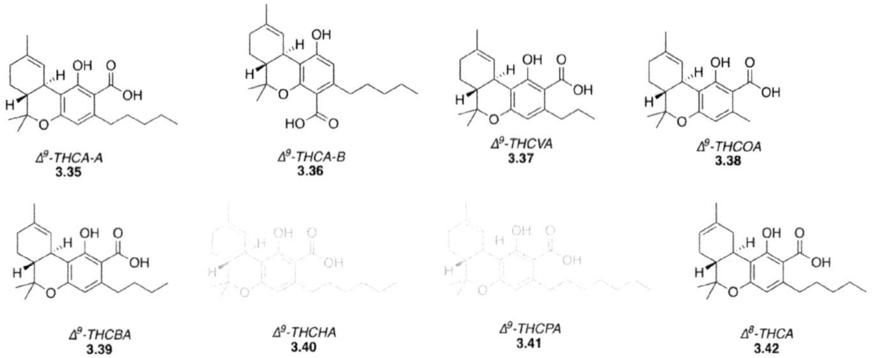

Δ^9-THCA-A
3.35

Δ^9-THCA-B
3.36

Δ^9-THCVA
3.37

Δ^9-THCOA
3.38

Δ^9-THCBA
3.39

Δ^9-THCHA
3.40

Δ^9-THCPA
3.41

Δ^8-THCA
3.42

FIGURE 3.12 Biogenic three-ring$_{[6,6,6]}$ type cannabinoid structures. Grayed-out structures indicate cannabinoids that have not yet been isolated but are assumed to exist due to the existence of related downstream cannabinoids.

reported by Korte et al. (1965a); Δ^9-THCA-A was found to be sensitive to light and could not be successfully crystallized.

A few years later, a second Δ^9-THC acid was discovered by Mechoulam et al. (1969). This positional isomer, called Δ^9-tetrahydrocannabinolic acid B (Δ^9-THCA-B, **3.36**), features the carboxylic acid group at C4 on the resorcinol ring, as opposed to the C2 substitution seen in nearly every other acidic cannabinoid. In contrast to the Δ^9-THCA-A isomer, Δ^9-THCA-B is readily crystallized, and X-ray crystallographic analysis has confirmed the proposed structure (Rosenqvist and Ottersen 1975). It is unclear how Δ^9-THCA-B is formed *in vivo*, as no evidence for enzymatic cyclization has been found, and a chemical rearrangement from Δ^9-THCA-A to Δ^9-THCA-B cannot be ruled out. However, it is noted that samples containing Δ^9-THCA-B had little to no Δ^9-THCA-A present, which may be due to biochemical variation, suggesting that the presence of Δ^9-THCA-B may be of chemotaxonomic importance (Mechoulam et al. 1969). All the reported analogs and variants of acidic Δ^9-THC exist as the Δ^9-THCA-A isomer.

As with the other cannabinoid types, three-ring$_{[6,6,6]}$ type cannabinoids with a range of alkyl chain lengths have been identified. The varinoid analog of Δ^9-THCA-A, Δ^9-tetrahydrocannabivarinic acid (Δ^9-THCVA, **3.37**) was first identified by Fetterman and Turner (1972) by spectroscopic analysis of an Indian varietal of *Cannabis sativa* L., and quickly confirmed with mass spectral data (Turner et al. 1973b). In 1976, Harvey detailed mass spectral studies that identified both methyl and butyl analogs of Δ^9-THCA-A, Δ^9-tetrahydrocannabiorcolic acid (Δ^9-THCOA, **3.38**), and Δ^9-tetrahydrocannabibutolic acid (Δ^9-THCBA, **3.39**), respectively (Harvey 1976). Analogs with longer alkyl chain lengths, such as Δ^9-tetrahydrocannabihexolic acid (Δ^9-THCHA, **3.40**) and Δ^9-tetrahydrocannabiphorolic acid (Δ^9-THCPA, **3.41**), have not been isolated, but are assumed to exist *in vivo* due to the isolation and characterization of their neutral counterparts (see Section 3.3.3.2).

Only one acidic three-ring$_{[6,6,6]}$ type cannabinoid with unsaturation at a position other than C9 has been reported. Hanus and Krejci (1975) isolated Δ^8-tetrahydrocannabinolic acid (Δ^8-THCA, **3.42**) from a Czechoslovakian strain of *Cannabis sativa*. It has yet to be determined if Δ^8-THCA is formed enzymatically by THCA synthase, or if it undergoes isomerization *in vivo* to the more thermodynamically stable Δ^8 isomers. Formation of the Δ^8 isomers during sample workup cannot be ruled out.

Unlike the other cannabinoid types discussed in this work, there has not yet been successful isolation of a monomethyl ether analog of Δ^9-THCA. In a report disclosing the identification of CBDM in hemp using a GC-MS assay, Bercht et al. (1973) suggest that the presence of Δ^9-tetrahydrocannabinol monomethyl ether (Δ^9-THCM) "seems likely."

3.3.3.2   Compounds Formed by Heat

Δ^9-Tetrahydrocannabinol (Δ^9-THC, **3.43**) is the primary psychoactive cannabinoid found in the cannabis plant and was first isolated by Gaoni and Mechoulam (1964b) (Figure 3.13). Subsequent X-ray crystallographic analysis by Archer et al. (1970) gave a detailed analysis of the molecular conformation of Δ^9-THC, which revealed it is nearly planar, with the cyclohexene ring existing predominantly in a half-chair

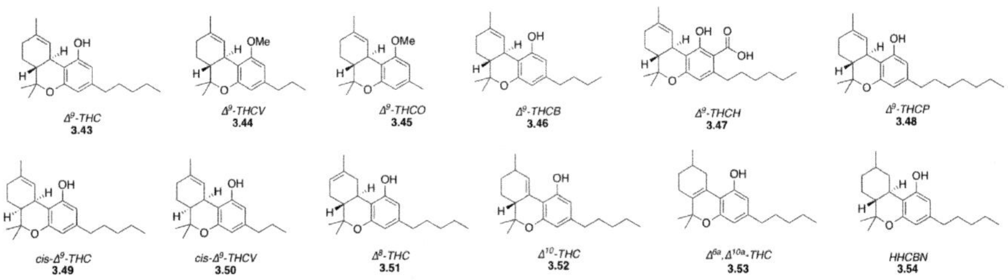

FIGURE 3.13 Neutral three-ring$_{[6,6,6]}$ type cannabinoid structures.

conformation. As a pure compound, Δ^9-THC is unstable and prone to undergo oxidative degradation, primarily through the abstraction of a hydrogen atom from C10a (see Figure **3.1**). It is estimated that the rate of Δ^9-THC degradation is 10% per month at room temperature (Hanuš et al. 2016a).

A range of alkyl chain length analogs of Δ^9-THC has been reported. Gill (1971) isolated the varinoid analog Δ^9-tetrahydrocannabinovarin (Δ^9-THCV, **3.44**) from a hashish extract. A year later, Vree et al. (1972a) isolated Δ^9-tetrahydrocannabiorcol (Δ^9-THCO, **3.45**) from a Brazilian strain of cannabis. The butyl analog of Δ^9-THC, Δ^9-tetrahydrocannabutol (Δ^9-THCB, **3.46**), was first identified by Harvey (1976). This early report was later unambiguously confirmed by Cannazza's isolation of Δ^9-THCB from the Italian FM2 cannabis strain (Linciano et al. 2019). The Cannazza group would go on to isolate both the C6-length variant Δ^9-tetrahydrocannabihexol (Δ^9-THCH, **3.47**) and C7-length variant Δ^9-tetrahydrocannabiphorol (Δ^9-THCP, **3.48**) from the same strain (Linciano et al. 2020; Citti et al. 2019b). Additionally, two *cis* diastereomers of THC, *cis*-Δ^9-THC (**3.49**) and *cis*-Δ^9-THCV (**3.50**) have been identified in cannabis extracts (Smith and Kempfert 1977; Hanuš et al. 2016b). Little is known of the origin of these *cis* diastereomers, though they appear to exist in higher concentrations in fiber hemp samples.

Several Δ^9-THC analogs with varied positions and degrees of unsaturation within the *p*-menthyl ring have been identified. The most common double bond isomer is Δ^8-tetrahydrocannabinol (Δ^8-THC, **3.51**), which was isolated from the flowering tops of the cannabis plant by Hively et al. (1966). Δ^8-THC is commonly formed as an isolation artifact during post-processing treatment of cannabis material where oxygen and/or trace acid promote a shift of the endocyclic double bond. A double bond at the C8 position is more thermodynamically stable than at the C9 position, which is the main driving force in isomerization (Razdan 1981). This thermodynamic discrepancy manifests in fascinating ways, such as in archeological findings from an Israeli burial tomb dating to the fourth century CE (Zias et al. 1993). Burned cannabis was likely used in a palliative manner, and analysis of the ashes revealed high levels of Δ^8-THC, which formed over the centuries from the gradual conversion of Δ^9-THC to the more stable Δ^8-THC.

Siegel (2020) employed 2D NMR experiments to identify two new double-bond isomers formed during the decarboxylation of a crude Δ^9-THCA distillate. The two isomers, Δ^{10}-tetrahydrocannabinol (Δ^{10}-THC, **3.52**) and Δ^{6a},Δ^{10a}-tetrahydrocannabinol

(Δ^{6a},Δ^{10a}-THC, **3.53**), have been previously observed as byproducts in cannabinoid syntheses and were likely formed due to the high heat needed for the decarboxylation reaction to proceed (Srebnik et al. 1984).

Finally, there is a single report of a fully saturated analog of Δ^9-THC. Qureshi et al. (2012) identified hexahydrocannabinol (HHCBN, **3.54**) by mass spectral analysis of several *Cannabis indica* strains from Pakistan. It is unclear if HHCBN is formed naturally in the plant or exists as an isolation artifact; this compound could form via disproportionation of a dihydrocannabinol intermediate, such as **3.56** (*vide infra*).

3.3.3.3 Aromatic Products of Oxidation

Δ^9-THC is known to be unstable, and prone to undergo oxidative degradation. One result of this oxidation reaction affords three-ring$_{[6,6,6]}$ type cannabinoids with a fully aromatized *p*-menthyl moiety (Figure 3.14). Oxidative aromatization of Δ^9-THC yields cannabinol (CBN, **3.55**), a compound first isolated by Wood et al. (1899), which represents the first phytocannabinoid ever isolated from cannabis material. Adams et al. (1940) would determine the correct structure of CBN over 40 years later. CBN and its analogs are considered isolation artifacts, not found in the living cannabis plant and only formed by oxidative aromatization of the corresponding Δ^9-THC analogs. This view is supported by the isolation of 7,8-dihydrocannabinol (**3.56**), a partially aromatized intermediate proposed to exist on the Δ^9-THC to CBN degradation pathway (Ross et al. 2005). CBN is quite stable and will not undergo further oxidation. It has been used as a marker for the identification of cannabis strains in archeological sites dating back to the 7th century BCE (Russo et al. 2008). The acidic form of CBN, cannabinolic acid (CBNA, **3.57**) has also been isolated from hashish (Mechoulam and Gaðni 1965). It is believed to be an oxidative degradation product of Δ^9-THCA-A (Turner et al. 1980).

A variety of alkyl homologs of CBN have been identified. Merkus (1971) isolated the varinoid analog cannabivarin (CBV, **3.58**) from Nepalese hashish. Five years later, Harvey (1976) identified both cannabiorcol (CBNO, **3.59**) and cannabibutol (CBNB, **3.60**) by mass spectral analysis of a mixed cannabis sample. The

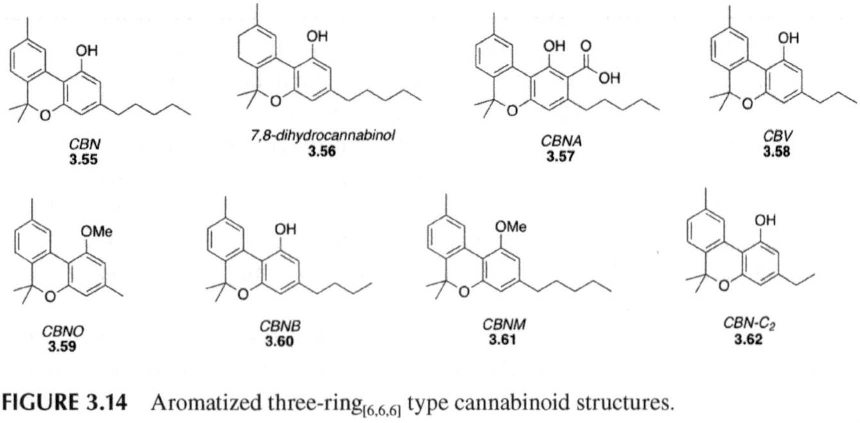

FIGURE 3.14 Aromatized three-ring$_{[6,6,6]}$ type cannabinoid structures.

monomethyl ether analog of CBN, cannabinol monomethyl ether (CBNM, **3.61**) has also been identified (Bercht et al. 1973).

Of note, there is a single reference in the literature to the isolation of an ethyl homolog of CBN (CBN-C_2, **3.62**). The report was given by Harvey (1985) at an Oxford symposium on cannabis and appears to detail the isolation of CBN-C_2 from a 140-year-old ethanolic extract of cannabis. The authors of this chapter could not access this reference, and CBN-C_2 has not been reported by any other investigations. This, combined with the fact that no ethyl variants of any cannabinoid have ever been isolated, including the hypothetical biosynthetic precursors CBGA-C_2 and Δ^9-THCA-A-C_2, suggests the report in question should be viewed with skepticism. If true, the existence of CBN-C_2 would make CBN the only cannabinoid to have alkyl chain analogs ranging from methyl to pentyl.

3.3.3.4 Hydroxylated Products of Oxidation

An alternate oxidative degradation pathway of Δ^9-THC yields three-ring$_{[6,6,6]}$ type cannabinoids that are hydroxylated at the C9- and C10- positions (Figure 3.15). The simplest hydroxylated Δ^9-THC analog is cannabitriol (CBT, **3.63**), which was first reported by Obata and Ishikama (1966). The structure of CBT was determined by Chan et al. (1976), and later X-ray crystallographic analysis by McPhail would determine the relative stereochemistry of the molecule (McPhail et al. 1984). However, this X-ray analysis could not determine which of the two enantiomers was dextrorotatory or levorotatory. Thus, CBT isolated by both Obata and Chan is designated (±)-*trans*-CBT; in this work, it is represented as a racemic mixture of the *trans* diastereomer. A handful of other CBT analogs have been reported in cannabis (Ross and ElSohly 1995), such (±)-*cis*-CBT (**3.64**), the trihydroxylated 8-OH-CBT-C_5 (**3.65**), and CBDA-C_5 9-O-CBT-C_5 ester (**3.66**), which is the only reported ester of a naturally occurring cannabinoid (Von Spulak et al. 1968). Two varinoid analogs have

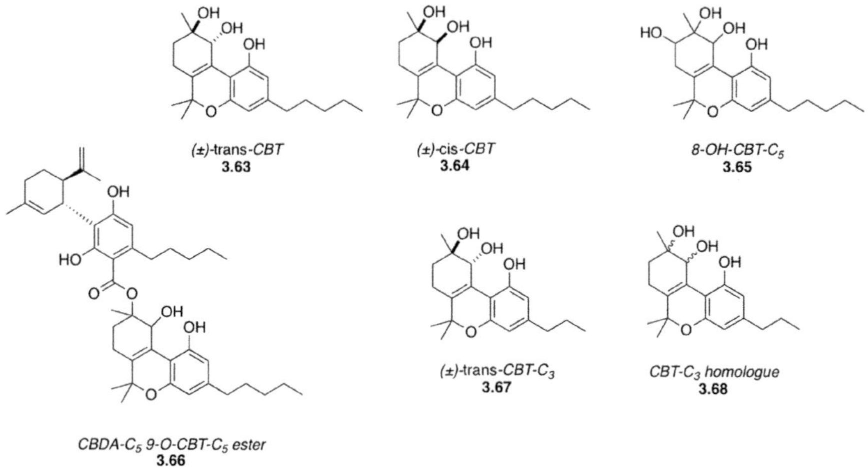

(±)-trans-*CBT*
3.63

(±)-cis-*CBT*
3.64

8-OH-CBT-C_5
3.65

(±)-trans-CBT-C_3
3.67

CBT-C_3 homologue
3.68

CBDA-C_5 9-O-CBT-C_5 ester
3.66

FIGURE 3.15 Hydroxylated three-ring$_{[6,6,6]}$ type cannabinoid structures.

also been identified: (±)-*trans*-CBT-C$_3$ (**3.67**), and a homolog of unknown stereo-chemistry (**3.68**). Of note, two previously reported CBT analogs have been omitted from this work, as the two ethoxy cannabitriols are most likely isolation artifacts formed via a ring-opening reaction between the ethanolic solvent and epoxide deriv-atives (ElSohly et al. 1978).

3.3.4 Two-Ring$_{[6,6]}$ Type

Two-ring$_{[6,6]}$ type cannabinoids are a class of cannabinoids that were first thought to form as isolation artifacts during cannabis processing (Figure 3.16). However, it has now been conclusively shown that two-ring$_{[6,6]}$ type cannabinoids are formed from the enzymatic reaction of the biogenic precursor CBGA (Morimoto et al. 1997). As with the biosynthesis of bridged two-ring and three-ring$_{[6,6,6]}$ type cannabinoids by the action of CBDA synthase and THCA synthase, respectively, the enzyme respon-sible for the formation of two-ring$_{[6,6]}$ type cannabinoids is named CBCA synthase, after the most prominent cannabinoid in the class. The defining structural feature of two-ring$_{[6,6]}$ type cannabinoids is a pyran ring, formed from an oxido-cyclization reaction that proceeds via a proposed dienone intermediate (Morimoto et al. 1998).

Cannabichromene (CBC, **3.69**) was the first two-ring$_{[6,6]}$ type cannabinoid discov-ered and was independently reported by both Claussen et al. (1966) and Gaoni and Mechoulam (1966). As with other cannabinoids, the neutral decarboxylated form was identified before the isolation of the naturally occurring acidic form; two years later, Shoyama et al. (1968) isolated cannabichromenic acid (CBCA, **3.70**) from an extract of hemp. The concentration of CBC and its analogs was found to be higher during the vegetative stage of cannabis when compared with the reproductive stage (Shoyama et al. 1977).

Alkyl chain analogs of CBC have also been isolated. Shoyama et al. isolated can-nabichromevarin (CBCV, **3.71**) and cannabichromevarinic acid (CBCVA, **3.72**), both from the "Meao variant" of Thai cannabis (Shoyama et al. 1975b; Shoyama et al. 1977). Additionally, a double-bond isomer of CBCV bearing a 4-methyl-2-pentenyl side chain (**3.73**) has been identified by Morita and Ando (1984); however, this is the only reference in the literature to this compound and may be the product of mis-identification. An orcinoid analog, cannabiorcochromene (CBCO, **3.74**), has recently

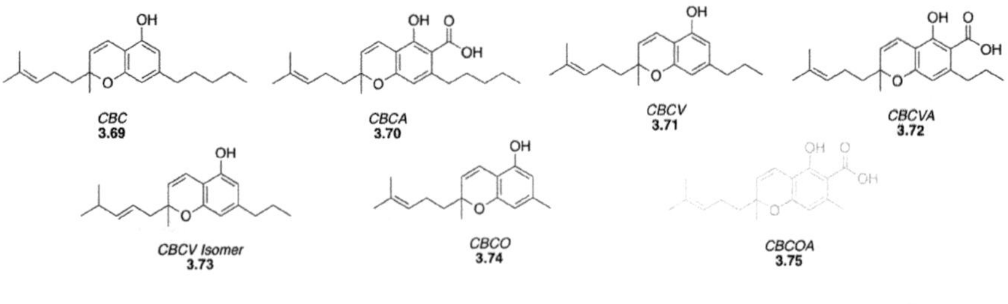

CBC
3.69

CBCA
3.70

CBCV
3.71

CBCVA
3.72

CBCV Isomer
3.73

CBCO
3.74

CBCOA
3.75

FIGURE 3.16 Two-ring$_{[6,6]}$ type cannabinoid structures. Grayed-out structures indicate cannabinoids that have not yet been isolated but are assumed to exist due to the existence of related downstream cannabinoids.

been identified as a component in seized hashish samples from Israel and the Czech Republic (Hanuš et al. 2016b). The acidic form of CBCO has yet to be reported in cannabis; interestingly, cannabiorcochromenic acid (CBCOA, **3.75**) has been identified as an active component in cultures of the fungus *Cylindrocarpon Olidum* (Quaghebeur et al. 1994). As with other neutral cannabinoids reasonably assumed to arise from decarboxylation of an acidic precursor, it is expected that CBCOA can exist *in vivo*, and thus, has been included in Figure 3.16.

3.3.5   FOUR-RING[5,4,6,6] TYPE CANNABINOIDS

This class of cannabinoids has a unique molecular skeleton that features a congested cyclobutane ring as one of four total rings (Figure 3.17). This highly unusual structure is believed to arise from the photoinduced stereoselective [2+2] cycloaddition between the two double bonds of CBC (Crombie et al. 1968) (see Section 3.2.1). Thus, all four-ring[5,4,6,6] type cannabinoids are considered artifacts formed during the storage of cannabis samples in the presence of light.

A limited number of these cannabinoids have been found. The first reported four-ring[5,4,6,6] type cannabinoid was cannabicyclol (CBL, **3.76**), which was detected by Korte and Sieper (1964) and isolated from mixed hashish samples a year later by the same group (Korte et al. 1965b). The complex structure of CBL was deduced by Begley et al. (1970) via X-ray crystallographic analysis of the dibromo derivative. Shoyama et al. (1972b) successfully isolated cannabicyclolic acid (CBLA, **3.77**) from the Kumamoto strain of cannabis, and confirmed it is formed during storage by the irradiation of CBCA. As with many other cannabinoid types, the varinoid analog, cannabicyclovarin (CBLV, **3.78**), was isolated from the "Meao variant" of Thai cannabis (Shoyama et al. 1981).

3.3.6   THREE-RING[6,5,6] TYPE

The final class of cannabinoids are three-ring[6,5,6] type cannabinoids, in which the *p*-menthyl and aromatic resorcinol rings are fused by a five-membered *O*-heterocycle (Figure 3.18). The first three-ring[6,5,6] type cannabinoid identified was cannabielsoin (CBE, **3.79**), which was reported by Bercht et al. (1973) through mass spectral analysis of a Lebanese hashish sample. Uliss et al. (1974) confirmed the structure of CBE via synthesis from a cannabidiol diacetate precursor. That same year, two different acidic isomers of CBE, cannabielsoic acid A (CBEA-A, **3.80**) and cannabielsoic acid

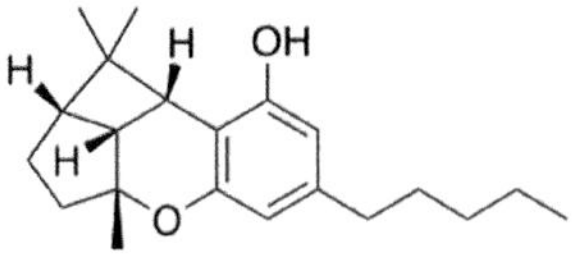

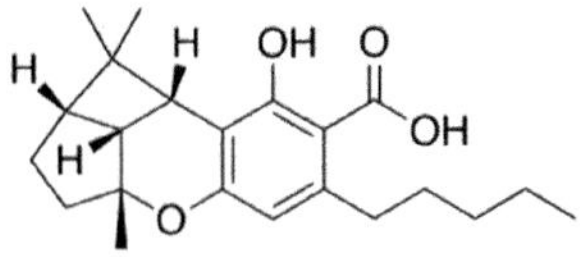

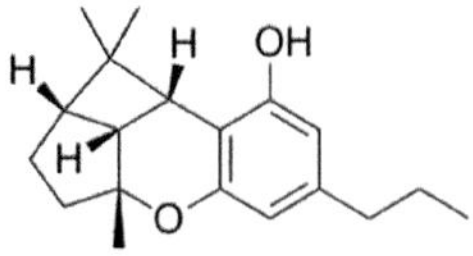

FIGURE 3.17   Four-ring[5,4,6,6] type cannabinoid structures.

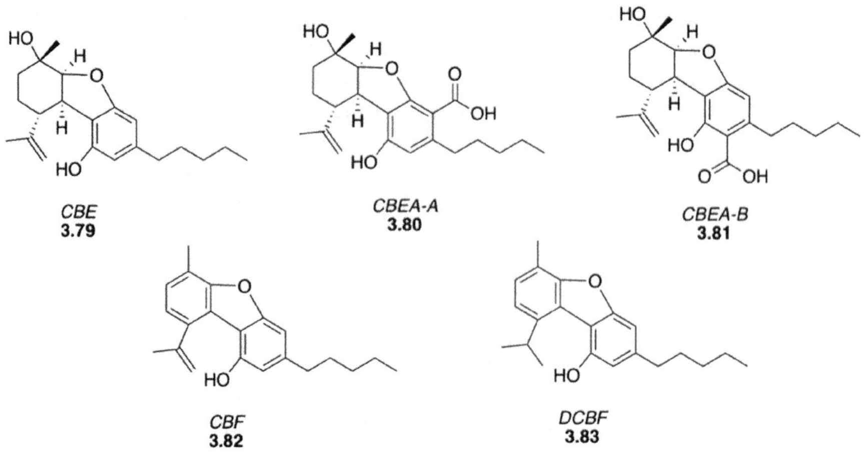

FIGURE 3.18   Three-ring$_{[6,5,6]}$ type cannabinoid structures.

B (CBEA-B, **3.81**) were isolated from Lebanese hashish by Shani and Mechoulam (1974). This report conclusively shows that CBEA is formed by an oxidative cyclization reaction of CBD and is promoted by the presence of both light and oxygen. Due to the *trans*-relationship of the oxygen functionalities on the *p*-menthyl moiety, it is proposed that the reaction occurs via a formal intramolecular ring-opening reaction of a CBD-epoxide intermediate (see Figure 3.1). The identification of two isomeric forms of CBEA is reminiscent of the two isomeric forms of THCA and suggests that the cyclization of the proposed CBD-epoxide intermediate is not selective for a particular –OH group on the resorcinol fragment. Thus, all three-ring$_{[6,5,6]}$ type cannabinoids are considered artifacts formed during the storage of cannabis in the presence of light and air.

CBE is proposed to undergo further degradation in the presence of oxygen. Freidrich-Fiechtl and Spiteller (1975) isolated and characterized two new three-ring$_{[6,5,6]}$ type cannabinoids, cannabifuran (CBF, **3.82**) and dehydrocannabifuran (DCBF, **3.83**). It is believed these two compounds are formed from CBE and have undergone oxidative aromatization of the *p*-menthyl moiety, analogous to how Δ^9-THC degrades into CBN in the presence of oxygen (see Section 3.3.3.3). Although Freidrich-Fiechtl's reported findings are the first official documentation of CBF, it is believed that Van Ginneken et al. (1972) first isolated CBF in 1972 but mistakenly believed it to be CBND (see Section 3.3.2.3). However, the findings of Freidrich-Fiechtl unambiguously confirm the existence of the CBE degradation products CBF and DCBF.

3.3.7   MISCELLANEOUS CANNABINOIDS

3.3.7.1   Unusual Structures

A handful of cannabinoids exist that feature molecular structures that cannot be classified by the six cannabinoid category types defined herein (Figure 3.19).

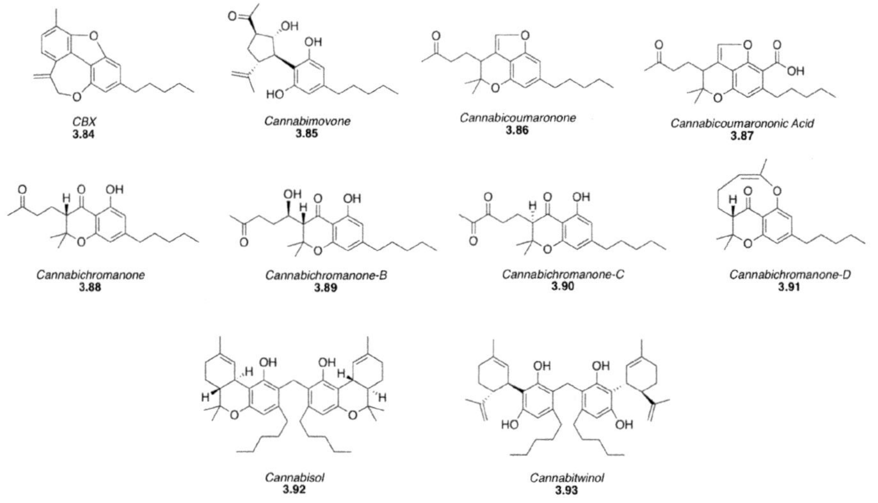

FIGURE 3.19 Cannabinoids with unusual molecular structures.

Cannabioxepane (CBX, **3.84**) was isolated from hemp by Pagani et al. (2011) and is the first cannabinoid to show a linkage between the oxygen atom at C5 and the pendant carbon atom C13. Due to its similarity to CBE and other three-ring[6,5,6] type cannabinoids, it is proposed that CBX is formed from the 7-*endo-tet* ring opening of an epoxidized CBE-like precursor. Taglialatela-Scafati et al. (2010) isolated and characterized cannabimovone (**3.85**) from the ancient "Carmagnola" variant of *Cannabis sativa*. This compound features an unprecedented *abeo*-menthane terpenoid structure and has unclear biosynthetic origins. Cannabicoumaronone (**3.86**) and cannabicoumarononic acid (**3.87**) have been isolated from high potency *Cannabis sativa* extracts (Grote and Spiteller 1978; Radwan et al. 2009). It is proposed these compounds arise from oxidative cleavage of the endocyclic double bond of Δ^9-THC, but it has yet to be determined if cannabicoumaronone and its acid are biological in origin or formed as isolation artifacts. Another proposed product of this oxidative cleavage is cannabichromanone (**3.88**), first isolated by Friedrich-Fiechtl and Spiteller (1975) from a degraded sample of hashish. An additional three derivatives (**3.89–3.91**) have been isolated from high potency *Cannabis sativa* L. (Ahmed et al. 2008a).

In recent years, a new class of dimeric cannabinoids has been discovered. First reported by Zulfiqar et al. (2012), cannabisol (**3.92**) is a dimer composed of two Δ^9-THC units connected by a single methylene bridge at the C2 position. An analogous CBD dimer, cannabitwinol (**3.93**), has also been reported, thus confirming that cannabisol is not a unique structural oddity (Chianese et al. 2020). Dimeric compounds linked via a methylene bridge are well documented in natural products, and it is proposed that these sterically congested dimers are formed enzymatically in cannabis, possibly mediated by a one-carbon transfer from methylene tetrahydrofolate on the monomeric cannabinoid acids. It is anticipated that other dimeric forms of

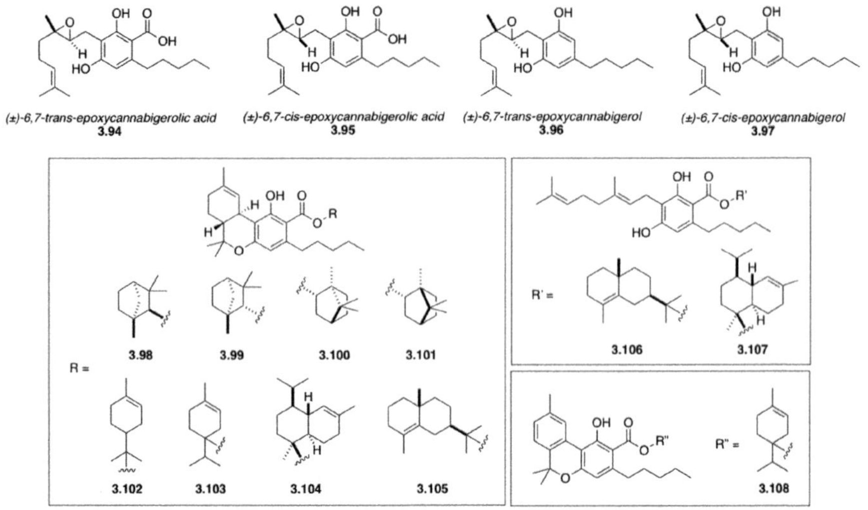

FIGURE 3.20 Cannabinoid epoxides and esters. For clarity, cannabinoid esters are represented with R-groups.

cannabinoids, such as those derived from CBG and CBC monomers or varinoid and orcinoid analogs, will be identified in the future.

3.3.7.2 Epoxides and Esters

Several cannabinoid epoxide and ester derivatives have been isolated from high potency strains of *Cannabis sativa* (Figure 3.20). Radwan et al. (2008) reported four racemic epoxides of CBG, with *cis* and *trans* diastereomers for both neutral and acidic forms of the molecule (**3.94–3.97**). Ahmed et al. (2008b) isolated 11 distinct cannabinoid esters (**3.98–3.108**) that feature mono- and sesquiterpene moieties attached by an ester linkage to three different cannabinoid units (THC, CBG, CBN). There has been no proposed biosynthesis of these compounds, and the authors posit that further investigations of high potency cannabis strains will reveal other new metabolites. Additional cannabinoids with unique oxidation and substitution patterns have been disclosed by Radwan et al. (2009).

3.4 CONCLUSION

There is more to cannabinoids than just THC and CBD. The cannabinoids discussed in this chapter are diverse. They show a wide range of chemical moieties, molecular scaffolds, and biosynthetic and/or chemical origins. As noted by ElSohly et al. (2017), the total number of known cannabinoids has increased each decade, a trend that is sure to persist in the coming years. The discovery of novel cannabinoids expands our knowledge of the cannabis metabolome, as each new substitution pattern, oxidation site, or molecular skeleton helps to elucidate the complex chemistry behind the cannabis plant. However, the gap between the number of known cannabinoids and their behavior *in vivo* is massive. Due to widespread regulations surrounding cannabis research, a mere handful of cannabinoids have been studied for potential therapeutic and medicinal applications, with the vast majority of studies focusing on Δ^9-THC (Hazekamp et al. 2010). Additionally, the cannabis metabolome includes hundreds of terpenes, flavonoids, and biologically relevant compounds, all of which could have unreported physiological effects in humans (Brenneisen 2007). Thus, Raphael Mechoulam's evocation of cannabis as a "neglected pharmacological treasure trove" is writ large: an ancient plant, which produces an ever-expanding array of chemically unique and biologically relevant compounds, has been largely locked away from scientific investigation due to restrictive legislation and ill-informed social stigmas. It is perhaps only time, and the persistence of the scientific community, that will be the key that unlocks the full potential of the cannabis plant.

REFERENCES

Adams, R., Baker, B. R., and R. B. Wearn. 1940. Synthesis of cannabinol, 1-hydroxy-3-*n*-amyl-6,6,9-trimethyl-6-dibenzopyran. *Journal of the American Chemical Society* 62:2204–7.

Ahmed, S. A., Ross, S. A., Slade, D., Radwan, M. M., Khan, I. A., and M. A. ElSohly. 2008a. Structure determination and absolute configuration of cannabichromanone derivatives from high potency *Cannabis sativa*. *Tetrahedron Letters* 49(42):6050–3.

Ahmed, S. A., Ross, S. A., Slade, D., Radwan, M. M., Zulfiqar, F., and M. A. ElSohly. 2008b. Cannabinoid ester constituents from high-potency *Cannabis sativa*. *Journal of Natural Products* 71:536–42.

Appendino, G., Giana, A., Gibbons, S., et al. 2008. A polar cannabinoid from *Cannabis sativa* var. *Carma Natural Product Communications* 3(12):1977–80.

Archer, R. A., Boyd, D. B., Demarco, P. B., Tyminski, I. J., and N. L. Allinger. 1970. Structural studies of cannabinoids: a theoretical and proton magnetic resonance analysis. *Journal of the American Chemical Society* 92(17):5200–6.

Begley, M. J., Clarke, D. G., Crombie, L., and D. A. Whiting. 1970. The x-ray structure of dibromocannabicyclol: structure of bicyclomahanimbine. *Journal of the Chemical Society D, Chemical Communications* 1547–8.

Bercht, C. A. L., Lousberg, R. J. J. Ch., Küppers, F. J. E. M., Salemink, C. A., Vree, T. B., and J. M. Van Rossum. 1973. Identification of cannabinol methyl ether from hashish. *Journal of Chromatography* 81:163–6.

Berman, P., Futoran, K., Lewitus, G. M., et al. 2018. A new ESI-LC/MS approach for comprehensive metabolic profiling of phytocannabinoids in *Cannabis*. *Scientific Reports* 8(1):14280–95.

Brenneisen, R. 2007. Chemistry and analysis of phytocannabinoids and other *Cannabis* constituents. In: ElSohly, M. A. (eds.), *Marijuana and the Cannabinoids: Forensic Science and Medicine*. Humana Press, Totowa, NJ. 17–49.

Carbone, M., Castelluccio, F., Daniele, A., et al. 2010. Chemical characterisation of oxidative degradation products of Δ^9-THC. *Tetrahedron* 66(49):9497–501.

Caprioglio, D., Mattoteia, D., Pollastro, F., et al. 2020. The oxidation of phytocannabinoids to cannabinoquinoids. *Journal of Natural Products* 83(5):1711–5.

Chan, W. R., Magnus, K. E., and H. A. Watson. 1976. The structure of cannabitriol. *Experientia* 32:283–4.

Chianese, G., Lopatriello, A., Schiano-Moriello, A., et al. 2020. Cannabitwinol, a dimeric phytocannabinoid from hemp, *Cannabis sativa* L., is a selective thermo-TRP modulator. *Journal of Natural Products* 83(9):2727–36.

Chuchev, K., and J. J. BelBruno. 2007. Mechanisms of decarboxylation of ortho-substituted benzoic acids. *Journal of Molecular Structure: THEOCHEM* 807:1–9.

Citti, C., Linciano, P., Forni, F., et al. 2019a. Analysis of impurities of cannabidiol from hemp: isolation, characterization and synthesis of cannabidibutol, the novel cannabidiol butyl analog. *Journal of Pharmaceutical and Biomedical Analysis* 175:112752–65.

Citti, C., Linciano, P., Russo, F., et al. 2019b. A novel phytocannabinoid isolated from *Cannabis sativa* L. with an in vivo cannabimimetic activity higher than Δ^9-tetrahydrocannabinol: Δ^9-tetrahydrocannabiphorol. *Scientific Reports* 9(1):20335–48.

Claussen, U., Spulak, F. V., and F. Korte. 1966. Cannabichromen, ein neuer haschisch-inhaltsstoff. *Tetrahedron* 22(4):1477–9.

Crombie, L., Ponsford, R., Shani, A., Yagnitinsky, B., and R. Mechoulam. 1968. Photochemical production of cannabicyclol from cannabichromene. *Tetrahedron Letters* 9:5771–2.

ElSohly, M. A., Boeren, E. G., and C. E. Turner. 1978. (±)-9,10-Dihydroxy-$\Delta^{6a(10a)}$-tetrahydrocannabinol and (±)-8,9-dihydroxy-$\Delta^{6a(10a)}$-tetrahydrocannabinol: 2 new cannabinoids from *Cannabis sativa* L. *Experientia* 34:1127–8.

ElSohly, M. A. 2002. Chemical constituents of Cannabis. In: Grotenhermen, F., Russo, E. (eds.), *Cannabis and Cannabinoids. Pharmacology, Toxicology, and Therapeutic Potential*. The Haworth Press, Inc., Binghamton, NY, 27–36.

ElSohly, M. A., Radwan, M. M., Gul, W., Chandra, S., and A. Galal. 2017. Phytochemistry of *Cannabis sativa* L. *Progress in the Chemistry of Organic Natural Products* 103:1–36.

Fellermeier, M., and M. H. Zenk. 1998. Prenylation of olivetolate by a hemp transferase yields cannabigerolic acid, the precursor of tetrahydrocannabinol. *FEBS Letters* 427: 283–5.

Fetterman, P. S., and C. E. Turner. 1972. Constituents of *Cannabis sativa* L.: propyl homologs of cannabinoids from an Indian variant. *Journal of Pharmaceutical Sciences* 61(9):1476–7.

Friedrich-Fiechtl, J., and G. Spiteller. 1975. Neue cannabinoide. *Tetrahedron* 31:479–87.

Gagne, S. J., Stout, J. M., Liu, E., Boubakir, Z., Clark, S. M., and J. E. Page. 2012. Identification of olivetolic acid cyclase from *Cannabis sativa* reveals a unique catalytic route to plant polyketides. *Proceedings of the National Academy of Sciences* 109(31):12811–6.

Gaoni, Y., and R. Mechoulam. 1964a. Structure and synthesis of cannabigerol, a new hashish constituent. *Proceedings of the Chemical Society* March, 82.

Gaoni, Y., and R. Mechoulam. 1964b. Isolation, structure, and partial synthesis of an active constituent of hashish. *Journal of the American Chemical Society* 86:1646–7.

Gaoni, Y., and R. Mechoulam. 1966. Cannabichromene, a new active principle in hashish. *Chemical Communications* 1:20–1.

Gill, E. W. 1971. Propyl homologue of tetrahydrocannabinol: its isolation from *Cannabis*, properties, and synthesis. *Journal of the Chemical Society C* 579–82.

Grlic, L. 1962. A comparative study on some chemical and biological characteristics of various samples of *Cannabis* resin. United Nations Office of Drugs and Crime. https://www.unodc.org/unodc/en/data-and-analysis/bulletin/bulletin_1962-01-01_3_page005.html (accessed on March 19, 2021).

Grote, H., and G. Spiteller. 1978. Die struktur des cannabicumaronons und analoger verbindungen. *Tetrahedron* 34:3207–13.

Hanus, L., and Z. Krejci. 1975. Isolation of two new cannabinoid acids from *Cannabis sativa* L. of Czechoslovak Origin. *Acta Universitatis Palackianae Olomucenis Facultatis Medicae* 74:161–7.

Hanuš, L. O., Meyer, S. M., Muñoz, E., Taglialatela-Scafati, O., and G. Appendino. 2016a. Phytocannabinoids: a unified critical inventory. *Natural Product Reports* 33(12):1357–92.

Hanuš, L. O., Levy, R., Vega, D. D. L., Katz, L., Roman, M., and P. Tomek. 2016b. The main cannabinoids content in hashish samples seized in Israel and Czech Republic. *Israel Journal of Plant Science* 63(3):182–90.

Harvey, D. J. 1976. Characterization of the butyl homologues of Δ^1-tetrahydrocannabinol, cannabinol and cannabidiol in samples cannabis by combined gas chromatography and mass spectrometry. *Journal of Pharmacy and Pharmacology* 28:280–5.

Harvey, D. J. 1985. Examination of a 140 year old ethanolic extract of *Cannabis*: identification of new cannabitriol homologues and the ethyl homologue of cannabinol. In: D. J. Harvey, W. Paton, and G. G. Hahas (eds.), *Marihuana '84: Proceedings of the Oxford Symposium on Cannabis: 9th International Congress of Pharmacology, 3rd Satellite Symposium on Cannabis*. Washington, DC, 1985, IRL, 23–30.

Hazekamp, A., Fischedick, J. T., Díez, M. L., Lubbe, A. and R. L. Ruhaak. 2010. Chemistry of *Cannabis*. In: L. Mander, and H.-W. Liu (eds.), *Comprehensive Natural Products II: Chemistry and Biology: Chemical Ecology*. Elsevier Science, Amsterdam, Netherlands, 3(24), 1033–84.

He, W., Foth, P. J., Roggen, M., Sammis, G. M., and P. Kennepohl. 2020. Why is THCA decarboxylation faster than CBDA? An in silico perspective. *ChemRxiv Preprint*.

Hillig, K. W., and P. G. Mahlberg. 2004. A chemotaxonomic analysis of cannabinoid variation in *Cannabis* (Cannabaceae). *American Journal of Botany* 91(6):966–75.

Hively, R. L., Mosher, W. A., and F. W. Hoffmann. 1966. Isolation of trans-d^6-tetrahydrocannabinol from marijuana. *Journal of the American Chemical Society* 8:1832–3.

Jacob, A., and A. Todd. 1940. Cannabidiol and cannabol, constituents of *Cannabis indica* resin. *Nature* 145:350.

Jones, P. G., Falvello, L., Kennard, O., and R. Mechoulam. 1977. Cannabidiol. *Acta Crystallographica, B* 33:3211–14.

Kajima, M. and M. Piraux. 1982. The biogenesis of cannabinoids in *Cannabis sativa*. *Phytochemistry* 21:67–9.

Korte, F., and H. Sieper. 1964. Untersuchung von haschisch-inhaltsstoffen durch dünnschichtchromatographie. *Journal of Chromatography A* 13:90–8.

Korte, F., Hagg, M., and U. Claussen. 1965a. Tetrahydrocannabinolcarboxylic acid, a component of hashish. *Angewandte Chemie International Edition in English* 4(10):872–3.

Korte, F., Sieper, H., and S. Tira. 1965b. New results on hashish-specific constituents. *Bulletin on Narcotics* 17:35.

Krejci, Z., and F. Santavy. 1955. The isolation of further substances from the leaves of Indian hemp (*Cannabis sativa* L., var. Indica). *Acta Universitatis Palackianae Olomucensis, Faculty of Medicine* 6:59–66.

Li, J., and T. B. Brill. 2003. Spectroscopy of hydrothermal reactions 23: the effect of OH substitution on the rates and mechanisms of decarboxylation of benzoic acid. *Journal of Physical Chemistry A* 107:2667–73.

Linciano, P., Citti, C., Luongo, L., et al. 2019. Isolation of a high-affinity cannabinoid for the human CB1 receptor from a medicinal *Cannabis sativa* variety: Δ^9-tetrahydrocannabutol, the butyl homologue of Δ^9-tetrahydrocannabinol. *Journal of Natural Products* 83(1):88–98.

Linciano, P., Citti, C., Russo, F., et al. 2020. Identification of a new cannabidiol n-hexyl homolog in a medicinal cannabis variety with an antinociceptive activity in mice: cannabidihexol. *Scientific Reports* 10(1):22019–30.

Lousberg, R. J. J. Ch., Bercht, C. A. L., Van Ooyen, R., and H. J. W. Spronck. 1977. Cannabinodiol: conclusive identification and synthesis of a new cannabinoid from *Cannabis sativa*. *Phytochemistry* 16(5):595–7.

McPhail, A. T., ElSohly, H. N., Turner, C. E., and M. A. ElSohly. 1984. Stereochemical assignments for the two enantiomeric pairs of 9,10-dihydroxy-$\Delta^{6a(10a)}$-tetrahydrocannabinols.

X-ray crystal structure analysis of (±)-*trans*-cannabitriol. *Journal of Natural Products* 47:138–42.

Mechoulam, R., and Y. Shvo. 1963. The structure of cannabidiol. *Tetrahedron* 19:2073–8.

Mechoulam, R., and Y. Gaoni. 1965. The isolation and structure of cannabinolic cannabidiolic and cannabigerolic acids. *Tetrahedron* 21(5):1223–9.

Mechoulam, R., and Y. Gaoni. 1967. Recent advances in the chemistry of hashish. *Fortschritte der Chemie Organischer Naturstoffe* 25:175–213.

Mechoulam, R.; Ben-Zvi, Z. and Y. Gaoni. 1968. Hashish--13. On the nature of the Beam test. *Tetrahedron* 24:5615–24.

Mechoulam, R., Ben-Zvi, Z., Yagnitinsky, B., and A. Shani. 1969. A new tetrahydrocannabinolic acid. *Tetrahedron Letters* 28:2339–41.

Mechoulam, R. 2005. Plant cannabinoids: a neglected pharmacological treasure trove. *British Journal of Pharmacology* 146(7):913–5.

Merkus, F. W. H. M. 1971. Cannabivarin and tetrahydrocannabivarin, two new constituents of hashish. *Nature* 232:579–80.

Miller, I. J., McCallum, N. K., Kirk, C. M., and B. M. Peake. 1982. The free radical oxidation of the tetrahydrocannabinols. *Experientia* 38:230–1.

Morimoto, S., Komatsu, K., Taura, F., and Y. Shoyama. 1997. Enzymological evidence for cannabichromenic acid biosynthesis. *Journal of Natural Products* 60:854–7.

Morimoto, S., Komatsu, K., Taura, F., and Y. Shoyama. 1998. Purification and characterization of cannabichromenic acid synthase from *Cannabis sativa*. *Phytochemistry* 49(6):1525–9.

Morita, M., and H. Ando. 1984. Analysis of hashish oil by gas chromatography/mass spectrometry. *Kagaku Keisatsu Kenkyujo Hokoku. Hogaku-Hen* 37(2):137–40.

Obata, Y., and Y. Ishikama. 1966. Constituents of hemp plant (*Cannabis sativa*). III. Isolation of a Gibbs-positive compound from Japanese hemp. *Agricultural and Biological Chemistry* 30:619–20.

Pagani, A., Fernando, S., Giuseppina, C., Gianpaolo, G., Appendino, G., and O. Taglialatela-Scafati. 2011. Cannabioxepane, a novel tetracyclic cannabinoid from hemp, *Cannabis sativa* L. *Tetrahedron* 67(19):3369–73.

Pellati, F., Borgonetti, V., Brighenti, V., Biagi, M., Benvenuti, S., and L. Corsi. 2018. *Cannabis sativa* L. and nonpsychoactive cannabinoids: their chemistry and role against oxidative stress, inflammation, and cancer. *BioMed Research International* 2018:1–15.

Perrotin-Brunel, H., Buijs, W., van Spronsen, J. et al. 2011. Decarboxylation of Δ⁹-tetrahydrocannabinol: kinetics and molecular modeling. *Journal of Molecular Structure* 987:67–73.

Pollastro, F., Taglialatela-Scafati, O., Allarà, M., et al. 2011. Bioactive prenylogous cannabinoid from fiber hemp (*Cannabis sativa*). *Journal of Natural Products* 74:2019–22.

Pollastro, F., Caprioglio, D., Marotta, P., et al. 2017. Iodine-promoted aromatization of p-menthane-type phytocannabinoids. *Journal of Natural Products* 81(3):630–3.

Quaghebeur, K., Coosemans, J., Toppet, S., and F. Compernolle. 1994. Cannabiorci- and 8-chlorocannabiorcichromenic acid as fungal antagonists from Cylindrocarpon Olidum. Phytochemistry 37(1):159–61.

Qureshi, M. N., Afridi, M. S., Kanwal, F., Inayat-ur-Rahman, and M. Akram. 2012. Estimation of biologically active cannabinoids in Cannabis indica by gas chromatography-mass spectrometry (GC-MS). *World Applied Sciences Journal* 19(7):918–23.

Radwan, M. M., Ross, S. A., Slade, D., Ahmed, S. A., Zulfiqar, F., and M. A. ElSohly. 2008. Isolation and characterization of new *Cannabis* constituents from a high potency variety. *Planta Medica* 74(3):267–72.

Radwan, M. M., ElSohly, M. A., Slade, D., Ahmed, S. A., Khan, I. A., and S. A. Ross. 2009. Biologically active cannabinoids from high-potency *Cannabis sativa*. *Journal of Natural Products* 72(5):906–11.

Razdan, R. K. 1981. The Total Synthesis of Cannabinoids. In *The Total Synthesis of Natural Products, Volume 4*, ed. J. ApSimon. John Wiley & Sons, Inc. 4:185–262.

Robertson, L. W., Lyle, M. A., and S. Billets. 1975. Biotransformation of cannabinoids by *Syncephalastrum racemosum*. *Biomedical Mass Spectrometry* 2:266–71.

Rosenqvist, E., and T. Ottersen. 1975. The crystal and molecular structure of d9-tetrahydro-cannabinolic acid B. *Acta Chemica Scandinavia B* B29(3):379–84.

Ross, S. A., and M. A. ElSohly. 1995. Constituents of *Cannabis sativa* L. XXVIII. A review of the natural constituents: 1980–1994. *Zagazig Journal of Pharmaceutical Science* 4:1–10.

Ross, S. A., and M. A. ElSohly. 1999. CBN and D^9-THC concentration ratio as an indicator of the age of stored marijuana samples. United Nations Office on Drugs and Crime. https ://www.unodc.org/unodc/en/data-and-analysis/bulletin/bulletin_1997-01-01_1_page0 08.html#fn (accessed on March 19, 2021).

Ross, S. A., ElSohly, M. A., Sultana, G. N. N., Mehmedic, Z., Hossain, C. F., and S. Chandra. 2005. Flavonoid glycosides and cannabinoids from the pollen of *Cannabis sativa* L. *Phytochemical Analysis* 16(1):45–8.

Ruelle, P. 1986. Theoretical study of the mechanism of thermal decarboxylation of salicylic and *p*-aminobenzoic acids; models for aqueous solution. *Journal of the Chemical Society, Perkin Transactions* 2(12):1953–9.

Russo, E. B. 2001. Hemp for headache: an in-depth historical and scientific review of cannabis in migraine treatment. *Journal of Cannabis Therapeutics* 1(2):21–92.

Russo, E. B. 2007. History of *Cannabis* and its preparations in saga, science, and sobriquet. *Chemistry & Biodiversity* 4(8):1614–48.

Russo, E. B., Jiang, H.-E., Li, X., et al. 2008. Phytochemical and genetic analyses of ancient *Cannabis* from central Asia. *Journal of Experimental Botany* 59(15):4171–82.

Shani, A., and R. Mechoulam. 1974. Cannabielsoic acids: isolation and synthesis by a novel oxidative cyclization. *Tetrahedron* 30(15):2437–46.

Shoyama, Y., Fujita, T., Tamauchi, T., and I. Nishioka. 1968. Cannabichromenic acid, a genuine substance of cannabichromene. *Chemical and Pharmaceutical Bulletin* 16(6):1158–9.

Shoyama, Y., Yamauchi, T., and I. Nishioka. 1970. Cannabigerolic monomethyl ether and cannabinolic acid. *Chemical and Pharmaceutical Bulletin* 18:1327–32.

Shoyama, Y., Kuboe, K., Nishioka, I., and T. Yamauchi. 1972a. Cannabidiol monomethyl ether – a new neutral cannabinoid. *Chemical and Pharmaceutical Bulletin* 20(9):2072.

Shoyama, Y., Oku, R., Yamauchi, T., and I. Nishioka. 1972b. Cannabicyclolic acid. *Chemical and Pharmaceutical Bulletin* 20(9):1927–30.

Shoyama, Y., Yagi, M., Nishioka, I., and T. Yamauchi. 1975a. Biosynthesis of Cannabinoid acids. *Phytochemistry* 14(10):2189–92.

Shoyama, Y., Hirano, H., Oda, M., Somehara, T., and I. Nishioka. 1975b. Cannabichromevarin and cannabigerovarin, two new propyl homologues of cannabichromene and cannabig-erol. *Chemical and Pharmaceutical Bulletin* 23(8): 1894–5.

Shoyama, Y., Hirano, H., Makino, H., Umekita, N., and I. Nishioka. 1977. The isolation and structures of four new propyl cannabinoid acids, THCVA, CBVA, CBCVA, and CBGVA from Thai cannabis, "Meao variant." Chemical and Pharmaceutical Bulletin 25(9):2306–11.

Shoyama, Y., Morimoto, S., and I. Nishioka. 1981. Two new ropyl cannabinoids, cannabi-cyclovarin and d^7-cis-iso-tetrahydrocannabivarin, from Thai *Cannabis*. *Chemical and Pharmaceutical Bulletin* 29(12):3720–3.

Siegel, A. 2020. Identification of manufacturing byproduct as synthetic cannabinoid Δ^{10} THC. *Presented at the 6th Annual Emerald Conference,* San Diego, CA.

Smith, R. M., and K. D. Kempfert. 1977. Δ^1-3,4-cis-Tetrahydrocannabinol in *Cannabis sativa*. *Phytochemistry* 16:1088–9.

Srebnik, M., Lander, N., Breuer, A., and R. Mechoulam. 1984. Base-catalysed double-bond isomerizations of cannabinoids: structural and stereochemical aspects. *Journal of the Chemical Society, Perkin Transactions* 1, 2881–6.

Taglialatela-Scafati, O., Pagani, A., Scala, F., et al. 2010. Cannabimovone, a cannabinoid with a rearranged terpenoid skeleton from hemp. *European Journal of Organic Chemistry* 2010(11):2067–72.

Taura, F., Morimoto, S., and Y. Shoyama. 1995a. Cannabinerolic acid, a cannabinoid from *Cannabis sativa*. *Phytochemistry* 39(2):457–8.

Taura, F., Morimoto, S., and Y. Shoyama. 1995b. First direct evidence for the mechanism of Δ^1-tetrahydrocannabinolic acid biosynthesis. *Journal of the American Chemical Society* 117:9766–7.

Taura, F., Morimoto, S., and Y. Shoyama. 1996. Purification and characterization of cannabidiolic-acid synthase from *Cannabis sativa* L. *Journal of Biological Chemistry* 271(29):17411–6.

Thomas, B. F., and M. A. ElSohly. 2016. Biosynthesis and pharmacology of phytocannabinoids and related chemical constituents. In: Thomas, B. F.; ElSohly, M. A. (eds.), *The Analytical Chemistry of Cannabis*; Elsevier, Waltham, MA. 27–41.

Turner, C. E., Hadley, K. W., Fetterman, P. S., Doorenbos, N. J., Quimby, M. W., and C. Waller. 1973a. Constituents of *Cannabis sativa* L.: IV. stability of cannabinoids in stored plant material. *Journal of Pharmaceutical Science* 62(10):1601–5.

Turner, C. E., Hadley, K., and P. S. Fetterman. 1973b. Constituents of *Cannabis sativa*: propyl homologs in samples of known geographical origin. *Journal of Pharmaceutical Sciences* 62(10):1739–41.

Turner, C. E., and M. A. Elsohly. 1979. Constituents of *Cannabis sativa* L. XVI. A possible decomposition pathway of Δ^9-tetrahydrocannabinol to cannabinol. *Journal of Heterocyclic Chemistry* 16(8):1667–8.

Turner, C. E., ElSohly, M. A., and E. G. Boeren. 1980. Constituents of *Cannabis sativa* L. A review of the natural constituents. *Journal of Natural Products* 43:169–234.

Uliss, D. B., Razdan, R. K., and H. C. Dalzell. 1974. Stereospecific intramolecular epoxide cleavage by phenolate anion. Synthesis of novel and biologically active cannabinoids. *Journal of the American Chemical Society* 96(23):7372–4.

Van Ginneken, C. A. M., Vree, T. B., Breimer, D. D., Thijssen H. W. H., and J. M. Van Rossum. 1972. Cannabinodiol, a new hashish constituent, identified by gas chromatography – mass spectrometry. In: Frigerio, A. (ed.), *Proceedings of the International Symposium on Gas Chromatography Mass Spectrometry*. Tamburini Editore, Isle of Elba, Milan, Italy, pp. 109–29.

Vollner, L., Bieniek, D., and F. Korte. 1969. Cannabidivarin ein neuer haschischinhaltsstoff. Ein Neuer Haschischinhaltsstoff. *Tetrahedron Letters* 3:145–7.

Von Spulak, F., Claussen, U., Fehlhaber, H. W., and F. Korte. 1968. Cannabidiol carbonsaure-tetrahydrocannabitrol-ester ein neuer haschisch-inhaltsstoff. *Tetrahedron* 24:5379–83.

Vree, T. B., Breimer, D. D., Ginneken, C. A. M., and J. M. Rossum. 1972a. Identification in hashish of tetrahydrocannabinol, cannabidiol and cannabinol analogues with a methyl side-chain. *Journal of Pharmacy and Pharmacology* 24(1):7–12.

Vree, T. B., Breimer, D. D., Van Ginneken, C. A. M., and J. M. Van Rossum. 1972b. Gas chromatography of *Cannabis* constituents and their synthetic derivatives. *Journal of Chromatography* 74(2):209–24.

Wang, M., Wang, Y.-H., Avula, B., et al. 2016. Decarboxylation study of acidic cannabinoids: a novel approach using ultra-high-performance supercritical fluid chromatography/photodiode array-mass spectrometry. *Cannabis and Cannabinoid Research* 1:262–71.

Webster, G. R. B., Sarna, L. P., and R. Mechoulam. 2008. Conversion of CBD to Δ^8-THC and Δ^9-THC. US Patent US-7399872-B2, filed February 25, 2004, and issued July 15, 2008.

Welling, M. T., Liu, L., Shapter, T., Raymond, C. A., and G. J. King. 2016. Characterisation of cannabinoid composition in a diverse *Cannabis sativa* L. germplasm collection *Euphytica* 208(3):463–75.

Wood, T. B., Spivey, W. T., and T. H. Easterfield. 1899. Cannabinol. Part I. *Journal of the Chemical Society* 75:20–36.

Yamauchi, T., Shoyama, Y., Matsuo, Y., and I. Nishioka. 1968. Cannabigerol monomethyl ether, a new component of hemp. *Chemical and Pharmaceutical Bulletin* 16:1164–5.

Zias, J., Stark, H., Seligman, J., et al. 1993. Early medical use of *Cannabis*. *Nature* 363:215.

Zulfiqar, F., Ross, S. A., Slade, D., et al. 2012. Cannabisol, a novel Δ^9-THC dimer possessing a unique methylene bridge, isolated from *Cannabis sativa*. *Tetrahedron Letters* 53(28):3560–2.

4 Use of Mass Spectrometry for the Analysis of *Cannabis sativa* spp.

Allegra Leghissa and Zacariah L. Hildenbrand

CONTENTS

4.1 INTRODUCTION

4.1.1 CANNABIS AND CANNABINOIDS

The *Cannabis sativa* plant belongs to the *Cannabaceae* family and is an herbaceous annual that can grow 8–12 feet tall. One likely origin of this unique plant is the Altai Mountains in southern Siberia (Russia) (ej Hanuš 2009; Leghissa et al. 2018), and the oldest evidence of human use dates back to the Gravettian settlements in Eastern Europe (29,000–22,000 years ago) (Leghissa et al. 2018). These tribes used *C. sativa* as cordage and textiles, while the first medical evidence was found with Emperor Chen Nung in China (5000 years ago), who is believed to have discovered medicinal plants (Leghissa et al. 2018).

There are more than 500 different natural products found in *C. sativa,* and among these, 100 are classified as cannabinoids, the main bioactive principles of the plant (Leghissa et al. 2018). They were first described in 1967 by Gaoni and Mechoulam as "the group of C21 compounds typical of and present in *Cannabis sativa*, their carboxylic acids, analogs, and transformation products" (Mechoulam and Gaoni

DOI: 10.1201/9780429274893-4

1967). Today, these compounds have been classified into ten categories based on their structures (ElSohly and Slade 2005), as shown in Figure 4.1, see also Chapter 1 and Table 1.1.

The first cannabinoid to have been isolated was cannabigerol (CBG), which showed antibacterial activity against Gram-positive bacteria (Mechoulam and Gaoni 1967). Currently, up to seven different variants of CBG have been discovered, with varying lengths of the carbon side chain (Leghissa et al. 2018). Another cannabinoid that was identified by Gaoni and Mechoulam (1971), and almost simultaneously by Claussen et al. (Claussen and Von Spulak 1968), was cannabichromene (CBC), which exists in five different forms. Additionally, Adams et al. (1940) discovered cannabidiol (CBD) in 1940, which exists in seven different structures, and has a wide variety of medical benefits (analgesic, anti-inflammatory, etc.) (Leghissa et al. 2018). The main psycho-active component, Δ^9-tetrahydrocannabinol (THC), was also discovered by Gaoni and Mechoulam (1971), and nine different forms have been identified, including its acid precursor (Δ^9-tetrahydrocannabinolic acid, THCA) (ElSohly and Slade 2005). An important, more stable isomer of Δ^9-THC is Δ^8-tetrahydrocannabinol (Δ^8-THC), which is reportedly 20% less psychoactive than THC (ElSohly and Slade 2005). Furthermore, other subclasses of cannabinoids include cannabinol (CBN), an oxida-tion byproduct of THC; cannabicyclol (CBL), which exists in three different forms and is produced via exposure of CBC to ultraviolet radiation; cannabielsoin (CBE) and its five structures; cannabinodiol (CBDN), the oxidation byproduct of CBD; and cannabitriol (CBT) (Leghissa et al. 2018).

Some cannabinoids, such as THC, Δ^8-THC, and CBD, share similarities in their metabolism, but THC is the most studied due to its elevated psychotropic activity compared with Δ^8-THC and CBD (Leghissa et al. 2018). In general, only 1% of this cannabinoid is eliminated from the human body in its original form once it reaches

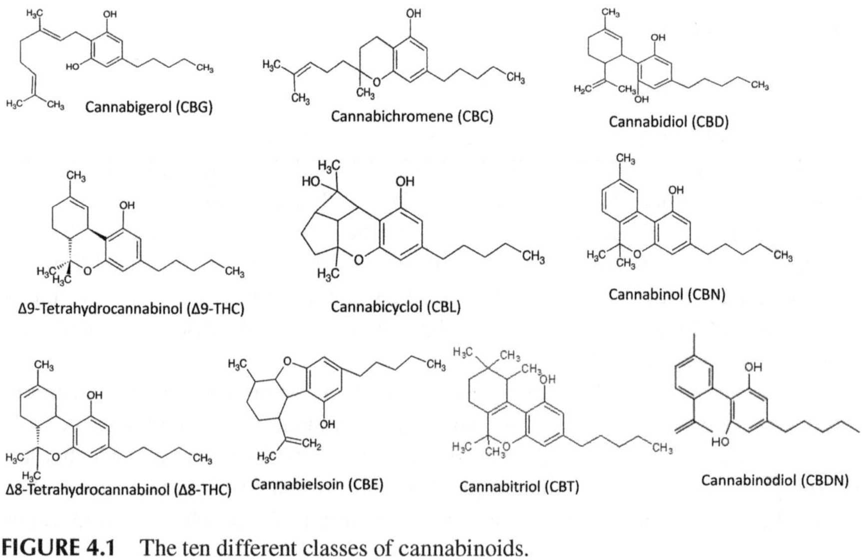

FIGURE 4.1 The ten different classes of cannabinoids.

the lungs, liver, or intestine. THC is primarily transformed into its hydroxylated metabolite, 11-hydroxy-Δ^9-tetrahydrocannabinol (THC-OH), which is also its most active metabolite. Subsequently, THC-OH is transformed into the carboxy metabolite 11-nor-9-carboxy-Δ^9-tetrahydrocannabinol (11-nor-9-carboxy-THC), which is inactive and can be detected in feces, urine, and plasma (Leghissa et al. 2018). The excretion time of cannabinoids varies on different parameters, but generally, 80–90% of cannabinoid load is eliminated within the first five days after consumption, mainly in feces (65%) (Leghissa et al. 2018). Also see Chapter 3 for an extensive overview of cannabinoid structures and Chapter 10 for more information about cannabinoid metabolism.

C. sativa can produce different types of products for human consumption, the most well-known being cannabis flowers, hashish, and liquid cannabis (United Nations Office on Drugs and Crime 2009). THC is primarily located in the cannabis resin and is produced in the glandular trichomes of *C. sativa* flowers, and it is usually extracted by hydraulic compression. On the other hand, what is referred to as "liquid cannabis" is a tincture, obtained by the extraction of the components into alcohol. There are three ways of extracting cannabinoids: room temperature method (the most traditional one), cold brew method, and accelerated hot method (Leghissa et al. 2018).

Different laws and regulations control the use and cultivation of *C. sativa* around the world. For instance, in Canada, South Africa, Georgia, and Uruguay, its recreational use is legal, while countries that have legalized its medical use include Argentina, Australia, Barbados, Bermuda, Brazil, Chile, Colombia, Croatia, Cyprus, Czech Republic, Denmark, Ecuador, Finland, Germany, Greece, Ireland, Italy, Jamaica, Lebanon, Lithuania, Luxemburg, Malawi, Malta, the Netherlands, New Zealand, North Macedonia, Norway, Peru, Poland, Portugal, Saint Vincent and the Grenadines, San Marino, Sri Lanka, Switzerland, Thailand, the United Kingdom, Uruguay, Vanuatu, Zambia, and Zimbabwe. As of June 25, 2019, 33 states of the United States, the District of Columbia, Guam, Puerto Rico, and the US Virgin Islands have legalized medical *C. sativa* programs, 14 of which legalized the recreational use as well, as depicted in Figure 4.2 (National Conference of State Legislatures, n.d.). In the United States, each state has its own regulations with respect to testing for state compliance and product safety, including analysis for pesticides, residual solvents, bacteria and fungi, metals, and cannabinoids (Leghissa et al. 2018).

A wide variety of analytical methods and tools are available for the identification and quantification of cannabinoids. In this chapter, we will focus on the use of mass spectrometry (MS), a universal detector that can be coupled with gas chromatography (GC), liquid chromatography (LC), or stand by itself.

4.1.2 GAS CHROMATOGRAPHY

GC is one of the most popular separative techniques in analytical chemistry. Its invention is attributed to Martin and James in 1952 (James and Martin 1952), and the first commercial instrument was introduced by PerkinElmer in 1955. In the following years, GC has garnered significant importance in the analysis of petrochemical

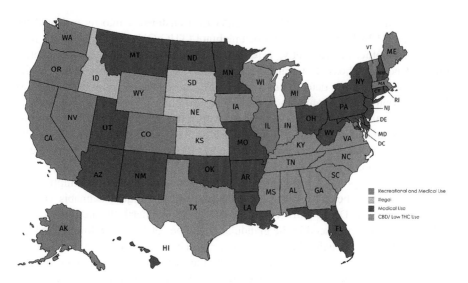

FIGURE 4.2   Legalization status in the United States.

products, whereas today it is utilized for food and beverages, pharmaceutical, and
environmental applications. This evolution has been facilitated by better separative
columns and more suited sample preparations (Weil and Willams 1950; Skoog et al.
2014).

The International Union of Pure and Applied Chemistry (IUPAC) defines GC
as "a separation technique in which the mobile phase is a gas. Gas chromatography
is always carried out in a column." (McNaught and Wilkinson 1997). To be more
precise, in this separation method, the components of a mixture need to be volatil-
ized, and therefore, need to have a boiling point of less than 400°C. Another analyte
cut-off for the use of this technique is the molecular weight; the upper limit is 500
g/mol. The separation among species is achieved by the different chemical affinities
for the solid (gas-solid) or liquid (gas-liquid) stationary phase of the column (Weil
and Willams 1950; Skoog et al. 2014).

In GC, the analytes are introduced into the system through a microsyringe and
will then pass into the analytical column. The carrier gas will move the molecules
through the separation column, but their passage is detained by their adsorption
either onto the column walls or onto the packing materials; the velocity of the analytes will depend on the level of adsorption, which depends on the chemical similarities between the molecules and the stationary phase (Weil and Willams 1950;
Skoog et al. 2014). Due to this phenomenon, the species of a mixture are separated
in the GC column, reaching its end at different times (retention time). After exiting
the column, the molecules enter a detector where they are identified and quantified
(Weil and Willams 1950).

There is an extensive list of detectors that can be coupled with the GC (Table 4.1).
The most commonly used detectors include MS, the flame ionization detector
(FID), followed by the thermal conductivity detector (TCD) (Harris 1999; Weil and

TABLE 4.1
Common Gas Chromatography Detectors

Detector	Selectivity	Sensitivity	Linearity
Thermal conductivity (TCD)	Universal	ng	10^{4-6}
Flame ionization (FID)	All organic substances	pg	10^7
Electron capture (ECD)	Molecules with electronegative/withdrawing elements	fg	10^4
Photoionization (PID)	Aromatic unsaturated; carboxyl acids; esters; aldehydes; iodoalkanes; bromoalkanes; silanes; amides; alkylamides	pg	10^6
Mass spectrometry (MS)	Universal	fg-pg	10^{4-7}
Vacuum ultraviolet (VUV)	Universal	pg	10^{4-7}

Willams 1950). The FID is mainly sensitive to hydrocarbons, while the latter is considered universal, given that the thermal conductivity of the analyte differs from that of the carrier gas at detector temperature. Furthermore, FID is a destructive detector, contrary to TCD, but both are quite robust. The FID consists of electrodes and a hydrogen/air fueled flame near the end of the column that will pyrolyze all the carbon-containing analytes once they exit the GC system. C-containing compounds form cations and electrons once pyrolyzed, and this creates a current between the electrodes; an increase in current is translated as a chromatographic peak (Harris 1999; Higson 2004). FID has low detection limits (pg/s), but it is not universal. The TCD uses a tungsten-rhenium filament with a current passing through it to calculate the thermal conductivity of compounds. The carrier gases are usually He or N due to their relatively high conductivity, which is able to keep the filament cool with constant resistivity and electrical efficiency. When the analytes, together with the carrier gas, exit the GC system, the thermal conductivity decreases and generates a response in the detector. The decrease in thermal conductivity, in fact, increases the filament temperature and resistivity causing voltage fluctuations (Harris 1999; Higson 2004; Skoog et al. 2014).

Another available detector is the electron capture detector (ECD), based on the use of a radioactive beta particle source to detect analytes with electronegative or withdrawing elements and functional groups such as halogens, carbonyl, nitrites, nitriles, and organometallics (Harris 1999; Higson 2004). Once the carrier gas passes between the two electrodes at the exit of the column, with the cathode carrying a radioactive foil (^{63}Ni), beta particles are emitted and collide with the ionized carrier gas, generating more ions that generate a current. The molecules with electronegative elements and the functional groups previously listed will decrease the current and generate a response in the detector (Harris 1999; Higson 2004; Skoog et al. 2014).

Other important detectors are the catalytic combustion detector (CCD), which measures combustible hydrocarbons and H, the discharge ionization detector (DID), which produces ions through a high-voltage electric discharge, and the flame photometric detector (FPD), which detects the spectral lines of compounds burning in the flame through a photomultiplier tube (Harris 1999; Higson 2004; Skoog et al. 2014).

The vacuum ultraviolet detector (VUV) is the most recent detector in gas chromatography. The VUV detects analytes that absorb in the 120–240 nm wavelength, giving unique sets of absorption profiles (Schug et al. 2014; Santos and Schug 2017). This detector has been used in the analysis of various compounds, including petrochemical analytes (Ling Bai et al. 2015), terpenes (Qiu et al. 2017), pesticides (Fan et al. 2015), cannabinoids (Leghissa et al. 2018), carbohydrates (Schenk et al. 2017), and new designer stimulants (Skultety et al. 2017), and it is currently gaining a lot of interest due to its capability for an absolute quantitation without calibration (Bai et al. 2017).

Other detectors include the helium ionization detector (HID), the Hall electrolytic conductivity detector (EICD), the infrared detector (IRD), the photoionization detector (PID), the pulsed discharge ionization detector (PDD), the thermionic ionization detector (TID), the atomic emission detector (AED), the alkali flame detector (AFD), the nitrogen-phosphorous detector (NPD), and the dry electrolytic conductivity detector (DELCD) (Harris 1999; Poole 2015; Skoog et al. 2014).

There is a long list of reasons for choosing a GC instrument for the analysis of *C. sativa*. One of them is the ability to perform identification and quantification of different classes of compounds with only one machine (cannabinoids, terpenes, some pesticides, and residual solvents) (Leghissa et al. 2018). Furthermore, GC has been reported to have better sensitivity and higher throughput than LC, with the only drawback of an extra sample preparation step (derivatization) to protect the carboxylic acids of the acidic cannabinoids from decarboxylation (Leghissa et al. 2018).

4.1.3 LIQUID CHROMATOGRAPHY

LC uses the interactions between the samples and the phases (mobile and stationary) to separate a sample into its components (Higson 2004). Its development started with the problem posed by analyzing polar high molecular weight biopolymers by GC. Cal Giddings and co. carried out different experiments between the 1960s and the 1970s to prove that the LC could be efficiently operated by reducing the packing-particle diameter and by pressure-increasing the mobile phase velocity (Karger 1997). During the 1970s, many researchers began using pumps and injectors, creating the first design of a high-performance liquid chromatography (HPLC) system (Karger and Berry 1971).

LC separates components based on their differential affinity for stationary and mobile phases, meaning that if their polarities are similar to the mobile phase, the analytes will move through the column faster than the others (Higson 2004). On the contrary, the components that are more comparable to the stationary phase will move slower than the former (Higson 2004). In any case, the separation efficacy depends on the chemistry of the adsorbent solid and the polarity of the mobile phase (Higson 2004).

Due to the various chemical properties of analytes, mobile phases, and stationary phases, a wide range of chromatographic techniques are used, including:

normal-phase chromatography, where the stationary phase on the column is more polar than the mobile phase (less polar components will elute faster); reversed-phase chromatography, where the mobile phases are highly polar solvents, such as water, methanol, and acetonitrile; and non-polar stationary phases are prepared by coating the silanized silica with non-polar liquids such as silicone and various hydrocarbons (more polar components will elute faster) (Higson 2004; Skoog et al. 2014; Meyer 2013). Other forms include flash chromatography, which is mainly controlled by gravity with the help of pressurized air or a vacuum; partition chromatography, where the stationary and the mobile phases are immiscible liquids; ion exchange chromatography, where the stationary phase has either positively or negatively charged groups that attract opposite ions in solution; size exclusion chromatography (SEC), where the silica (or polymers) of the stationary phase are packed to form uniform pores that will then separate molecules by size; affinity chromatography, based on the retention of only analytes that have been previously bound to a specific ligand; and chiral chromatography, which separates enantiomers using a chiral additive to either the mobile or stationary phases (Meyer 2013).

Similar to GC, various detectors are available for LC (Skoog et al. 2014), which are summarized in Table 4.2. The most commonly used are MS and absorbance detectors such as the ultraviolet-visible absorbance detector (UV-Vis) and the photodiode array detector (PDA) (Swartz 2010). These are able to detect all light-absorbing compounds and they are easy to operate. Once eluted from the column, analytes pass through a clear colorless flow cell and are irradiated with light, absorbing part of it causing a difference in the intensity of the UV-Vis light transmitted by the mobile phase (no sample) and the eluent containing the analytes (Skoog et al. 2014; Swartz 2010). Measuring this difference allows detection and quantification of the sample. It is crucial to appropriately choose the wavelength prior to analysis as the UV-Vis absorbance differs based on this selection. The wavelength range of UV-Vis detectors typically ranges from 195–700 nm, and the most commonly used wavelength is 254 nm (Higson 2004; Swartz 2010). PDA detectors, on the other hand, allow the simultaneous detection of the entire spectrum, adding a third dimension (wavelength) to the UV-Vis spectra (transmittance and time) (Swartz 2010). For this reason, the PDA is suited for the determination of the most appropriate wavelength without the need to repeat the analysis (Swartz 2010).

TABLE 4.2
Common Liquid Chromatography Detectors

Detector	Selectivity	Sensitivity	Linear Range
Ultraviolet-visible absorption (UV-Vis)	Universal to chromophores	pg	10^{3-4}
Photodiode array (PDA)	Universal to chromophores	pg	10^{3-4}
Fluorescence	Fluorescent compounds	fg	10^{5}
Refractive index (RID)	Universal	ng	10^{3}
Mass spectrometry (MS)	Universal	fg-pg	10^{4-7}
Evaporative light scattering (ELSD)	Universal	ng	10^{5}

The refractive index (RI) detector measures the changes in the refractive index using a glass cell consisting of two parts: the sample cell containing the HPLC effluent and the reference cell containing only the mobile phase (Swartz 2010; Skoog et al. 2014). When the effluent in the sample cell does not contain any analyte, a beam irradiated on the cell will be straight, but when the sample cell contains dissolved analytes, the incident beam will bend due to a difference in the refractive index between the two liquids (Swartz 2010; Skoog et al. 2014).

Other detectors include the evaporative light scattering detector (ELSD), which measures the scattered radiation emitted from an evaporated sample once radiated with a laser beam (suited for lipids, sugars, and high molecular weight analytes); the multi-angle light scattering detector (MALS), allowing the quantitation through SEC analysis without the creation of a calibration curve; the conductivity detector, which measures the electronic resistance of ionic components to quantify analytes separated through ion chromatography; and the fluorescence detector, in which analytes absorb light and then emit light at a higher wavelength by fluorescence, which is then used to quantify the analytes of interest (Swartz 2010). Less common detectors include the chemiluminescence detector, the optical rotation detector, and the electro-chemical detector (Swartz 2010).

Just as for the GC, the use of LC systems for analyzing *C. sativa* has many advantages. For example, the same system may be used for the analysis of cannabinoids, some pesticides, and mycotoxins (Leghissa et al. 2018). Most significant is its ability to directly analyze acid cannabinoids without the need for derivatization to protect the carboxy groups, given the temperatures seen in LC are not elevated enough to cause decarboxylation of these species (Leghissa et al. 2018).

4.1.4 MASS SPECTROMETRY

MS is a detection technique used to quantify known analytes, identify unknown targets, and clarify the structural and chemical properties of compounds (Skoog et al. 2014). The process is based on the formation of gaseous ions from the compound molecules, which are then analyzed based on their mass-to-charge ratios (m/z) and relative abundances (Skoog et al. 2014).

The initial inventions of MS date back to 1886 when Eugene Goldstein observed the so-called "canal rays" (Kanalstrahlen), the rays in gas discharges that, under low pressures, travel from an anode to a cathode (Griffiths 2008). After that, Wilheim Wien found that these rays could be deflected through a strong electric or magnetic field, and in 1899, he constructed a device with perpendicular magnetic and electric fields to separate the positive rays based on their charge-to-mass ratio (Q/m) (Griffiths 2008). The modern version of the MS was developed by Arthur Jeffrey Dempster and Francis W. Aston in 1918 and 1919, respectively (Downard 2007; Griffiths 2008). The most recent developments in MS were recognized in 2002 when John Bennet Fenn and Koichi Tanaka were awarded the Nobel Prize in Chemistry for the development of electrospray ionization (ESI) and soft laser desorption (SLD) (The Nobel Foundation, n.d.).

The principle of the MS is the generation of multiple ions from the sample, their separation according to the m/z ratio, and the recording of the relative abundance of each generated ion (de Hoffman and Stroobant 2001; Gross 2017; Skoog et al. 2014; Higson 2004). This process is achieved through three major parts: the ion source, which produces gaseous ions from the sample; the analyzer, which resolves the ions according to their *m/z*; and the detector, which detects the formed ions and records their relative absorbance (de Hoffman and Stroobant 2001; Gross 2017). Furthermore, a sample introduction system and a computer are necessary.

The ion source is therefore the first part of the MS, which creates ions that are then transported (via magnetic or electric fields) to the mass analyzer (de Hoffman and Stroobant 2001; Gross 2017). Various sources can be used based on the nature of the sample and its physical state; for example, electron impact (EI) and chemical ionization (CI) are used for gases, while ESI, atmospheric-pressure chemical ionization (APCI), and SLD are suited for liquid and solid samples (de Hoffman and Stroobant 2001; Gross 2017).

In general, the most common classifications of ion sources are *soft* and *hard* ionization. *Soft* ionization imparts little residual energy onto the molecule, resulting in negligible fragmentation, allowing for the detection of the molecular ion and the measurement of the molecular weight of the analyte. Soft ionization techniques include ESI, APCI, CI, fast atom bombardment (FAB), desorption electrospray ionization (DESI), and matrix-assisted laser desorption ionization (MALDI) (de Hoffman and Stroobant 2001; Gross 2017). On the other hand, *hard* ionization techniques, such as EI, impart high quantities of residual energy onto the molecule, resulting in a high degree of fragmentation that provides more opportunities for structure elucidation (de Hoffman and Stroobant 2001; Gross 2017). Other ion sources include inductively coupled plasma (ICP), wherein a plasma is used to atomize the molecules and eliminate the outer electrons from the resulting atoms (de Hoffman and Stroobant 2001); photoionization, where a high energy photon dissociates stable gaseous molecules (used to study chemical kinetics mechanisms and the branching between isomers; de Hoffman and Stroobant 2001); ambient ionization, where the source is outside the mass spectrometer (DESI); glow discharge; field desorption; thermospray; desorption ionization on silicon (DIOS); direct analysis in real time (DART); secondary ion mass spectrometry (SIMS); spark ionization; and thermal ionization (TIMS) (de Hoffman and Stroobant 2001).

The mass analyzer is the second major part of the MS used to separate and measure ions based on their *m/z*. There are a wide variety of analyzers, using either a static or dynamic field and a magnetic or electric field, summarized in Table 4.3. Many mass spectrometers use multiple analyzers for so-called tandem MS (MS/MS). Several important characteristics need to be considered while choosing the analyzer: the mass resolving power, which is the ability to distinguish neighboring *m/z*; the mass accuracy, which is the ratio between measured and theoretical *m/z*; the mass range, which is the window of analyzable *m/z*: the linear dynamic range, which is the range over which the intensity is linear with the sample concentration; and the speed, which is the number of spectra per unit of time that can be generated (Gross 2017; de Hoffman and Stroobant 2001).

The most common analyzer is the quadrupole mass filter, which uses two pairs of parallel rods charged with radio frequency (RF) and DC voltage to create an

TABLE 4.3

Common Mass Spectrometry Analyzers

Analyzer	*m/z* Range	Resolution	Mass accuracy*
Quadrupole	Up to 4000	2000	100
Time-of-flight (TOF)	Up to 30,000 or more	10,000	10 (Reflection)
Ion trap	Up to 2000	4000	100
Orbitrap	Up to 6000	100,000	<5
Fourier transform ion cyclotron resonance (FTMS)	Unlimited	$10^{5\text{-}6}$	<5

* = ppm.

oscillating electric field that stabilizes or destabilizes the paths of ions passing through to where only the ions in a certain range of *m/z* will be allowed to pass through the system and reach the detector to be analyzed. A common variation of the quadrupole is its MS/MS version, the triple quadrupole, with three quadrupoles in series. The first and the third ones working as mass filters, whereas the second one serves as a collision chamber (de Hoffman and Stroobant 2001; Gross 2017).

Another common analyzer is the time-of-flight (TOF) mass spectrometer, which uses an electric field to accelerate ions through the same potential, and then measures the time they take to reach the detector (de Hoffman and Stroobant 2001). When the ions have the same charge, their kinetic energies will be identical, and therefore their velocities will depend only on their masses; lower masses will reach the detector first (de Hoffman and Stroobant 2001). Due to the fact that the initial velocity does not often depend on the mass of the ion, ions with the same *m/z* may reach the detector at different times, generating broader peaks. To address this problem, modern TOF-MS uses the delayed extraction technique. Using a delay, slower ions receive enough potential energy to "catch" the faster ones toward the detector (de Hoffman and Stroobant 2001).

Other analyzers include the sector field, which uses a static electric and/or magnetic field to change the path and/or velocity of ions; the ion trap, which functions like a quadrupole but by trapping and sequentially ejecting the ions; Fourier transform ion cyclotron resonance (FTMS), which measures mass by detecting the image current produced by ions in a circular acceleration in the presence of a magnetic field; and the orbitrap, where ions are electrostatically trapped in an orbit around an electrode, generating an image current in the detector plates (de Hoffman and Stroobant 2001; Gross 2017).

Finally, the last part of the MS is the detector, which either records the charge or current produced by an ion passing by or hitting its surface (de Hoffman and Stroobant 2001). Typically, an electron multiplier is used, but Faraday cups and ion-to-photon detectors have seen usage as well. Considering that the number of ions exiting the mass filter is usually small, considerable amplification is needed (de Hoffman and Stroobant 2001; Gross 2017).

MS detectors provide valuable information about molecular weights and structures. Even if their cost is higher than for more basic detectors, MS is considered vital in the understanding and discovery of molecules. For this reason, cannabinoids are widely analyzed via MS or MS/MS in research and development (R&D) laboratories, rather than commercial potency testing (Leghissa et al. 2018). Furthermore, not only is it universal and specific, allowing for the analysis of almost all types of analyte, the attainable LODs and LOQs make the MS one of the most sensitive available detectors (Leghissa et al. 2018).

4.2 CANNABINOID ANALYSIS BY GAS CHROMATOGRAPHY-MASS SPECTROMETRY

Cannabinoids can be analyzed through a wide variety of techniques including gas chromatography-mass spectrometry (GC-MS). This technique often relies on the use of EI, which is able to fragment the ions consistently through the application of ionization energy of 70 eV (Traeger 2015), allowing the creation and the use of a compound library for the identification. The main advantage of using GC-MS as a means for analyzing cannabinoids is that these species contain functional groups, such as phenols and carboxylic acids, that are not efficiently ionized by ESI or APCI, allowing for a better sensitivity via GC-MS (Leghissa et al. 2018). On the other hand, the presence of carboxylic acids is what causes the disadvantages of using a GC-MS for analyzing acid cannabinoids. The high temperatures of the injector can degrade this functional group unless they are protected via derivatization (such as silanization or methylation and esterification) (Leghissa et al. 2018). Nevertheless, it needs to be highlighted that silanization of cannabinoids will make these species more volatile, leading to an improvement in chromatographic separation and peak shape (Leghissa et al. 2018). A list of published works based on the use of GC-MS for the analysis of cannabinoids is listed in Table 4.4.

Generally, the GC-MS analysis of cannabinoids is carried out through the use of a low polarity stationary phase column, such as 5% diphenyl 95% dimethyl polysiloxane, leading to short analytical run times (<25 min) and elutions at <300°C (Leghissa et al. 2018). An important aspect of GC-MS analysis is the proper extraction of cannabinoids from the matrix.

Omar et al. (2013) compared ultrasound-assisted extraction (UAE) and supercritical fluid extraction (SFE) for the analysis of three cannabinoids (Δ^9-THC, CBD, and CBC) and three terpenes (α-pinene, β-pinene, and limonene) from 13 different cannabis cultivars and found UAE to be more efficient after the first extraction with an 80% recovery of terpenes and cannabinoids, but the SFE was considered to be more advantageous due to its ability to differentiate extracted compounds (Omar et al. 2013). For instance, the extraction of terpenes is attained using solely supercritical CO_2, while an ethanol co-solvent allows the extraction of cannabinoids. A notable achievement for their method of SFE coupled with retention time-locking GC-MS was that it allowed for the classification of the samples based on the type of plant, growing area, and growing season (Omar et al. 2013).

TABLE 4.4

Published Work Utilizing Gas Chromatography-Mass Spectrometry (GC-MS)

Analytes	Technique	Matrix	Other	Reference
Cannabinoids	GC-MS	Plant	–	(Ross et al. 2000; Leghissa 2016; Cardenia et al. 2018)
Cannabinoids	GC-MS	Plant	SFE	(Omar et al. 2013)
Cannabinoids	GC-MS	Plant	Headspace solid-phase microextraction	(Ilias et al. 2005)
Cannabinoids	GC-TOF-MS	Plant	–	(Delgado-Povedano et al. 2019)
Cannabinoids	GC-MS	Plant	MRM database	(Leghissa et al. 2018)
Cannabinoids	GC-MS	Plant	DPX extraction	(Horne et al. 2020)
Cannabinoids	GC-MS	Plant	2D-GC-MS	(Omar et al. 2014; Franchina et al. 2020)
Cannabinoids	GC-MS	Hemp food	–	(Pellegrini et al. 2005)
Cannabinoids	GC-MS	Hemp food	Headspace solid-phase microextraction	(Lachenmeier et al. 2004)
Cannabinoids	GC-MS	Hair	–	(Villamor et al. 2004; Baptista et al. 2002; Rodrigues et al. 2018)
Cannabinoids	GC-MS	Hair	Headspace	(Emidio et al. 2010; de Oliveira et al. 2007; Musshoff et al. 2003)
Cannabinoids	GC-MS	Air	In-injector thermal desorption	(Chou et al. 2007)
Δ^9-THC metabolites	GC-MS	Urine, plasma	MRM	(Leghissa et al. 2018)
Δ^9-THC metabolites	GC-MS	Urine	–	(Tsai et al. 2000; Abraham et al. 2007; Kala and Kochanowski 2006; Kemp et al. 1995)
Δ^9-THC metabolites	GC-MS	Blood serum	–	(Steinmeyer et al. 2002; Kala and Kochanowski 2006; Purschke et al. 2016; Fabritius et al. 2013; Van der Linden et al. 2014)
Δ^9-THC metabolites	GC-MS	Plasma	–	(Kemp et al. 1995; Nadulski et al. 2005)
Δ^9-THC metabolites	GC-MS	Hair	–	(Baptista et al. 2002; Han et al. 2011)
Δ^9-THC metabolites	GC-MS	Oral fluids	–	(Van der Linden et al. 2014; Fabritius et al. 2013)
Δ^9-THC metabolites	GC-MS	Oral fluids, plasma	GC×GC-MS	(Lowe et al. 2007; Schwilke et al. 2009; Lee et al. 2015; Milman et al. 2010)

Another extraction approach was taken by Horne et al. (2020), who based their research on the fact that simple solvent extraction, such as with methanol, would also extract chlorophyll and other non-volatile compounds that would ruin the injection port liner and column. Their approach was therefore to use pipette tip solid-phase extraction (DPX) for the analysis of THC and THCA, as described in Figure 4.3. This technique is performed with an automated liquid handler, which allows the manipulation of up to 24 samples in <11 minutes, with no human involvement (Horne et al. 2020). To complete the sample preparation, prior to GC-MS analysis, a derivatization step is required to protect the carboxylic acid groups on any acid cannabinoid species.

Nuapia et al. (2020) used pressurized hot water extraction (PHWE) for the removal of polar and semi-polar compounds from plant matrices, in this case *C. sativa* seeds. After having investigated the extraction time, extraction temperature, and collector vessel temperature for the extraction of THC, CBN, CBG, CBC, and CBD, identification and semi-quantification were performed on a GC/GC-TOFMS.

Ross et al. (2000) compared the amount of THC in cannabis and hemp seeds using GC-MS. In their classification, cannabis seeds were those with a higher amount of THC (35.6–124 μg/g), whereas, in the hemp seeds, THC was almost absent (0–12 μg/g). The sample preparation consisted of extraction with chloroform and methanol (99:1), followed by homogenization and centrifugation. An important conclusion that

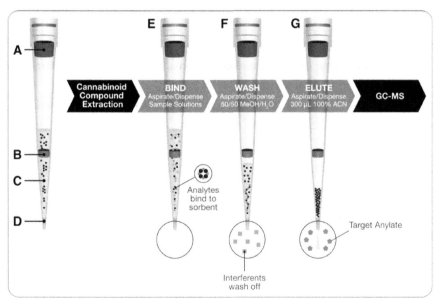

DPX tips include an upper porous barrier (A) and a lower frit barrier (D), between which is a freely moving styrene divinyl benzene sorbent (C). A baffle system contained within the tip disrupts the flow of liquid sample aspirated into the pipette tip and encourages turbulent mixing when binding sample to sorbent (B). Sample binding (E), washing (F), and elution (G) are all accomplished within a single DPX tip. Black circles indicate divinyl binding sorbent, gray squares represent interferent, and gray pentagons depict target analyte.

FIGURE 4.3 Schematization of the pipette tip-based solid-phase extraction (DPX).

they drew was that the highest concentration of THC was found on the seed's surface, probably due to adherence from the flowers onto the seeds (Ross et al. 2000).

Leghissa et al. (2018) developed the first GC-MS method based on the use of the multiple reaction monitoring (MRM) mode for both normal and silylated cannabinoids (THCV, CBC, CBD, Δ^8-THC, THC, CBG, CBN, and THCA) using a triple quadrupole (QQQ) MS. The MRM transitions are listed in Table 4.5. They identified the MS/MS fragmentation patterns of the radical cations formed by each underivatized and derivatized cannabinoids (Leghissa et al. 2018). Their method was validated using hops as a surrogate matrix; this plant is extremely similar to *C. sativa* as they both belong to the *Cannabaceae* family, and it is more available to researchers (*C. sativa* is a Schedule 1 controlled substance under the United States Controlled Substances Act) (Leghissa et al. 2018). The two resulting techniques have both advantages and disadvantages: the specific MRM mode leads to low LODs (low pg on-column), and even though the underivatized analysis indicates slightly lower LODs, the silylated one allows for the analysis of acidic cannabinoids and an improved chromatographic separation due to the lower volatility (Leghissa et al. 2018).

With respect to the different derivatization techniques, Leghissa et al. (Leghissa 2016) developed a SIM analysis on GC-MS of nine different cannabinoids (THCV, CBD, CBC, Δ^8-THC, THC, THC-TMS, CBG, CBN, and THCA-2TMS) using two different silylation agents, N,O-bis(trimethylsilyl)trifluoroacetamide + 1% chlorotrimethylsilane (BSTFA +1% TMCS) and N-methyl-N-trimethylsilyltrifluoroacetam

TABLE 4.5
GC-MS Multiple Reaction Monitoring Database for Seven Underivatized and Eight Derivatized Cannabinoids

Compound	Quantitative ion	Qualitative ion 1	Qualitative ion 2
THCV	203.00 > 174.10	286.00 > 271.20	271.00 > 189.20
CBD	231.00 > 174.10	231.00 > 145.10	232.00 > 175.20
CBC	231.00 > 174.20	231.00 > 173.10	232.00 > 175.10
Δ^8-THC	231.00 > 174.00	314.00 > 231.00	314.00 > 174.30
Δ^9-THC	231.00 > 174.10	231.00 > 145.10	231.00 > 147.30
CBG	231.00 > 174.10	193.00 > 123.10	193.00 > 137.10
CBN	295.00 > 238.00	295.00 > 223.20	296.00 > 224.10
THCV-TMS	315.00 > 73.10	343.00 > 73.10	358.00 > 343.20
CBD-2TMS	301.00 > 73.10	390.00 > 73.10	337.00 > 73.10
CBC-TMS	303.00 > 246.10	303.00 > 73.10	303.00 > 174.10
Δ^8-THC-TMS	303.00 > 246.10	303.00 > 73.10	386.00 > 303.20
Δ^9-THC-TMS	315.00 > 73.10	315.00 > 81.10	386.00 > 371.20
CBG-2TMS	337.00 > 73.10	338.00 > 73.10	391.00 > 73.10
CBN-TMS	367.00 > 310.10	367.00 > 295.10	382.00 > 367.20
Δ^9-THCA-2TMS	487.00 > 147.20	487.00 > 365.10	487.00 > 73.20

ide (MSTFA), and they concluded that BSTFA +1% TMCS led to better results when analyzing cannabinoids. A different approach for the analysis of silylated cannabinoids was taken by Madea et al. (Lachenmeier et al. 2004; Musshoff et al. 2003). They quantified four different silylated cannabinoids (THC-TMS, CBD-2TMS, CBN-TMS, and CBC-TMS) from different matrices, and developed a fully automated method using HS solid-phase dynamic extraction followed by the GC-MS analysis for the characterization of hair samples and hemp food. Another study performed on hair samples from CBD-rich *C. sativa* users (from the same producer) was carried out by Rodrigues et al. (2018), where they analyzed THC, CBN, and CBD from 14 people (seven males and seven females) who self-declared the consumption of 4–128 mg CBD/day. The sample preparation was performed by pulverizing the hair with a ball mill of type MM2 and extracting the cannabinoids with a polymeric reversed-phase extraction cartridge. The cartridge was previously conditioned with methanol and water and then washed with sodium hydroxide and acetone. The elution was carried out using dichloromethane as a solvent, and the derivatization was performed with MSTFA (Rodrigues et al. 2018). In the samples, CBD was detected between 10 and 325 pg/mg of hair, THC was detected in one sample but with a concentration lower than the cut-off, and CBN was not detected (Rodrigues et al. 2018).

Additionally, Cardenia et al. (2018) used a GC-MS SIM mode to analyze ten cannabinoids (THCV, CBC, CBD, CBDA, Δ^8-THC, Δ^9-THC, CBG, CBGA, CBN, and THCA) in hemp flowers. Their extraction was carried out with methanol:chloroform (9:1), and they compared two different internal standards: 5α-cholestane, and THC-d_3. Furthermore, they compared the derivatization efficiency between methylation, using diazomethane and silylation, as well as MSTFA+1%TMCS. Even though methylation increased the signal-to-noise (S/N) for almost all acid cannabinoids, with the exception of CBGA, the silylation reaction was routinely performed for the validation of the method. This is because diazomethane is not commercially available and requires a one-day synthesis (Cardenia et al. 2018). Concerning the recoveries, at the low spiking level (0.25 ng), THC-d_3 was found between 80.3 and 103.3%, whereas 5α-cholestane was between 89.3 and 103.3%. Similar results were obtained when spiking the hemp flowers with 25 ng that showed that the use of a more cost-effective internal standard, such as 5α-cholestane, can be used for routine analysis (Cardenia et al. 2018).

A more exhaustive complex approach for the analysis of *C. sativa* by GC-MS is the use of a GC/GC-MS. Franchina et al. (2020) used stir bar sorptive extraction (SBSE) to preconcentrate analytes from *C. sativa* flowers for subsequent desorbtion into the GC/GC-TOFMS. The optimized parameters were shown to be a 60 min extraction time at 50°C using water:methanol:acetonitrile (5:4:1). The work can be divided into two parts, the first one using a low-resolution TOF-MS (LR-TOFMS) for the quantification of known targets, and the second one using a high-resolution TOF-MS (HR-TOFMS) for untargeted analysis and identification of unknowns. In the former, the analysis was based on the coupling of a first non-polar column (Rxi-5MS, Restek, Bellefonte [PA]) with a second mid-polar one (Rxi-17Sil MS, Restek) through a lab-made differential flow modulator (Franchina, Dubois, and Focant 2020). The identity of cannabinoids was confirmed using a NIST 2017 library

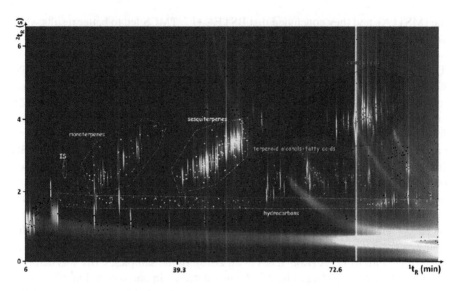

FIGURE 4.4   SBSE-GCxGC-LR-TOF-MS analysis in a representative 2D chromatogram, with highlighted regions of components.

(minimum of 70% similarity) and RI (±20 RI) in a SIM mode. Figure 4.4 shows that there were six different elution areas: monoterpenes, sesquiterpenes, hydrocarbons, cannabinoids, terpenoid alcohols, and fatty acids (Franchina et al. 2020). The method was validated with $R^2>0.98$ for CBD, CBN, and THC, with a %RSD of 9–19% for the lowest point, and 13–17% for the highest. In the GC/GC-HRTOFMS part, on the other hand, the two columns were coupled through a cryogenic modulator, and in this analysis, the pesticides chlorothalonil and cyprodinil were detected and confirmed in one sample, while the plasticizer additive bisphenol G was confirmed in all samples. Furthermore, the authors screened for synthetic cannabinoids and metabolites, finding in one sample the cannabinoid quinone HU-331 resulting from the oxidation of CBD (Franchina et al. 2020). Finally, even the decarboxylation of CBDA and THCA was studied, proving that the inlet causes decarboxylation of 56–61% (Franchina et al. 2020).

The GC/GC approach was also taken by Moore et al. (2006), Karschner et al. (Karschner et al., n.d.), and Lowe et al. (2007) for the analysis of metabolites of THC. Another analysis of metabolites was performed by Kemp et al. (1995) and Steinmeyer et al. (2002), who extracted the molecules from biological samples (urine and blood) and derivatized them via methylation prior to SIM analysis via GC-EI-MS due to the ability of the EI source to create consistent fragmentations and ions that can be matched with an existing database. Kala et al. (Kala and Kochanowski 2006), on the other hand, used a GC-MS with a negative CI (NCI) ionization source, which provides favorable responses to the analysis of targeted compounds, but less qualitative information than the EI-MS. Finally, Leghissa et al. (2018) developed an MRM method on a GC-QQQ-MS for silylated THC-OH and 11-nor-9-carboxy-THC and validated the analysis on spiked urine and plasma. This approach leads to better sensitivity and specificity of the metabolites in complex biological samples.

4.3 CANNABINOID ANALYSIS BY LIQUID CHROMATOGRAPHY-MASS SPECTROMETRY

Laboratories that routinely analyze cannabinoids in *C. sativa* for its potency generally prefer using LC due to this technique's ability to directly analyze acid cannabinoids without derivatization. The most widely used columns are non-polar, such as C18 or biphenyl variants, and the mobile phases are water and methanol with 0.1% formic acid (Leghissa et al. 2018). A list of published works based on the use of LC-MS for the analysis of cannabinoids is listed in Table 4.6.

In their approach, Calvi et al. (2018) analyzed two different matrices of *C. sativa*, the plant and the oil. In both cases, they extracted the molecules with superfine grinding followed by accelerated solvent extraction (ASE), testing five different solvents for the plant material, methanol, methanol:chloroform 9:1, hexane, acetonitrile, ethanol, and olive oil at different volumes for the oil. The ASE technique is based on high temperatures and pressure for an improved extraction from a solid matrix, saving time and solvent. They used a full scan data-dependent acquisition (FS-dd-MS2) on an orbitrap for the quantification of THC, CBD, CBN, CBG, THCA, CBDA, and CBGA and the qualification of untargeted cannabinoids with the same molecular ions but different retention times, as shown in Figure 4.5.

A similar orbitrap approach was taken by Citti et al. (2019), who used a negative and positive FS-dd-MS2 for analyzing metabolites and identifying cannabinoids by LC-MS. They created an empty matrix by washing hemp seeds with ethanol (96%) and subsequently cold squeezing them to obtain an oil with cannabinoids below the LODs. The samples, on the other hand, were extracted with isopropyl alcohol. The novelty of the work is not only the study of the fragmentation of different groups of cannabinoids but is also the first identification of 30 cannabinoids in hemp seed oil (Citti et al. 2019).

Pavlovic et al. (2019), on the other hand, used different technologies to perform a comprehensive analysis of *C. sativa*: evaluating cannabinoids, polyunsaturated fatty acids (GC-FID), protein profiles (LC-MS/MS and SDS-PAGE), and terpenes (HS-SPME and GC-MS). Much like in the research performed by Calvi et al. (2018), Pavlovic performed a superfine grinding followed by an ASE for the extraction of *C. sativa* flowers. The quantification was performed on 14 cannabinoids (THC, CBD, CBN, CBC, CBG, THCV, CBDV, THCA, CBDA, CBGA, CBNA, THCVA, CBDVA, and CBCA), and was followed by the qualitative identification of cannabinoids, flavonoids, lignans, stilbenoids, and alkaloids (Pavlovic et al. 2019).

Another untargeted analysis was performed by Delgado-Povedano et al. (2019), who analyzed leaves and inflorescences from 17 different cultivars by extracting the powdered material using hexane for the GC-TOF-MS analysis (non-polar extracts), and methanol for their LC-QTOF-MS analysis (polar extracts). Their findings concluded in the matching of 169 compounds, as shown in Figure 4.6.

TABLE 4.6

Published Work Utilizing LC-MS

Analytes	Technique	Matrix	Other	Reference
Cannabinoids	LC-IT-MS	*C. sativa* products	–	(Stolker et al. 2004)
Cannabinoids	LC-MS	Oral fluids, plasma, urine	–	(Teixeira et al. 2004; Concheiro et al. 2013; Andersson et al. 2016)
Cannabinoids	LC-MS-MS	Plant	–	(Pellati et al. 2018; Palmieri et al. 2019; Protti et al. 2019)
Cannabinoids	LC-MS-MS	Honey	–	(Brighenti et al. 2019)
Cannabinoids	LC-MS-MS	Plant	Orbitrap	(Calvi et al. 2018; Citti et al. 2019; Pavlovic et al. 2019)
Cannabinoids	LC-MS-MS	Oral fluids, plasma, urine	–	(Grauwiler et al. 2007; Jung et al. 2009; Andersson et al. 2016; Desrosiers et al. 2015; Laloup et al. 2005; Sergi et al. 2013; Abbara et al. 2006)
Cannabinoids	LC-QTOF	Plant	–	(Delgado-Povedano et al. 2019)
Cannabinoids	LC-QTOF	Urine	–	(Jung et al. 2009)
Cannabinoids	SFC-MS	Plant	–	(Bäckström et al. 1997; Wang et al. 2017)
Δ^9-THC metabolites	LC-MS-MS	Urine	–	(Jung et al. 2009; Stolker et al. 2004; Weinmann et al. 2001; Andersson et al. 2016; Hädener et al. 2017; Fernández et al. 2009)
Δ^9-THC metabolites	LC-MS-MS	Plant	SPE	(Escrivá et al. 2017)
Δ^9-THC metabolites	LC-MS-MS	Liver tissues	SPE	(Escrivá et al. 2017)
Δ^9-THC metabolites	LC-MS-MS	Milk	SPE	(Escrivá et al. 2017)
Δ^9-THC metabolites	LC-MS-MS	Plasma	–	(Grauwiler et al. 2007; Ferreirós et al. 2013)
Δ^9-THC metabolites	LC-MS-MS	Oral fluids	–	(Desrosiers et al. 2015; Sergi et al. 2013; Fabritius et al. 2013; Van der Linden et al. 2014; Scheidweiler et al. 2017)
Δ^9-THC metabolites	LC-MS-MS	Oral fluids	Microflow	(Concheiro et al. 2013)
Δ^9-THC metabolites	LC-MS-MS	Oral fluids	Orbitrap	(He et al. 2012)
Δ^9-THC metabolites	LC-MS-MS	Hair	–	(Park et al. 2014; Kuwayama et al. 2015; Thieme et al. 2014)
Δ^9-THC metabolites	LC-MS-MS	Blood	–	(Mercolini et al. 2013; Simoes et al. 2011; König et al. 2011)

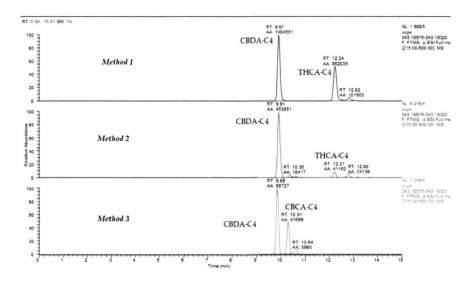

FIGURE 4.5 Untargeted cannabinoids with the same *m/z* but different retention times.

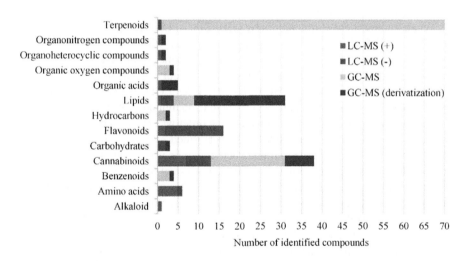

FIGURE 4.6 Classification of untargeted compounds found with different techniques.

A similar Q-TOF approach was used by Aizpurua-Olaizola et al. (2014), who analyzed six cannabinoids (CBD, THCV, CBG, CBN, THC, and THCA) in 30 different strains of *C. sativa*. The use of a Q-TOF detector allowed not only for an MS/MS analysis but also for a higher mass accuracy due to its high resolving power. Furthermore, they were able to differentiate between indoor and outdoor-grown plants, with the former having higher concentrations of CBD, THC, and CBN (Aizpurua-Olaizola et al. 2014).

Pellati et al. (2018) performed a comprehensive analysis of *C. sativa* using different extraction methods: dynamic maceration at room temperature using methanol for cannabinoids, hexane for flavonoids, and HS-SPME for volatile compounds. CBG, CBD, CBGA, and CBDA were analyzed by HPLC-UV/DAD and HPLC-MS/MS using the positive and negative modes. They focused on the analysis of fragmentation pathways through MS/MS, whereas the quantification was performed and validated via HPLS-UV/PDA (Pellati et al. 2018). Palmieri et al. (2019) used an HPLC-MS/MS system for identifying nine cannabinoids (THC, CBD, CBN, CBC, CBG, CBDV, THCA, CBDA, and CBGA) in 161 different cultivars of hemp. Their findings showed that acid cannabinoids have a lower capacity of discrimination than neutral forms and that all hemp cultivars showed the same profile of high CBD and CBDA content.

Brighenti et al. (2019) analyzed three different matrices of *C. sativa* using two different extraction methods and analytical techniques. Hashish "pollen" and inflorescences were extracted through dynamic maceration with ethanol and analyzed via HPLC-DAD, and a cannabis "honey" was extracted through a liquid–liquid extraction (LLE) with water and hexane, and analyzed via HPLC-MS/MS. In the latter, they quantified CBDA, CBGA, THCA, CBD, CBG, and THC, obtaining $R^2>0.975$, LOD = 0.3 ng/g, and LOQ = 0.5 ng/g. No matrix effect was observed, and the most abundant cannabinoid was found to be CBDA, while THCA and THC were not detected in the honey (Brighenti et al. 2019). Wang et al. (2017) used ultra-high performance supercritical chromatography (UHPSFC)-PDA/MS for the determination of CBD, Δ^8-THC, THCV, THC, CBN, CBG, THCA, CBGA, and CBDA by extracting them from plant matrices using 80:20 acetonitrile:methanol. Analyzing at a fixed wavelength at 220 nm with eight-point calibration curves, favorable linearity and precision were obtained ($R^2>0.994$, RSD<6.9%). An LOD between 1 and 3 µg/mL and an LOQ of 5 µg/mL was achieved for acid cannabinoids (Wang et al. 2017). An extremely interesting finding is that the elution order was inverted between UHPLC and UHSFC. Backstrom et al. (1997) also performed an SFC analysis of cannabinoids using 2% methanol as a modifier. Their detection was based on APCI-MS, and they used a cyanopropyl silica-based column. The use of SFC-MS for the analysis of cannabinoids is increasing due to the reduced number of solvents required, and the comparable efficiency and specificity to the HPLC (Leghissa et al. 2018).

Protti et al. (2019) used an HPLC-DAD-MS/MS system to analyze THC, THCA, CBD, CBDA, and CBN in herbal samples extracted by UAE with the following solvents: ethanol, methanol, acetonitrile, and mixtures thereof. Methanol was found to be the most effective in drying and reconditioning in acetonitrile:water (50:50) + 0.1% FA. The method was validated with $R^2>0.9992$, RSD<6%, and accuracies >92.1%, and different LOQs and LODs were obtained for different cannabinoids; 0.1 and 0.03 ng/mL for Δ^9-THC and CBD, 0.2 and 0.06 ng/mL for THCA and CBDA, and 0.5 and 0.15 ng/mL for CBN, respectively (Protti et al. 2019).

Finally, Stolker et al. (2004) used an LC-ion trap-MS system for determining five spiked cannabinoids in hop matrices. This coupling system has not been widely used for the analysis of cannabinoids, but it can be powerful for qualitative analysis due to its multistage fragmentation. On the other hand, it may be less efficient in quantitation than a QQQ system due to its limited dynamic range (Stolker et al. 2004). In this study, LOQs were found as 9.9 g/kg for Δ^9-THCA, 0.28 g/kg for Δ^9-THC, 0.1 g/kg for CBD, 0.04 g/kg for CBDA, and 0.03 g/kg for CBN (Stolker et al. 2004).

With respect to the analysis of Δ^9-THC metabolites, the LC-MS has been found to be a precise and viable method as well. For example, Escriva et al. (2017) used LC-MS to analyze Δ^9-THC and its two metabolites Δ^9-THC-OH and 11-nor-9-carboxy-THC in different matrices (13 samples of milk, five junior formulas, ten hemp seeds, and ten liver tissues). The extraction was carried out by adding 10 mL of MeOH, and sonicating, centrifuging, and performing an SPE extraction with an OASIS HLB cartridge. The cartridge was activated with 1 mL of HCl at 0.1 mM, and then the samples were passed and re-washed with MeOH. The liver samples, on the other hand, had the additional step of adding 5 mL of 0.1 M potassium phosphate buffer at pH 6.8, 200 µL of β-glucuronidase, and incubation at 37°C for 16 hours (Escrivá et al. 2017). The validation of the method was concluded by obtaining seven-point calibration curves with $R^2 > 0.99$ and recoveries between 70 and 120%; furthermore, no matrix effect was pointed out (Escrivá et al. 2017).

Grauwiler et al. (2007) used an APCI method of an LC-QQQ-MS for the analysis of CBD, CBN, Δ^9-THC, Δ^9-THC-OH, and 11-nor-9-carboxy-THC in human plasma and urine. The LOQs obtained in urine were of 0.2 ng/mL in 25 min, leading to a reliable quantitation when considering that regular *C. sativa* users exhibit an 11-nor-9-carboxy-THC concentration >75 ng/mL in the first eight days after consumption, whereas occasional users were below 5 ng/mL (Grauwiler et al. 2007). Always using an APCI approach, Weinmann et al. (2001) solely detected nor-9-carboxy-THC in urine samples, preceded by automated SPE, showing an LOD of 2.0 ng/mL. Other approaches were taken by Park et al. (2014) and Mercolini et al. (2013), who used an LC-MS system but based on the use of an ESI. Park et al. (2014) prepared samples through LLE and used a three-column system (precolumn, trap column, and analytical column) for the analysis. The LOQ for Δ^9-nor-9-carboxy-THC was 0.1 pg/mg, making this a reliable solution considering the concentration in human samples was found between 0.13 and 15.75 pg/mg (Park et al. 2014). On the other hand, Mercolini et al. (2013), performed the analysis of Δ^9-THC, Δ^9-THC-OH, and 11-nor-9-carboxy-Δ^9-THC in human dried blood spot, creating a reliable method for roadside testing. This approach avoids the issues linked to the transportation and storage of samples usually associated with police road tests (Mercolini et al. 2013).

4.4 CANNABINOID ANALYSIS BY MASS SPECTROMETRY

In some cases, research into the detection, characterization, and quantification of cannabinoids has been exclusively performed using an MS detector without prior coupling it to a GC or LC. One example is given by Beasley et al. (2016), who used a MALDI-MS to identify and image cannabinoids in hair samples. The greatest advantage of this technique is the absence of sample preparation; hair samples were directly placed on the target with a matrix. Furthermore, the MALDI-MS was able to detect Δ^9-THC and its metabolites in a single analysis and at low concentrations. Unfortunately, its irreproducibility is a key drawback because matrix deposition can vary across the sample and from sample to sample, and the required derivatization prior to analysis performed via the addition of an *N*-methylpyridium group (Beasley et al. 2016).

Furthermore, Borille et al. (2017) used an electrospray ionization coupled to a Fourier transform ion cyclotron resonance mass spectrometer (ESI-FT-ICR-MS) for the analysis of *C. sativa*, identifying 123 cannabinoids and metabolites and eight non-cannabinoid constituents. This detector allows for the highest mass resolving power and mass accuracy, and a wide mass range (MW = 200–3000 Da), providing reliable analysis of complex mixtures without prior extraction or separation (Borille et al. 2017). Through this technique, researchers are able to define the composition of $C_cH_hN_nO_oS_s$ based on single charged ions and define double bond equivalent (DBE), facilitating the categorization of molecules through their heteroatom contents and degrees of aromacity (Borille et al. 2017). In their research, Borille et al. analyzed *C. sativa* plants that were grown in different conditions, using positive and negative ESI. They observed that ESI(+) had a higher number of assigned signals than ESI(–), as shown in Figure 4.7, probably due to the highest abundance of adducts, a wider *m/z* range (*m/z* = 160–1250 for ESI(+) and *m/z* = 180–850 for ESI (–)), and in ESI (–), the signal obtained by species with carboxyl groups can be increased by lower pK_a values, leading to ion suppression for other species (Borille et al. 2017).

Dong et al. (2019), on the other hand, performed a thermal desorption direct analysis in real-time MS (TD-DART-MS) on hemp cultivars. Their 15-min method (8 min for data acquisition and 7 min for cooling down the thermal stage) required no sample preparation or chromatographic separation, and the obtained classification accuracy was 99.3 ± 0.3%. Some of the advantages of a TD-DART analysis include the flexibility of sample types and sizes, easy sample immobilization, less ion suppression and MS contamination, and additional chemical volatility information (Dong et al. 2019); for these reasons, it has been used to overcome the problems witnessed with on-axis and off-axis DART, such as irreproducibility and unstable positioning of the sample. In DART, the compounds are desorbed from plant matrices with a temperature gradient due to their volatility, leading to good reproducibility and sensitivity. This technique, on the other hand, was not able to resolve Δ^9-THC and CBD, and THCV and CBDV, and may cause decarboxylation of acidic cannabinoids (Dong et al. 2019).

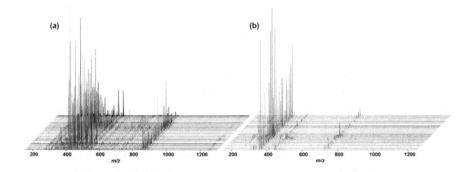

FIGURE 4.7 Mass spectra via positive (a) and negative (b) ESI-FT-ICR.

Finally, Yousefi-Taemeh and Ifa (2019) analyzed Δ^9-THC in chocolate samples by coupling thin-layer chromatography (TLC) to DESI. The samples were extracted with QuEChERS, and different solvents were tested to check the best ionization in DESI and the best development in TLC. The solvent optimization is crucial in DESI because polar analytes are enhanced by aqueous solvents and non-polar by high organic solvents (Yousefi-Taemeh and Ifa 2019). The chosen solvents were hexane for TLC and acetonitrile:methanol (8:2) + 1% ammonium hydroxide for DESI. The obtained LOQs and LODs for 1.5 µL of the extracted sample were 30 µg/mL and 20 µg/mL, respectively (Yousefi-Taemeh and Ifa 2019).

4.5 CONCLUSIONS

The *C. sativa* legalization process that is evolving all around the world provides an impetus for novel research and analysis to better understand *C. sativa* composition and its corresponding effects on human physiology. New cannabinoids and terpenes are continuously analyzed and discovered, which synergistically contribute to the apparent or potential medicinal and pharmaceutical benefits of the plant. Hopefully, the legalization process will lead to more funding opportunities for unraveling the mysteries associated with *C. sativa*, especially for creating universal methods for the comprehensive detection of all analytes of interest, including contaminants. Furthermore, more appropriate methods for field testing and forensic applications are needed, together with a better understanding of how the human body reacts to and metabolizes the administration of cannabinoids and related molecules. Other analytical challenges will come while dealing with more complex matrices such as edibles; however, these adversities will lead to more research opportunities and efforts, making this area extremely interesting. The path for having a comprehensive methodology for the analysis of all *C. sativa* components and matrices is still challenging and long, but it is of common interest to better understand the medicinal and pharmaceutical benefits that cannabis expresses.

REFERENCES

Abbara, C, R. Galy, A. Benyamina, M. Reynaud, and L. Bonhomme-Faivre. 2006. "Development and Validation of a Method for the Quantitation of Δ^9 Tetrahydrocannabinol in Human Plasma by High Performance Liquid Chromatography after Solid-Phase Extraction." *Journal of Pharmaceutical and Biomedical Analysis* 41: 1011–16.

Abraham, T. T., R. H. Lowe, S. O. Pirnay, W. D. Darwin, and M. A. Huestis. 2007. "Simultaneous GC–EI-MS Determination of Δ^9-Tetrahydrocannabinol, 11-Hydroxy-Δ^9-Tetrahydrocannabinol, and 11-Nor-9-Carboxy-Δ^9-Tetrahydrocannabinol in Human Urine Following Tandem Enzyme-Alkaline Hydrolysis." *Journal of Analytical Toxicology* 31: 477–85.

Adams, R., M. Hunt, and J. H. Clark. 1940. "Structure of Cannabidiol, a Product Isolated from the Marihuana Extract of Minnesota Wild Hemp." *Journal of the American Chemical Society* 62: 196–200.

Aizpurua-Olaizola, Oier, Jone Omar, Patricia Navarro, Maitane Olivares, Nestor Etxebarria, and Aresatz Usobiaga. 2014. "Identification and Quantification of Cannabinoids in Cannabis Sativa L. Plants by High Performance Liquid Chromatography-Mass Spectrometry." *Analytical and Bioanalytical Chemistry* 406: 7549–60. doi:10.1007/s00216-014-8177-x.

Andersson, M., K. B. Scheidweiler, C. Sempio, A. J. Barnes, and M. A. Huestis. 2016. "Simultaneous Quantification of 11 Cannabinoids and Metabolites in Human Urine by Liquid Chromatography Tandem Mass Spectrometry Using WAX-S Tips." *Analytical and Bioanalytical Chemistry* 408: 6461–71.

Bäckström, B., M. D. Cole, M. J. Carrott, D. C. Jones, G. Davidson, and K. Coleman. 1997. "A Preliminary Study of the Analysis of Cannabis by Supercritical Fluid Chromatography with Atmospheric Pressure Chemical Ionisation Mass Spectroscopic Detection." *Science & Justice* 37: 91–7.

Bai, L., J. Smuts, P. Walsh, C. Qiu, H.M. McNair, and K.A Schug. 2017. "Pseudo-Absolute Quantitative Analysis Using Gas Chromatography–Vacuum Ultraviolet Spectroscopy: A Tutorial." *Analytica Chimica Acta* 953: 10–22.

Bai, Ling, Jonathan Smuts, Phillip Walsh, Hui Fan, Zacariah Hildenbrand, Derek Wong, David Wetz, and Kevin A. Schug. 2015. "Permanent Gas Analysis Using Gas Chromatography with Vacuum Ultraviolet Detection." *Journal of Chromatography A* 1388: 244–50. doi:10.1021/ac5018343.

Baptista, M. J., P. V. Monsanto, E. G. P. Marques, A. Bermejo, S. Ávila, A. M. Castanheira, C. Margalho, M. Barroso, and D. N. Vieira. 2002. "Hair Analysis for Δ^9-THC, Δ^9-THC-COOH, CBN and CBD, by GC/MS–EI: Comparison with GC/MS–NCI for Δ^9-THC-COOH." *Forensic Science International* 128: 66–78.

Beasley, E., S. Francese, and T. Bassindale. 2016. "Detection and Mapping of Cannabinoids in Single Hair Samples through Rapid Derivatization and Matrix-Assisted Laser Desorption Ionization Mass Spectrometry." *Analytical Chemistry* 88: 10328–34.

Borille, Bruna T., Rafael S. Ortiz, Kristiane C. Mariotti, Gabriela Vanini, Lilian V. Tose, Paulo R. Filgueiras, Marcelo C.A. Marcelo, et al. 2017. "Chemical Profiling and Classification of Cannabis through Electrospray Ionization Coupled to Fourier Transform Ion Cyclotron Resonance Mass Spectrometry and Chemometrics." *Analytical Methods* 9 (27): 4070–81. doi:10.1039/c7ay01294b.

Brighenti, Virginia, Manuela Licata, Tatiana Pedrazzi, Davide Maran, Davide Bertelli, Federica Pellati, and Stefania Benvenuti. 2019. "Development of a New Method for the Analysis of Cannabinoids in Honey by Means of High-Performance Liquid Chromatography Coupled with Electrospray Ionisation-Tandem Mass Spectrometry Detection." *Journal of Chromatography A* 1597. Elsevier B.V.: 179–86. doi:10.1016/j.chroma.2019.03.034.

Calvi, L., R. Pavlovic, S. Panseri, L. Giupponi, V. Leoni, and A. Giorgi. 2018. "Quality Traits of Medical Cannabis Sativa L. Inflorescences and Derived Products Based on Comprehensive Mass-Spectrometry Analytical Investigation." In Williard James Costain and Robert Brad Laprairie (ed.), *Recent Advances in Cannabinoid Research*. London: InTechOpen. 55–78.

Cardenia, Vladimiro, Tullia Gallina Toschi, Simona Scappini, Rosamaria Cristina Rubino, and Maria Teresa Rodriguez-Estrada. 2018. "Development and Validation of a Fast Gas Chromatography/Mass Spectrometry Method for the Determination of Cannabinoids in Cannabis Sativa L." *Journal of Food and Drug Analysis* 26 (4). Elsevier Ltd: 1283–92. doi:10.1016/j.jfda.2018.06.001.

Chou, S. L., Y. C. Ling, M. H. Yang, and C. Y. Pai. 2007. "Determination of Δ^9-Tetrahydrocannabinol in Indoor Air as an Indicator of Marijuana Cigarette Smoking Using Adsorbent Sampling and in-Injector Thermal Desorption Gas Chromatography–Mass Spectrometry." *Analytica Chimica Acta* 598: 103–9.

Citti, Cinzia, Pasquale Linciano, Sara Panseri, Francesca Vezzalini, Flavio Forni, Maria Angela Vandelli, and Giuseppe Cannazza. 2019. "Cannabinoid Profiling of Hemp

Seed Oil by Liquid Chromatography Coupled to High-Resolution Mass Spectrometry." *Frontiers in Plant Science* 10 (February): 1–17. doi:10.3389/fpls.2019.00120.

Claussen, U., and K. F. Von Spulak. 1968. "Hashish. XIV. Information on the Substance of Hashish." *Tetrahedron* 24: 1021–23.

Compiled by A. D. McNaught and A. Wilkinson. 1997. *IUPAC. Compendium of Chemical Terminology*. 2nd ed. Oxford: Blackwell Scientific Publications.

Concheiro, Marta, Dayong Lee, Elena Lendoiro, and Marilyn A. Huestis. 2013. "Simultaneous Quantification of Δ^9-Tetrahydrocannabinol, 11-nor-9-Carboxy-Tetrahydrocannabinol, Cannabidiol and Cannabinol in Oral Fluid by Microflow-Liquid Chromatography-High Resolution Mass Spectrometry." *Journal of Chromatography A* 1297: 123–30. doi:10.1016/j.chroma.2013.04.071.

Delgado-Povedano, M. M., C. Sánchez-Carnerero Callado, F. Priego-Capote, and C. Ferreiro-Vera. 2019. "Untargeted Characterization of Extracts from Cannabis Sativa L. Cultivars by Gas and Liquid Chromatography Coupled to Mass Spectrometry in High Resolution Mode." *Talanta* 208 (July 2019). Elsevier B.V.: 120384. doi:10.1016/j.talanta.2019.120384.

Desrosiers, N. A., K. B. Scheidweiler, and M. A. Huestis. 2015. "Quantification of Six Cannabinoids and Metabolites in Oral Fluid by Liquid Chromatography–Tandem Mass Spectrometry." *Drug Testing and Analysis* 7: 684–94.

Dong, Wen, Jian Liang, Isabella Barnett, Paul C. Kline, Elliot Altman, and Mengliang Zhang. 2019. "The Classification of Cannabis Hemp Cultivars by Thermal Desorption Direct Analysis in Real Time Mass Spectrometry (TD-DART-MS) with Chemometrics." *Analytical and Bioanalytical Chemistry* 411 (30): 8133–42. doi:10.1007/s00216-019-02200-7.

Downard, Kevin M. 2007. "Francis William Aston: The Man Behind the Mass Spectrograph." *European Journal of Mass Spectrometry* 13: 3177–90.

ej Hanuš, Ondř. 2009. "Pharmacological and Therapeutic Secrets of Plant and Brain (Endo) Cannabinoids." *Medicinal Research Reviews* 29 (2): 213–71. doi:10.1002/med.20135.

ElSohly, Mahmoud A., and Desmond Slade. 2005. "Chemical Constituents of Marijuana: The Complex Mixture of Natural Cannabinoids." *Life Sciences* 78: 539–48. doi:10.1016/j.lfs.2005.09.011.

Emidio, E. S., V. D. Prata, and H. S. Dorea. 2010. "Validation of an Analytical Method for Analysis of Cannabinoids in Hair by Headspace Solid-Phase Microextraction and Gas Chromatography– Ion Trap Tandem Mass Spectrometry." *Analytica Chimica Acta* 610: 63–71.

Escrivá, Úrsula, María Jesús Andrés-Costa, Vicente Andreu, and Yolanda Picó. 2017. "Analysis of Cannabinoids by Liquid Chromatography–Mass Spectrometry in Milk, Liver and Hemp Seed to Ensure Food Safety." *Food Chemistry* 228: 177–85. doi:10.1016/j.foodchem.2017.01.128.

Fabritius, M., H. Chtioui, G. Battistella, J. M. Annoni, K. Dao, B. Favrat, E. Fornari, E. Lauer, P. Maeder, and C. Giroud. 2013. "Comparison of Cannabinoid Concentrations in Oral Fluid and Whole Blood between Occasional and Regular Cannabis Smokers Prior to and after Smoking a Cannabis Joint." *Analytical and Bioanalytical Chemistry* 405: 9791–803.

Fan, Hui, Jonathan Smuts, Phillip Walsh, Dale Harrison, and Kevin A. Schug. 2015. "Gas Chromatography-Vacuum Ultraviolet Spectroscopy for Multiclass Pesticide Identification." *Journal of Chromatography A* 1389: 120–27. doi:10.1016/j.chroma.2015.02.035.

Fernández, M. D. M. R., S. M. Wille, N. Samyn, M. Wood, M. López-Rivadulla, and G. De Boeck. 2009. "On-Line Solid-Phase Extraction Combined with Liquid Chromatography–Tandem Mass Spectrometry for High Throughput Analysis of 11-nor-Δ^9-Tetrahydrocannabinol-9-Carboxylic Acid in Urine." *Journal of Chromatography B* 877: 2153–7.

Ferreirós, N., S. Labocha, C. Walter, J. Lötsch, and G. Geisslinger. 2013. "Simultaneous and Sensitive LC–MS/MS Determination of Tetrahydrocannabinol and Metabolites in Human Plasma." *Analytical and Bioanalytical Chemistry* 405: 1399–1406.

Franchina, Flavio A., Lena M. Dubois, and Jean-François Focant. 2020. "In-Depth Cannabis Multiclass Metabolite Profiling Using Sorptive Extraction and Multidimensional Gas Chromatography with Low-and High-Resolution Mass Spectrometry." *Analytical Chemistry* 15: 10512–20.

Gaoni, Y., and R. Mechoulam. 1971. "The Isolation and Structure of Delta-1-Tetrahydrocannabinol and Other Neutral Cannabinoids from Hashish." *Journal of American Chemical Society* 93: 217–24.

Grauwiler, Sandra B., André Scholer, and Jürgen Drewe. 2007. "Development of a LC/MS/MS Method for the Analysis of Cannabinoids in Human EDTA-Plasma and Urine after Small Doses of Cannabis Sativa Extracts." *Journal of Chromatography B: Analytical Technologies in the Biomedical and Life Sciences* 850: 515–22. doi:10.1016/j.jchromb.2006.12.045.

Griffiths, Jennifer. 2008. "A Brief History of Mass Spectrometry." *Analytical Chemistry* 80 (15): 5678–83.

Gross, Jürgen H. 2017. *Mass Spectrometry: A Textbook*. Third. Berlin Heidelberg: Springer International Publishing.

Hädener, M, W. Weinmann, D. R. van Staveren, and S. König. 2017. "Rapid Quantification of Free and Glucuronidated THCCOOH in Urine Using Coated Well Plates and LC–MS/MS Analysis." *Bioanalysis* 9: 485–96.

Han, E., Y. Park, E. Kim, S. In, W. Yang, S. Lee, H. Choi, S. Lee, H. Chung, and J. Myong Song. 2011. "Simultaneous Analysis of Δ^9-Tetrahydrocannabinol and 11-nor-9-Carboxy-Tetrahydrocannabinol in Hair without Different Sample Preparation and Derivatization by Gas Chromatography–Tandem Mass Spectrometry." *Journal of Pharmaceutical and Biomedical Analysis* 55: 1096–103.

Harris, Daniel C. 1999. "Gas Chromatography." In *Quantitative Chemical Analysis*, Fifth, 675–712. New York: W. H. Freeman and Company.

He, X., M. Kozak, and S. Nimkar. 2012. "Ultra-Sensitive Measurements of 11-Nor-Delta(9)-Tetrahydrocannabinol-9-Carboxylic Acid in Oral Fluid by Microflow Liquid Chromatography-Tandem Mass Spectrometry Using a Benchtop Quadrupole/Orbitrap Mass Spectrometer." *Analytical Chemistry* 84: 7643–7.

Higson, Seamus P.J. 2004. *Analytical Chemistry*. Oxford: Oxford University Press.

Hoffman, E de, and V Stroobant. 2001. *Mass Spectrometry: Principles and Applications*. 2nd ed. Hoboken, NJ: John Wiley and Sons.

Horne, Melissa, Kaylee R. Mastrianni, Gray Amick, Rachel Hardy, Elissa Renneker, and Kevin W.P. Miller. 2020. "Fast Discrimination of Marijuana Using Automated High-Throughput Cannabis Sample Preparation and Analysis by Gas Chromatography–Mass Spectrometry." *Journal of Forensic Sciences* 65 (5): 1709–15. doi:10.1111/1556-4029.14525.

Ilias, Y., S. Rudaz, P. Mathieu, P. Christen, and J. L. Veuthey. 2005. "Extraction and Analysis of Different Cannabis Samples by Headspace Solid-Phase Microextraction Combined with Gas Chromatography–Mass Spectrometry." *Journal of Separation Science* 28: 2293–300.

James, Allen T., and Archer J.P. Martin. 1952. "Gas-Liquid Partition Chromatography: The Separation and Micro-Estimation of Volatile Fatty Acids from Formic Acid to Dodecanoic Acid." *The Biochemical Journal* 50 (5): 679–90.

Jung, J, M. R. Meyer, H. H. Maurer, C. Neusüß, W. Weinmann, and V. Auwärter. 2009. "Studies on the Metabolism of the Δ^9-Tetrahydrocannabinol Precursor

Δ^9-Tetrahydrocannabinolic Acid A (Δ^9-THCA-A) in Rat Using LC–MS/MS, LC–QTOF MS and GC–MS Techniques." *Journal of Mass Spectrometry* 44: 1423–33.

Kala, M., and M. Kochanowski. 2006. "Determination of Delta(9)-Tetrahydrocannabinol (9THC) and 11-nor-9-Carboxy-Delta(9)-Tetrahydrocannabinol (THCCOOH) in Blood and Urine Using Gas Chromatography Negative Ion Chemical Ionization Mass Spectrometry (GC-MS-NCI)." *Chemia Analityczna Warsaw* 51: 65–78.

Karger, Barry L. 1997. "HPLC: Early and Recent Perspectives." *Journal of Chemical Education* 74 (1): 45.

Karger, Barry L, and Laverne V. Berry. 1971. "Rapid Liquid-Chromatographic Separation of Steroids on Columns Heavily Loaded with Stationary Phase." *Clinical Chemistry* 17 (8): 757–64.

Karschner, Erin L., Eugene W. Schwilke, Ross H. Lowe, W. David Darwin, Ronald I. Herning, Jean Lud Cadet, and Marilyn A. Huestis. n.d. "Implications of Plasma Δ^9-Tetrahydrocannabinol, 11-Hydroxy-THC, and 11-nor-9-Carboxy-THC Concentrations in Chronic Cannabis Smokers." *Journal of Analytical Toxicology* 33: 469–77.

Kemp, P.M., I. K. Abukhalaf, J. E. Manno, B. R. Manno, D. D. Alford, and G. A. Abusada. 1995. "Cannabinoids in Humans. I. Analysis of Δ^9-Tetrahydrocannabinol and Six Metabolites in Plasma and Urine Using GC–MS." *Journal of Analytical Toxicology* 19: 285–91.

König, S., B. Aebi, S. Lanz, M. Gasser, and W. Weinmann. 2011. "On-Line SPE LC-MS/MS for the Quantification of Δ^9-Tetrahydrocannabinol (THC) and Its Two Major Metabolites in Human Peripheral Blood by Liquid Chromatography Tandem Mass Spectrometry." *Analytical and Bioanalytical Chemistry* 400: 9–16.

Kuwayama, K., H. Miyaguchi, T. Yamamuro, K. Tsujikawa, T. Kanamori, Y. T. Iwata, and H. Inoue. 2015. "Micro-Pulverized Extraction Pretreatment for Highly Sensitive Analysis of 11-nor-9-Carboxy-Δ^9-Tetrahydrocannabinol in Hair by Liquid Chromatography/Tandem Mass Spectrometry." *Rapid Communications in Mass Spectrometry* 29: 2158–66.

Lachenmeier, D.W., L. Kroener, F. Musshoff, and B. Madea. 2004. "Determination of Cannabinoids in Hemp Food Products by Use of Headspace Solid-Phase Microextraction and Gas Chromatography–Mass Spectrometry." *Analytical and Bioanalytical Chemistry* 378: 183–9.

Laloup, M., M. D. M. R. Fernandez, M. Wood, G. De Boeck, C. Henquet, V. Maes, and N. Samyn. 2005. "Quantitative Analysis of Δ^9-Tetrahydrocannabinol in Preserved Oral Fluid by Liquid Chromatography–Tandem Mass Spectrometry." *Journal of Chromatography A* 1082: 15–24.

Lee, D., M. M. Bergamaschi, G. Milman, A. J. Barnes, R. H. Queiroz, R. Vandrey, and M. A. Huestis. 2015. "Plasma Cannabinoid Pharmacokinetics after Controlled Smoking and Ad Libitum Cannabis Smoking in Chronic Frequent Users." *Journal of Analytical Toxicology* 39: 580–7.

Leghissa, A., Zacariah L. Hildenbrand, Frank W. Foss, and Kevin A. Schug. 2018. "Determination of Cannabinoids from a Surrogate Hops Matrix Using Multiple Reaction Monitoring Gas Chromatography with Triple Quadrupole Mass Spectrometry." *Journal of Separation Science* 41: 459–68. doi:10.1002/jssc.201700946.

Leghissa, A., Zacariah L. Hildenbrand, Frank W. Foss Jr., and Kevin A. Schug. 2018. "Determination of the Metabolites of Δ^9-tetrahydrocannabinol in Urine and Plasma Using Multiple Reaction Monitoring Gas Chromatography with Triple Quadrupole Mass Spectrometry." *Separation Science Plus* 1: 43–7.

Leghissa, Allegra. 2016. "Method Development for Qualification and Quantification of Cannabinoids and Terpens in Extracts by Gas Chromatography-Mass Spectrometry." PhD Thesis. University of Texas at Arlington.

Leghissa, Allegra, Zacariah L. Hildenbrand, and Kevin A. Schug. 2018. "A Review of Methods for the Chemical Characterization of Cannabis Natural Products." *Journal of Separation Science* 41: 398–415. doi:10.1002/jssc.201701003.

Leghissa, Allegra, Jonathan Smuts, Changling Qiu, Zacariah L. Hildenbrand, and Kevin A. Schug. 2018. "Detection of Cannabinoids and Cannabinoid Metabolites Using Gas Chromatography-Vacuum Ultraviolet Spectroscopy." *Separation Science Plus* 1: 37–42.

Linden, T. Van der, P. Silverans, and A.G. Verstraete. 2014. "Comparison between Self-Report of Cannabis Use and Toxicological Detection of THC/THCCOOH in Blood and THC in Oral Fluid in Drivers in a Roadside Survey." *Drug Testing and Analysis* 6: 137–42.

Lowe, R. H., E. L. Karschner, E. W. Schwilke, A. J. Barnes, and M. A. Huestis. 2007. "Simultaneous Quantification of Δ^9-Tetrahydrocannabinol, 11-Hydroxy-Δ^9-Tetrahydrocannabinol, and 11-nor-Δ^9-Tetrahydrocannabinol-9-Carboxylic Acid in Human Plasma Using Two-Dimensional Gas Chromatography, Cryofocusing, and Electron Impact-Mass Spectrome." *Journal of Chromatography A* 1163: 318–27.

Mechoulam, R., and Y. Gaoni. 1967. "Recent Advances in the Chemistry of Hashish." *Fortschritte der Chemie organischer Naturstoffe* 25: 175–213.

Mercolini, L., R. Mandrioli, V. Sorella, L. Somaini, D. Giocondi, G. Serpelloni, and M. A. Raggi. 2013. "Dried Blood Spots: Liquid Chromatography–Mass Spectrometry Analysis of Δ^9-Tetrahydrocannabinol and Its Main Metabolites." *Journal of Chromatography A* 1271: 33–40.

Meyer, Veronica R. 2013. Practical High-Performance Liquid Chromatography. Fifth. Hoboken, NJ: John Wiley & Sons.

Milman, G., A. J. Barnes, R. H. Lowe, and M. A. Huestis. 2010. "Simultaneous Quantification of Cannabinoids and Metabolites in Oral Fluid by Two-Dimensional Gas Chromatography Mass Spectrometry." *Journal of Chromatography A* 1217: 1513–21.

Moore, C., C. Coulter, S. Rana, M. Vincent, and J. Snares. 2006. "Analytical Procedure for the Determination of the Marijuanametabolite 11-nor-Δ^9-Tetrahydrocannabinol-9-Carboxylic Acid in Oral Fluid Specimens." *Journal of Analytical Toxicology* 30: 409–12.

Musshoff, F., D. W. Lachenmeier, L. Kroener, and B. Madea. 2003. "Automated Headspace Solid-Phase Dynamic Extraction for the Determination of Cannabinoids in Hair Samples." *Forensic Science International* 133: 32–8.

Nadulski, T., F. Sporkert, M. Schnelle, A. M. Stadelmann, P. Roser, T. Schefter, and F. Pragst. 2005. "Simultaneous and Sensitive Analysis of THC, 11-OH-THC, THC-COOH, CBD, and CBN by GC-MS in Plasma after Oral Application of Small Doses of THC and Cannabis Extract." *Journal of Analytical Toxicology* 29: 782–9.

National Conference of State Legislatures. n.d. "State Medical Marijuana Laws." www.ncsl.org/research/health/state-medical-marijuana-laws.aspx

Nuapia, Yannick, Hlanganani Tutu, Luke Chimuka, and Ewa Cukrowska. 2020. "Selective Extraction of Cannabinoid Compounds from Cannabis Seed Using Pressurized Hot." *Molecules* 25: 1335–50.

Oliveira, C. D. R. de, M. Yonamine, and R. L. D. Moreau. 2007. "Headspace Solid-Phase Microextraction of Cannabinoids in Human Head Hair Samples." *Journal of Separation Science* 30: 128–34.

Omar, J., M. Olivares, J. M. Amigo, and N. Etxebarria. 2014. "Resolution of Co-Eluting Compounds of Cannabis Sativa in Comprehensive Two-Dimensional Gas Chromatography/Mass Spectrometry Detection with Multivariate Curve Resolution-Alternating Least Squares." *Talanta* 121: 273–80.

Omar, Jone, Maitane Olivares, Mikel Alzaga, and Nestor Etxebarria. 2013. "Optimisation and Characterisation of Marihuana Extracts Obtained by Supercritical Fluid Extraction and Focused Ultrasound Extraction and Retention Time Locking GC-MS." *Journal of Separation Science* 36: 1397–404. doi:10.1002/jssc.201201103.

Palmieri, Sara, Marcello Mascini, Antonella Ricci, Federico Fanti, Chiara Ottaviani, Claudio Lo Sterzo, and Manuel Sergi. 2019. "Identification of Cannabis Sativa L. (Hemp) Retailers by Means of Multivariate Analysis of Cannabinoids." *Molecules* 24 (19). doi:10.3390/molecules24193602.

Park, M., J. Kim, Y. Park, S. In, E. Kim, and Y. Park. 2014. "Quantitative Determination of 11-nor-9-Carboxy-Tetrahydrocannabinol in Hair by Column Switching LC–ESI-MS." *Journal of Chromatography B* 947: 179–85.

Pavlovic, Radmila, Sara Panseri, Luca Giupponi, Valeria Leoni, Cinzia Citti, Chiara Cattaneo, Maria Cavaletto, and Annamaria Giorgi. 2019. "Phytochemical and Ecological Analysis of Two Varieties of Hemp (Cannabis Sativa L.) Grown in a Mountain Environment of Italian Alps." *Frontiers in Plant Science* 10 (October): 1–20. doi:10.3389/fpls.2019.01265.

Pellati, Federica, Virginia Brighenti, Johanna Sperlea, Lucia Marchetti, Davide Bertelli, and Stefania Benvenuti. 2018. "New Methods for the Comprehensive Analysis of Bioactive Compounds in Cannabis Sativa L. (Hemp)." *Molecules* 23 (10). doi:10.3390/molecules23102639.

Pellegrini, Manuela, Emilia Marchei, Roberta Pacifici, and Simona Pichini. 2005. "A Rapid and Simple Procedure for the Determination of Cannabinoids in Hemp Food Products by Gas Chromatography-Mass Spectrometry." *Journal of Pharmaceutical and Biomedical Analysis* 36: 939–46. doi:10.1016/j.jpba.2004.07.035.

Poole, Colin F. 2015. "Ionization-Based Detectors for Gas Chromatography." *Journal of Chromatography A* 1421: 137–53.

Protti, Michele, Virginia Brighenti, Maria Rita Battaglia, Lisa Anceschi, Federica Pellati, and Laura Mercolini. 2019. "Cannabinoids from Cannabis Sativa L.: A New Tool Based on HPLC-DAD-MS/MS for a Rational Use in Medicinal Chemistry." *ACS Medicinal Chemistry Letters* 10 (4): 539–44. doi:10.1021/acsmedchemlett.8b00571.

Purschke, K., S. Heinl, O. Lerch, F. Erdmann, and F. Veit. 2016. "Development and Validation of an Automated Liquid–Liquid Extraction GC/MS Method for the Determination of THC, 11-OH-THC, and Free THC-Carboxylic Acid (THC-COOH) from Blood Serum." *Analytical and Bioanalytical Chemistry* 408: 4379–88.

Qiu, Changling, Jonathan Smuts, and Kevin A. Schug. 2017. "Analysis of Terpenes and Turpentines Using Gas Chromatography with Vacuum Ultraviolet Detection." *Journal of Separation Science* 40: 869–77. doi:10.1002/jssc.201601019.

Rodrigues, Anaïs, Michel Yegles, Nicolas Van Elsué, and Serge Schneider. 2018. "Determination of Cannabinoids in Hair of CBD Rich Extracts Consumers Using Gas Chromatography with Tandem Mass Spectrometry (GC/MS–MS)." *Forensic Science International* 292. Elsevier Ireland Ltd: 163–6. doi:10.1016/j.forsciint.2018.09.015.

Ross, S. A., Z. Mehmedic, T. P. Murphy, and M. A. ElSohly. 2000. "GC–MS Analysis of the Total Δ^9-THC Content of Both Drug-and Fiber-Type Cannabis Seeds." *Journal of Analytical Toxicology* 24: 715–17.

Santos, I. C., and K. A. Schug. 2017. "Recent Advances and Applications of Gas Chromatography Vacuum Ultraviolet Spectroscopy." *Journal of Separation Science* 40: 138–51.

Scheidweiler, K. B., M. Andersson, M. J. Swortwood, C. Sempio, and M. A. Huestis. 2017. "Long-Term Stability of Cannabinoids in Oral Fluid after Controlled Cannabis Administration." *Drug Testing and Analysis* 9: 143–7.

Schenk, Jamie, Gabe Nagy, Nicola L.B. Pohl, Allegra Leghissa, Jonathan Smuts, and Kevin A. Schug. 2017. "Identification and Deconvolution of Carbohydrates with Gas Chromatography-Vacuum Ultraviolet Spectroscopy." *Journal of Chromatography A* 1513 (September): 210–21. doi:10.1016/j.chroma.2017.07.052.

Schug, Kevin A, Ian Sawicki, Doug D Carlton, Hui Fan, Harold M Mcnair, John P Nimmo, Peter Kroll, Jonathan Smuts, Phillip Walsh, and Dale Harrison. 2014. "Vacuum Ultraviolet Detector for Gas Chromatography." *Analytical Chemistry* 86: 8329–35. doi:10.1021/ac5018343.

Schwilke, E. W., D. M. Schwope, E. L. Karschner, R. H. Lowe, W. D. Darwin, D. L. Kelly, R. S. Goodwin, D. A. Gorelick, and M. A. Huestis. 2009. "Δ^9-Tetrahydrocannabinol (THC), 11-Hydroxy-THC, and 11-nor-9-Carboxy-THC Plasma Pharmacokinetics during and after Continuous High-Dose Oral THC." *Clinical Chemistry* 55: 2180–9.

Sergi, M, C. Montesano, S. Odoardi, L. M. Rocca, G. Fabrizi, D. Compagnone, and R. Curini. 2013. "Micro Extraction by Packed Sorbent Coupled to Liquid Chromatography Tandem Mass Spectrometry for the Rapid and Sensitive Determination of Cannabinoids in Oral Fluids." *Journal of Chromatography A* 1301: 139–46.

Simoes, S. S., A. C. Ajenjo, and M. J. Dias. 2011. "Qualitative and Quantitative Analysis of THC, 11-Hydroxy-THC and 11-nor-9-Carboxy-THC in Whole Blood by Ultra-Performance Liquid Chromatography/Tandem Mass Spectrometry." *Rapid Communications in Mass Spectrometry* 25: 2603–10.

Skoog, Douglas A., Donald M. West, F. James Holler, and Stanley R. Crouch. 2014. *Fundamentals of Analytical Chemistry*. 9th ed. Belmont, CA: Brooks/Cole Pub Co.

Skultety, Ludovit, Petr Frycak, Changling Qiu, Jonathan Smuts, Lindsey Shear-Laude, Karel Lemr, James X. Mao, et al. 2017. "Resolution of Isomeric New Designer Stimulants Using Gas Chromatography – Vacuum Ultraviolet Spectroscopy and Theoretical Computations." *Analytica Chimica Acta* 971: 55–67. doi:10.1016/j.aca.2017.03.023.

Steinmeyer, S., D. Bregel, S. Warth, T. Kraemer, and M. R. Moeller. 2002. "Improved and Validated Method for the Determination of Δ^9-Tetrahydrocannabinol (THC), 11-Hydroxy-THC and 11-nor-9-Carboxy-THC in Serum, and in Human Liver Microsomal Preparations Using Gas Chromatography–Mass Spectrometry." *Journal of Chromatography B* 772: 239–48.

Stolker, A A M., J. Van Schoonhoven, A. J. De Vries, I. Bobeldijk-Pastorova, W. H. J. Vaes, and R. Van Den Berg. 2004. "Determination of Cannabinoids in Cannabis Products Using Liquid Chromatography–Ion Trap Mass Spectrometry." *Journal of Chromatography A* 1058: 143–51. doi:10.1016/j.chroma.2004.08.089.

Swartz, Michael. 2010. "HPLC Detectors: A Brief Review." *Journal of Liquid Chromatography & Related Technologies* 33: 1130–50.

Teixeira, H., P. Proença, A. Castanheira, S. Santos, M. López-Rivadulla, F. Corte-Real, E. P. Marques, and D. N. Vieira. 2004. "Cannabis and Driving: The Use of LC–MS to Detect Δ^9-Tetrahydrocannabinol (Δ^9-THC) in Oral Fluid Samples." *Forensic Science International*. 146 (Supplement): S61–63.

The Nobel Foundation. n.d. "No TitleThe Nobel Prize in Chemistry 2002: Information for the Public."www.nobelprize.org/prizes/chemistry/2002/popular-information/

Thieme, D., H. Sachs, and M. Uhl. 2014. "Proof of Cannabis Administration by Sensitive Detection of 11-nor-Delta(9)-Tetrahydrocannabinol-9-Carboxylic Acid in Hair Using Selective Methylation and Application of Liquid Chromatography-Tandem and Multistage Mass Spectrometry." *Drug Testing and Analysis* 6: 112–18.

Traeger, John C. 2015. "The Development of Ion Production Methods The Development of Electron Ionization." *The Encyclopedia of Mass Spectrometry*, 9: 77–82. doi:10.1016/B978-0-08-043848-1.00008-0.

Tsai, J. S., M. A. ElSohly, S. F. Tsai, T. P. Murphy, B. Twarowska, and S. J. Salamone. 2000. "Investigation of Nitrite Adulteration on the Immunoassay and GC–MS Analysis of Cannabinoids in Urine Specimens." *Journal of Analytical Toxicology* 24: 708–14.

United Nations Office on Drugs and Crime. 2009. *Mended Methods for the Identification and Analysis of Cannabis and Cannabis Products*. New York: United Nations Publications.

Villamor, J. L., A. M. Bermejo, M. J. Tabernero, and P. Fernandez. 2004. "Determination of Cannabinoids in Human Hair by GC/MS." *Analytical Letters* 37: 517–28.

Wang, Mei, Yan Hong Wang, Bharathi Avula, Mohamed M. Radwan, Amira S. Wanas, Zlatko Mehmedic, John van Antwerp, Mahmoud A. ElSohly, and Ikhlas A. Khan. 2017. "Quantitative Determination of Cannabinoids in Cannabis and Cannabis Products Using Ultra-High-Performance Supercritical Fluid Chromatography and Diode Array/Mass Spectrometric Detection." *Journal of Forensic Sciences* 62 (3): 602–11. doi:10.1111/1556-4029.13341.

Weil, Herbert, and Trevor I. Willams. 1950. "History of Chromatography." *Nature* 166 (4232): 1000–1. doi:10.1038/1661000b0.

Weinmann, W, M. Goerner, S. Vogt, R. Goerke, and S. Pollak. 2001. "Fast Confirmation of 11-nor-9-Carboxy-Δ^9-Tetrahydrocannabinol (THC-COOH) in Urine by LC/MS/MS Using Negative Atmospheric-Pressure Chemical Ionisation (APCI)." *Forensic Science International* 121: 103–7.

Yousefi-Taemeh, Maryam, and Demian R. Ifa. 2019. "Analysis of Tetrahydrocannabinol Derivative from Cannabis-Infused Chocolate by QuEChERS-Thin Layer Chromatography-Desorption Electrospray Ionization Mass Spectrometry." *Journal of Mass Spectrometry* 54 (10): 834–42. doi:10.1002/jms.4436.

5 New Trends in the Analysis of Cannabis-Based Products

Laura Mercolini, Roberto Mandrioli
and Michele Protti

CONTENTS

5.1 INTRODUCTION

As one of the first plants to be cultivated by humans, probably since at least 8000–5000 BCE, hemp (*Cannabis sativa* L.) has been for millennia a source of textile, building, writing and food/feed materials, as well as being used for religious and recreational purposes. Only in relatively recent times has this plant been considered in a mostly negative light by state authorities; probably the first documented legislation restricting cannabis was passed in Arabia in the 1300s CE. More recently, international restrictions to cannabis trade were first applied in 1925 (International Opium Convention), but hemp cultivation mainly for fibre use continued both in Europe and in the United States until at least World War II, and primarily for recreational use in several Asian countries. Severe restrictions on cultivation have been applied at least since 1961 (Single Convention on Narcotic Drugs), and widely diffused with the "War on Drugs" in the United States during the 1970s and 1980s.

However, since the 1970s, several countries started making hemp cultivation and use easier, both for fibre and recreational purposes. Since then, restricting

DOI: 10.1201/9780429274893-5

legislation has been relaxed in several parts of the world, and medical uses for cannabis products have also been found, finding widespread application in the last ten years. Currently, great emphasis is being put on the difference between "fibre-type" (or "hemp-type") and "marijuana-type" cannabis. The main difference between the two types resides in the different contents of the two main bioactive compounds: Δ^9-tetrahydrocannabinol (THC, Figure 5.1a) and cannabidiol (CBD, Figure 5.1b). The former is considered responsible for the pleasant and recreational psychotropic effects of cannabis, while the latter can have muscle-relaxing and antiemetic properties while being devoid of psychotropic activity. Both are formed in the plant and during recreational use by decarboxylation of the corresponding acids, Δ^9-tetrahydrocannabinolic acid (THCA; Figure 5.1c) and cannabidiolic acid (CBDA, Figure 5.1d).

The United Nations Office on Drugs and Crime (UNODC) (Drugs 2009) and the American Herbal Pharmacopoeia (2013) define hemp-type cannabis as having a "total THC"/"total CBD" ratio (i.e., [THC+THCA]/[CBD+CBDA] ratio) lower than one, marijuana-type cannabis as having a total THC/total CBD ratio higher than one and intermediate cannabis as having a ratio close to one.

This renewed interest in traditional and new uses for cannabis also brings with itself the need for suitably accurate and selective analytical methods to certify the quality of hemp products and steer their use according to their detailed composition. In particular, cannabis-derived food and food supplements, beverages, cosmetics and perfumes need to be characterised in detail, since they are intended for relatively widespread use without any recreational overtones.

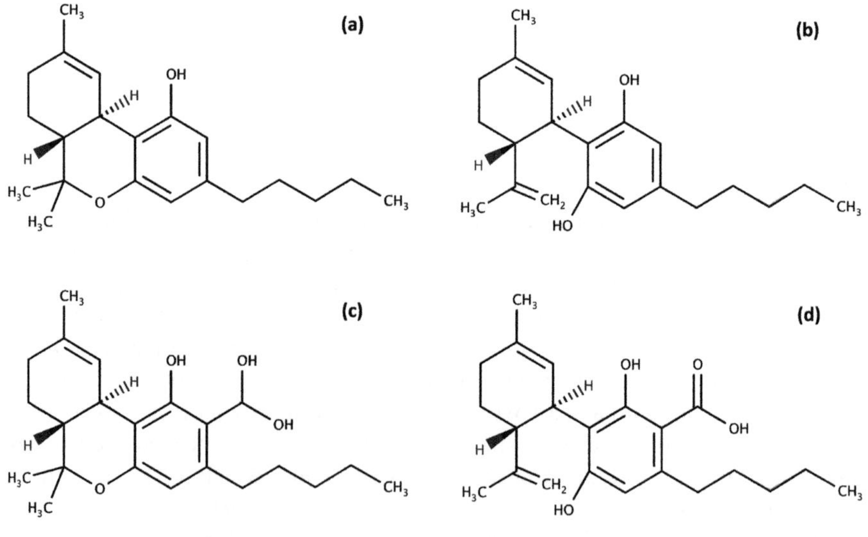

FIGURE 5.1   Chemical structures of (a) Δ^9-tetrahydrocannabinol (THC); (b) cannabidiol (CBD); (c) tetrahydrocannabinolic acid (THCA); and (d) cannabidiolic acid (CBDA).

As a consequence, the situation is being reflected in increased interest from the scientific community. Reviews of new trends for the chemical characterisation of natural cannabis products (Leghissa et al. 2018) (Citti et al. 2020) have recently underscored a lack of scientifically reliable data. Among the causes of this situation, which starkly contrasts with the human use of the cannabis plant since time immemorial, restricting legislation (especially in the United States) is cited. Judging from the relative wealth and diversity of new publications in this field, however, the scientific situation seems to be gradually improving. In this chapter, only methods published in the last five years (2016–February 2021) are reported and described.

5.2 ANALYSIS OF CANNABIS PRODUCTS: ANALYTE CLASSES

The analysis of cannabis product components is mainly directed by their possible biological activity. While non-bioactive product components can arguably have great importance for their effects on technical uses of cannabis (e.g., for fabrics, paper, building materials), this chapter is not concerned with these kinds of compounds. Instead, in the following sections, we will describe the latest trends in the analysis of three main classes of substances that can have important biological effects when cannabis products are consumed internally: cannabinoids, other specialised metabolites and contaminants.

5.2.1 CANNABINOIDS

Cannabinoids are specialised metabolites sharing a common biological origin from cannabigerolic acid (CBGA, Figure 5.2a), a cyclic terpenoid, and cannabigerol (CBG, Figure 5.2b). For more information regarding the structures of cannabinoids, please see Chapter 3.

The best-known cannabinoid is of course THC, which is considered the most important psychoactive compound contributing to the pleasant effects sought after by recreational cannabis users. Like most other cannabinoids, THC is formed in the plant (and in the products obtained from it) from the decarboxylation of the corresponding THCA, which occurs by the action of heat, light, time and other stressing conditions. On the other hand, CBD is currently considered the main bioactive, non-psychoactive component of cannabis, which is currently being used for therapeutic purposes in the treatment of emesis and muscle spasms.

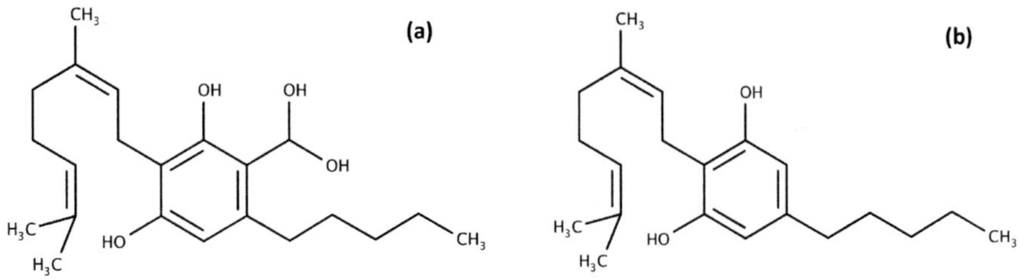

FIGURE 5.2 Chemical structures of (a) cannabigerolic acid (CBGA) and (b) cannabigerol (CBG).

5.2.1.1 Analysis of Δ⁹-Tetrahydrocannabinol and Other Psychoactive Cannabinoids

An analytical procedure obtained First Action Official Method of Analysis (OMA 2018.10) status from the Association of Official Analytical Communities (AOAC) International (Mudge and Brown 2020). This method uses 80% methanol and ultra-sound-assisted extraction (UAE) to extract six significant cannabinoids (THC, CBD, CBG, cannabinol [CBN], Figure 5.3a; cannabichromene [CBC], Figure 5.3b; and tetrahydrocannabivarin [THV], Figure 5.3c) and two related acids (THCA and CBDA) from dried *Cannabis* flowers and seed oils. Subsequent analysis is carried out by reversed-phase high-performance liquid chromatography with ultraviolet detection (RP-HPLC-UV). The method was fully validated; moreover, it can be extended to comply with standard method performance requirements (SMPR) with the inclusion of cannabidivarinic acid (CBDVA, Figure 5.4d) and CBG.

5.2.1.1.1 LC-MS Methods

HPLC coupled to some kind of mass spectrometric (MS) detection is by far the most important method class. In fact, the use of MS allows the unambiguous identification

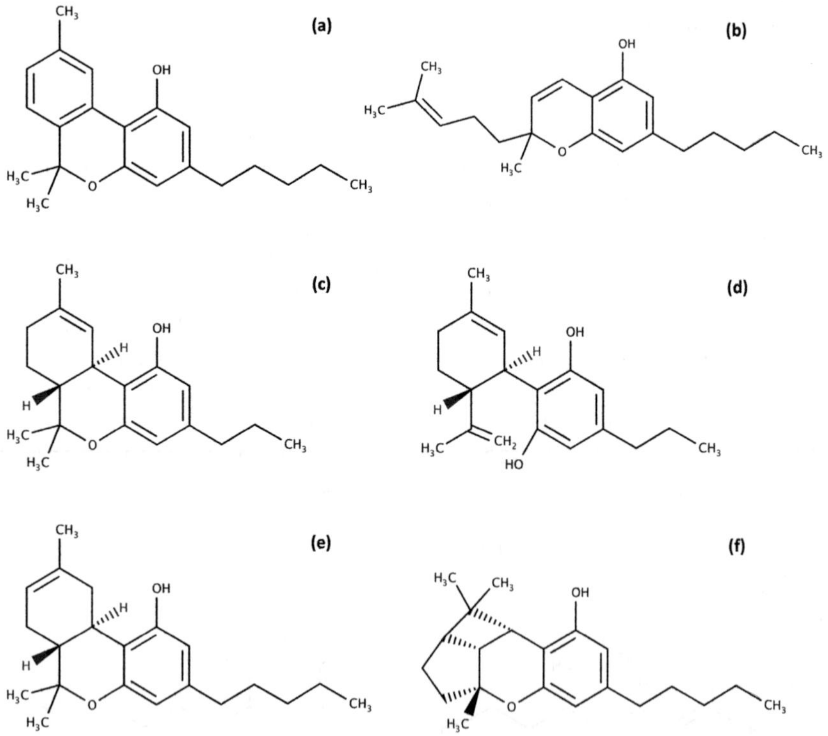

FIGURE 5.3 Chemical structures of (a) cannabinol (CBN); (b) cannabichromene (CBC); (c) tetrahydrocannabivarin (THV); (d) cannabidivarin (CBDV); (e) Δ⁸-tetrahydrocannabinol (Δ⁸-THC); and (f) cannabicyclol (CBL).

of the analytes, which can then be used for forensic purposes and presented before a court of law with a high degree of confidence. For example, an HPLC-tandem mass (MS/MS) method with electrospray ionisation (ESI) and triple quadrupole (TQ) detection has been developed to determine 17 psychoactive and non-psychoactive cannabinoids: nine neutral cannabinoids (THC, CBD, CBG, CBN, CBC, THV, cannabidivarin [CBDV] Figure 5.3d; Δ^8-tetrahydrocannabinol [Δ^8-THC], Figure 5.3e; and cannabicyclol [CBL], Figure 5.3f) and eight corresponding acidic forms (THCA, CBDA, CBGA, CBNA, CBCA, THVA, CBDVA and CBLA, Figures 5.1c, 5.1d, 5.2a, 5.4a–e) (McRae and Melanson 2020). The method was applied to dried *Cannabis* flowers after cryogenic grinding and vortex-assisted extraction (VAE) with 80% methanol.

HPLC coupled to both UV and MS/MS detection in series has been used to analyse eight cannabinoids (CBD, CBDA, THC, THCA, CBG, CBGA, CBDV, CBN) in a specific subset of cannabis products, i.e., CBD-rich ones: oils, ointments, hydrophilic liquids, plant material and gummy candy (Nemeškalová et al. 2020). In this case, UV detection was used to quantify CBD present at very high concentrations, while

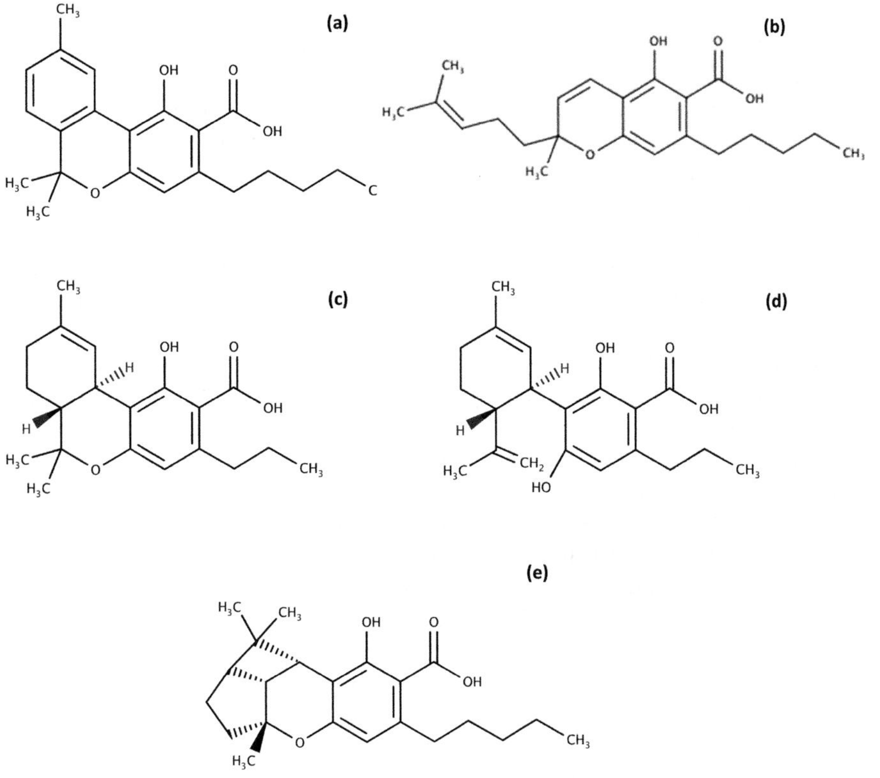

FIGURE 5.4 Chemical structures of (a) cannabinolic acid (CBNA); (b) cannabichromenic acid (CBCA); (c) tetrahydrocannabivarinic acid (THVA); (d) cannabidivarinic acid (CBDVA); and (e) cannabicyclolic acid (CBLA).

MS/MS was used for all other, minor components. Different solvents were applied for the extraction, according to the different matrices considered in the study.

An LC-MS/MS method developed by Waters for the analysis of THC, THCA and the hydroxylated metabolite of THC in human plasma (Zhang, Danaceau and Chambers) was adapted and applied to the determination of seven neutral (THC, CBD, CBG, CBN, CBC, Δ^8-THC and THV) and four acid cannabinoids (THCA, CBDA, CBGA and CBCA) in different industrial hemp samples: whole plants (without roots), leaves, stalks, flowers, seed heads, chaff (after seed harvest) and exhausted flowers (after industrial cannabinoid extraction) (Kleinhenz et al. 2020). In this case, cannabinoids were extracted from all matrices with 2% formic acid in acetonitrile in the presence of QuEChERS (quick, easy, cheap, effective, rugged, safe)-method salts and then purified by solid phase extraction (SPE) on a mixed-mode, strong anion-exchange (SAX) sorbent before LC-MS/MS analysis. The cannabinoids of interest, except Δ^8-THC, were found in all matrices; THC was found in all samples, but always at levels lower than 0.3%.

LC-MS/MS with a Q-Trap (QT) analyser was used to determine nine cannabinoids (THC, THCA, CBD, CBDA, CBG, CBGA, CBN, Δ^8-THC and THV) in cannabis-derived foods and beverages. QT is a hybrid of TQ and linear ion trap (LIT), coupling the outstanding quantitative performance of TQ with the superior mass accuracy of LIT. Different foods (flour, pasta, bread and other bakery products) and beverages (beers, energy drinks) not including any cannabis derivatives were spiked with the analytes and used for method validation; food samples were homogenised and extracted with a 9/1 (V/V) methanol/chloroform mixture, while beverage samples were diluted before injection into the LC-MS/MS system. The authors claim to have also carried out the analysis of foods and beverages containing cannabis seeds, flour and oil; however, neither the kind of products nor the analysis results are specified (they were submitted to the local Ministry of Health for evaluation) (Di Marco Pisciottano et al. 2018).

Another LC-MS/MS method was developed for the analysis of THC, THCA, CBD and CBDA in olive oil galenic preparations from *Cannabis* flowers (Carcieri et al. 2018). It has also been applied to the comparison of different galenic cannabis oils and decoctions to find the most advantageous means of bioactive compound extraction (Baratta et al. 2019).

A simple LC-MS/MS method was applied to the analysis of 40 different commercial hemp products (including oils, plant materials, and creams/cosmetics) to check compliance with regulatory restrictions by determining THC, THCA, CBD and CBDA levels (Meng et al. 2018); sample dilution with 95% methanol containing 0.005% formic acid and homogenisation were the only pre-treatment steps employed.

The first report of cannabinoid analysis in cannabis roots used LC-MS/MS after extraction with 80/20 (V/V) acetonitrile/methanol and found the presence of ten main cannabinoids (THC, THCA, CBD, CBDA, CBG, CBGA, CBN, Δ^8-THC, CBC and THV) in the matrix (Gul et al. 2018).

Quantitation of THC at trace levels in perfume has also been reported. THC identification was carried out by LC with high-resolution MS (HRMS) using an Orbitrap analyser, while quantitation was carried out by directly injecting perfume samples in LC-MS/MS(TQ) (Thalhamer et al. 2017). Finally, 11 cannabinoids were determined in leaves, flower buds and hashish from different *Cannabis* strains by UHPLC-UV-single quadrupole (SQ) after extraction with 80/20 (V/V) acetonitrile/methanol (Wang Yan-Hong et al. 2018).

5.2.1.1.2   (U)HPLC-UV and (U)HPLC-PDA Methods

HPLC-UV (or HPLC-PDA) has been used for different applications, including forensic science, although its limited selectivity cannot ensure analyte identification, so the certainty of results could be challenged in a legal setting.

For example, the assessment of the cannabinoid content of 922 flower samples from "light *Cannabis*" farms was performed (Dei Cas et al. 2020). After vortex-assisted extraction (VAE) with methanol, 11 cannabinoids (THC, THCA, CBD, CBDA, CBG, CBGA, CBN, CBC, Δ^8-THC, THV and CBDV) were separated with a dedicated CBX for Potency (Nexleaf) column, which contains a superficially porous sorbent with proprietary modifications to the silica matrix that provides high selectivity and resolution geared specifically toward cannabinoids. Five diagnostic cannabinoids (THC, THCA, CBD, CBDA, CBN) were quantified. Quite surprisingly, 82% of the samples were found to contain more than the legal limit of 0.20% total THC (THC+THCA). Another HPLC-UV application for the analysis of ten cannabinoids (THC, THCA, CBD, CBDA, CBG, CBGA, CBN, CBC, Δ^8-THC and THV) in *Cannabis* flowers has been reported, after UAE-assisted extraction with methanol-chloroform (9/1, V/V) (Mandrioli et al. 2019).

Other HPLC or UHPLC methods coupled to UV or PDA detection have been published: HPLC-UV for THC, THCA, CBD and CBDA determination in plant material after methanol/hexane extraction and separation in a general purpose core-shell C8 column (Hädener et al. 2019); UHPLC-UV for eight cannabinoids (THC, THCA, CBD, CBDA, CBG, CBGA, CBN and CBDV) after acetonitrile/water extraction using another core-shell column, with C18 chemistry (Zivovinovic et al. 2018); HPLC-UV (C18 column) again for THC and CBD in *Cannabis* extracts and an oro-mucosal spray (Saingam and Sakunpak 2018); HPLC-PDA on a mixed-mode C18-aromatic column after ethanol extraction for the determination of 11 cannabinoids in consumer and traditional products from cannabis (Ciolino et al. 2018); a study on the decarboxylation kinetics of CBDA and analysis of seven cannabinoids in hemp oil by HPLC-UV (Citti et al. 2018); the analysis of different cannabinoids in plant material by HPLC-PDA after grinding with dry ice and extraction with methanol/chloroform (9/1, V/V), drying and re-dissolving in a methanol/organic-pure water mixture (Patel et al. 2017); concentration and stability assessment of five cannabinoids in cannabis-based medicinal extracts by HPLC-UV (Citti et al. 2016); and HPLC-PDA for the analysis of THC, CBD and CBN in cannabis plants (Fu et al. 2016).

5.2.1.1.3   GC Methods

A simple gas-chromatographic method with flame ionisation detection (GC-FID) has been developed and applied to the simultaneous analysis of both cannabinoids and terpenes without derivatisation in stemless buds of industrial hemp (Zekič and Križman 2020). A total of six cannabinoids (THC, CBD, CBG, CBN, CBC and 8THC) and six terpenes (α-pinene, β-pinene, myrcene, limonene, β-caryophyllene and α-humulene, Figure 5.5a–f) were quantified after UAE with "acetone or ethyl acetate" (it is unclear which solvent was really used, or if each solvent was used to extract one class of compounds). A wide temperature gradient was used due to the much higher volatility of terpenes in comparison to cannabinoids, and all analytes could be detected within the same injection, despite cannabinoids being about 10–15 times more concentrated than terpenes. It should be noted that the high temperatures required to volatilise cannabinoids for GC separation also produce the decarboxylation of most of their acidic forms, so the latter cannot be separately analysed with this method. This has been confirmed by the comparison between the results of UHPLC-MS/MS and GC-MS for the analysis of twelve different samples of "light *Cannabis*", i.e. *Cannabis* products (usually dried flower tops) containing 0.20% (w/w) or less of THC, which are freely tradeable under local (Italian) law, although up to 0.60% THC is "tolerated" (Marchei et al. 2020). Both THC and CBD were extracted with cyclohexane and UAE. All samples had less than 0.20% THC, however this increased up to 0.34 in some of them if THCA was considered (since it can become THC upon heating); however, the law does not prescribe the determination of THCA when assessing compliance with "light *Cannabis*" regulations. As usual, CBD and CBDA content was highly variable and unrelated to THC content.

A detailed survey of cannabinoids found in marijuana-type *Cannabis* plants has been recently carried out by GC-MS after trimethylsyslylation to increase volatility; it found 43 cannabinoids, 16 of which had not been described before (Basas-Jaumandreu and De Las Heras 2020).

Fast GC/MS has been applied for the analysis of several cannabinoids in dried flowers: In comparison to "traditional" techniques, Fast GC uses shorter columns, faster oven temperature ramp rates, high carrier gas speeds, narrower i.d. columns and lower film thicknesses to obtain robust separations in shorter times. In order to avoid the thermal decarboxylation of acidic cannabinoids, different kinds of derivatisation were tested, and trimethylsilylation was applied (Cardenia et al. 2018).

Finally, a GC-FID method has been published with trymethylsilylation for the analysis of 10 neutral and acidic cannabinoids in different parts (buds, leaves, roots and stems) of *Cannabis* plants (Ibrahim et al. 2018).

5.2.1.1.4 *Other Analytical Methods*

UHP supercritical fluid chromatography (UHPSFC)-PDA-MS has been used for the analysis of nine cannabinoids (THC, THCA, CBD, CBDA, CBG, CBGA, CBN, Δ^8-THC and THCV) in cannabis flowering bud, hashish and leaf samples (CBC and CBL were only identified, not quantified) after UAE with an 8/2 (V/V) acetonitrile/methanol mixture. Chemometric analysis by PCA and partial least squares-discriminant analysis (PLS-DA) was applied to differentiate different sample types (Wang Mei et al. 2017).

An extremely fast screening method to evaluate the THC/CBD ratio of *Cannabis* flowers used two kinds of organic thin-film transistors (OTFT) in an electronic device: one OTFT was based on a p-type copper phthalocyanine (CuPc) organic semiconductor (OSC), while the other OTFT was based on an n-type copper hexadecafluorophthalocyanine (F16-CuPc) OSC (Comeau et al. 2019). Both OTFT also included a fast blue BB (FBBB) layer: this pigment is known to react covalently and non-selectively with both THC and CBD under alkaline conditions, producing a green colour. The use of OTFTs, however, allowed the differential detection of the two analytes because they produced different field effect mobilities in the OTFT. Thus, the electric readout of the instrument could be linked to the THC/CBD ratio. Moreover, the corresponding acidic forms (THCA and CBDA) also produced very similar readouts to the neutral cannabinoids, thus the devices were able to correctly assess (THC+THCA)/(CBD+CBDA) ratios as well, which are much more relevant to predict the biological effects of the samples. This fast procedure can be applied directly to an acetonitrile extract from the flowers.

Fast determination of THC, CBD, CBG, CBN, CBC, Δ^8-THC, THCV and CBDV (no acidic form was included) was carried out by direct dispersive near-infrared (dNIR) spectroscopy in reflectance mode (400–2498 nm) and by Fourier Transform NIR (FT-NIR) spectroscopy in diffuse reflectance mode (4000–12,500 cm^{-1}, 800–2500 nm) (Callado et al. 2018). The results were in good agreement with those of an established GC method.

A particularly original, very fast means of cannabinoid extraction from plant material was the use of a hard-cap espresso machine (HCEM) with 2-propanol as the solvent (Leiman et al. 2018). Before extraction, the homogenised sample was mixed with a dispersing agent, and the extraction procedure itself lasted 40 s, followed by GC-MS analysis. Alternatively, the extract could be absorbed on a PTFE filter and then be analysed by thermal desorption-ion mobility spectrometry (TD-IMS) with radioactive ionisation. In this case, the GC-MS method was applied to THC, CBD and CBN, while the IMS method did not detect CBN, and did not discriminate in any way THC from CBD. A similar result was obtained using another TD-IMS method (del Mar Contreras et al. 2018), where no single signal was assigned to individual cannabinoids, but statistical analysis of global signals by PCA-linear discriminant analysis (LDA) allowed individuating different clusters corresponding to different *Cannabis* varieties and also allowed discrimination from other plant species (including tobacco).

5.2.1.2 Analysis of Non-Psychoactive Cannabinoids

Many of the methods described previously for psychoactive cannabinoids are also suitable for non-psychoactive cannabinoids and allow their simultaneous determination. A method has recently been published (Tzimas et al. 2021) for the extraction of CBD and its precursor CBDA from three different fibre hemp varieties by UAE with methanol. UAE performance was compared with that of microwave-assisted extraction (MAE) and dynamic maceration (DM) using the same solvent, and UAE resulted in consistently providing the best yields for both analytes. The UAE procedure was then optimised with experimental design-response surface methodology (ExDe-RSM) to obtain the maximum extraction yield. Subsequent analysis and quality control of the extracts was carried out by reversed-phase ultra-high-performance liquid chromatography coupled with photodiode array detection (RP-UHPLC-PDA).

HPLC-UV has been used to assess the quality of CBD purified isolates to be used in commercial products (topicals, edibles, and beverages) by quantifying the main component as well as six other cannabinoids (THC, CBG, CBN, CBC, THCV and CBDV) (Layton and Aubin 2018); no acidic cannabinoids were assayed.

A carbon black-modified glassy carbon electrode has been developed as an electrochemical sensor for the detection and quantitation of CBD in different plant extracts, in particular, in cannabis seed oil and leaves. Optimal electrochemical conditions were determined by using phenyl derivatives much simpler than CBD but containing the same electroactive catechol function. Quantitation was carried out by means of the standard addition method (Cirrincione et al. 2021). CBD has also been analysed, together with 29 different terpenes, in flowers and apical leaves by GC-FID after UAE with absolute ethanol (Bakro et al. 2020).

CBN can be found in sediments as the main degradation products of most cannabinoids, thus enabling the identification of historical hemp-processing (retting) sites. In this case, CBN has been identified and quantified by high-performance thin-layer chromatography (HPTLC) combined with direct ESI-MS detection (Schmidt et al. 2020).

In recent times, green methods using non-polluting solvents and procedures, or very small amounts of solvents, are coming to the forefront of scientific research. In this regard, a method has been developed for CBD and CBDA extraction from cannabis seed oils using just 500 µL of acetonitrile and an oil freezing protocol to ease phase separation. The analytes were then determined by HPLC-PDA (Madej et al. 2020).

The LC-MS/MS analysis of CBD, CBDA, CBG, CBGA, THC and THCA in hemp honey has been carried out after acetonitrile extraction and partition with QuEChERS salts (Brighenti et al. 2019). Since cannabinoids levels in honey are very low, a linear quadrupole ion trap (QTRAP) MS setup was chosen to maximise selectivity and sensitivity. THC and THCA were below the limit of detection (LOD) of the method (0.3 ng/g for all analytes).

Recently, ^{13}C quantitative nuclear magnetic resonance (qNMR) spectroscopy has been used for the direct determination of CBD, CBDA, CBG and CBGA in flowers of fibre-type *Cannabis* without previous separation, with satisfactory sensitivity results (LOQ < 750 µg/mL) (Marchetti et al. 2019).

5.2.2 Analysis of Other Specialised Metabolites

As reported previously, some methods allow the determination of other specialised metabolites, in addition to cannabinoids; for example, terpenes. The terpene profile of hemp-, marijuana- and intermediate-type cannabis has been evaluated for possible use in identifying the three classes without directly determining cannabinoids (Rocha et al. 2020). Thirty different terpenes were identified and quantified, and nine of them were present in all samples; of these, the most abundant ones were α-pinene, β-myrcene and β-caryophyllene. Principal component analysis (PCA) showed that hemp-type samples had either β-myrcene or β-caryophyllene as the main terpene, while no clear pattern was found for marijuana-type samples. Terpenes were extracted directly from the solid, pulverised samples by headspace solid phase microextraction (HS-SPME) upon heating to 50°C and using a 100% polydimethylsiloxane (PDMS) fibre. Analysis was carried out by GC-MS after direct desorption from the fibre in the injection port.

GC-MS was used again for the analysis of ten common terpenes (α-pinene, β-pinene, myrcene, limonene, β-caryophyllene, α-humulene, terpinolene, linalool,

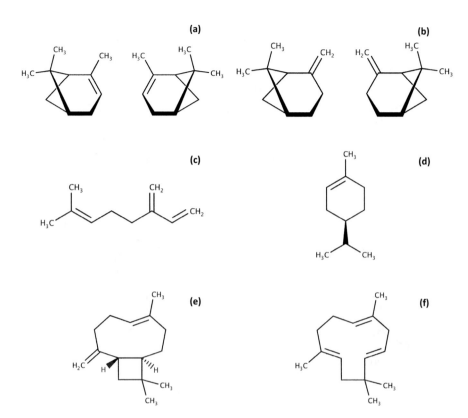

FIGURE 5.5 Chemical structures of (a) α-pinene; (b) β-pinene; (c) myrcene; (d) limonene; (e) β-caryophyllene; and (f) α-humulene.

α-terpineol and caryophyllene oxide; Figures 5.5a–f, 5.6a–d) in plant materials with a method validated according to AOAC International guidelines (Ibrahim et al. 2019). Analyte extraction was carried out with ethyl acetate.

An assessment of fat-soluble vitamin levels in hemp seed oil has been carried out by fast SFC-PDA (Tyśkiewicz et al. 2018). After studying different stationary phases, a high-strength silanophilic interaction C18 sorbent with additional selectivity for bases (HSS C18 SB) was chosen. This kind of sorbent is non-endcapped and has a low density of C18 coverage to enhance silanol-group interactions. After an established pre-treatment by saponification to increase vitamin concentration (O'Keefe and Ackman 1986), cis- and trans-retinyl palmitate, cis- and trans-retinyl acetate, retinol, α-, β-, γ-, δ-tocopherol, ergocalciferol (D_2), cholecalciferol (D_3), cis- and trans-phylloquinone (K_1) and menaquinone-4 (K_2-MK4) were determined (structures in Figure 5.7a–n).

Another paper reports the evaluation of flavonoids in different plants, including *C. sativa*, by HPLC-UV. The tested flavonoids were rutin, myricetin, luteolin, naringenin, apigenin, catechin, epicatechin and naringin; all of them excluding the last three were found in *Cannabis* after continuous Soxhlet extraction with 65% ethanol for 24 h (Gür et al.).

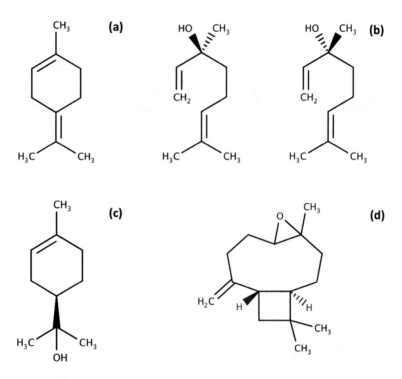

FIGURE 5.6 Chemical structures of (a) terpinolene; (b) linalool; (c) α-terpineol; and (d) caryophyllene oxide.

Twenty polyphenols belonging to different classes (several subclasses of phenolic acids and flavonoids) have been determined in cold-pressed oil from the Finola cultivar of *C. sativa* by HPLC-DAD-fluorescence (FL). Extraction was carried out by VAE with methanol/water (8/2, V/V), concentration under vacuum and nitrogen flow until syrupy in consistency, acetonitrile addition and washing with n-hexane to remove lipids (Smeriglio et al. 2016). Antioxidant activity was also assayed by the Folin-Ciocalteu, $AlCl_3$, ABTS, DPPH, β-carotene bleaching, ferrozine, FRAP and ORAC methods, and tocopherol content was assessed by HPLC-FL.

Qualitative, non-selective chemical assays have been used to detect the presence of alkaloids, glycosides, terpenoids, steroids, flavonoids, flavones, tannins, phenols and saponins in different cannabis leaf extracts. They found every compound class in at least one extract; hexane was the solvent where most classes were identified (six: alkaloids, glycosides, steroids, flavonoids, flavones, and saponins; Ahmed et al. 2019). The non-selective quantitation of total phenols, total flavonoids and antioxidant activity was carried out in the same study by the Folin–Ciocalteu, $AlCl_3$ and DPPH methods, respectively. Methanol resulted as the best solvent for extracting phenols, followed by water and ethyl acetate; flavonoids were best extracted with methanol or ethanol. On the other hand, antioxidant power as assessed by the DPPH assay was highest in the acetone extract, followed by hexane and water.

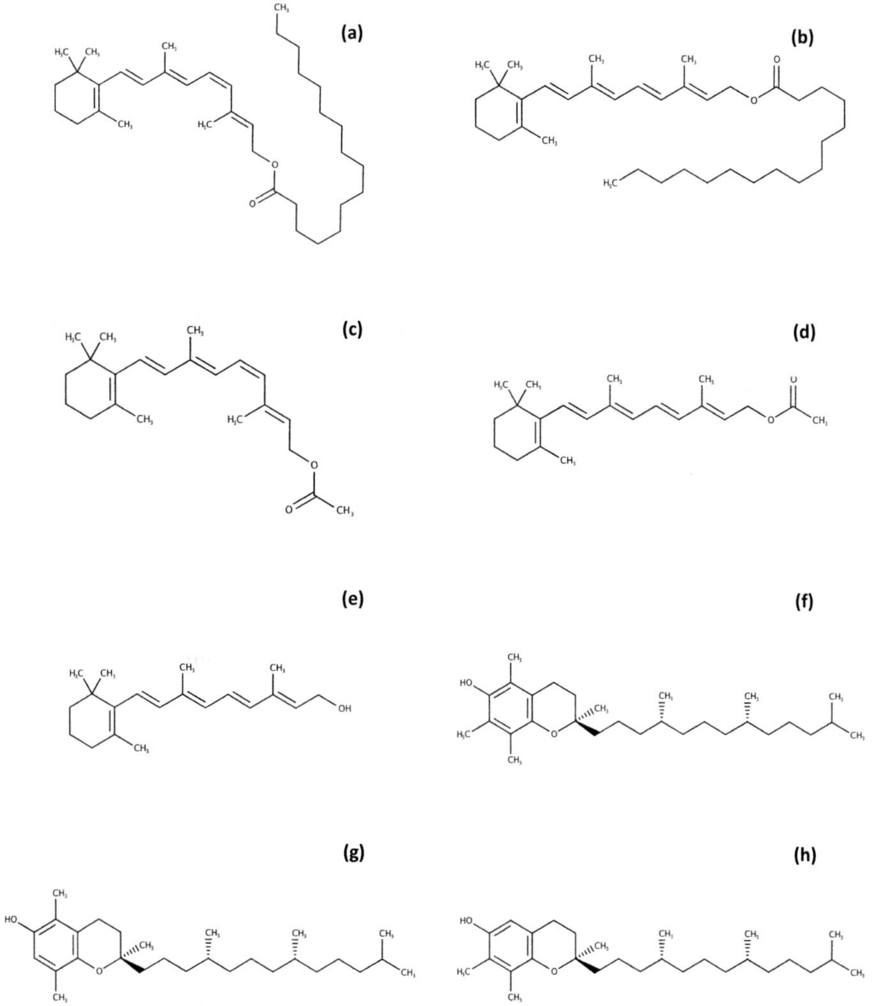

FIGURE 5.7A–H Chemical structures of (a) *cis*-retinyl palmitate; (b) *trans*-retinyl palmitate; (c) *cis*-retinyl acetate; (d) *trans*-retinyl acetate; (e) retinol; (f) α-tocopherol; (g) β-tocopherol; and (h) γ-tocopherol.

5.2.3 CONTAMINANTS

5.2.3.1 Herbicides and Other Pesticides

A method has recently been proposed for the simultaneous determination of cannabinoids, pesticides and mycotoxins, all in one analytical run, by LC-MS/MS. The main complication in this approach is the widely different concentrations of the three analyte classes in the plant: usually, cannabinoids are in the low per cent range, whereas pesticides are in the tens of ppb range and mycotoxin in the ppb range. The

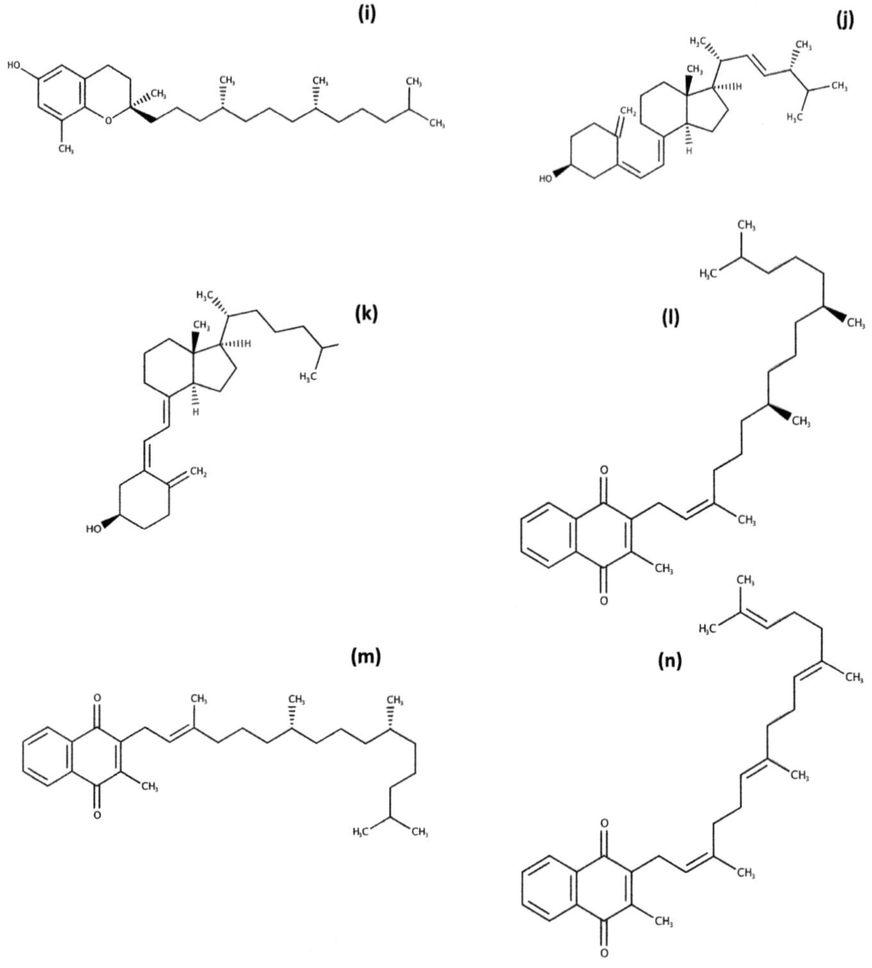

FIGURE 5.7I–N Chemical structures of (i) δ-tocopherol; (j) ergocalciferol; (k) cholecalciferol; (l) *cis*-phylloquinone; (m) *trans*-phylloquinone; and (n) menaquinone-4.

problem was solved by measuring high-intensity ^{12}C mass transitions for pesticides and mycotoxins while measuring low-intensity ^{13}C mass transitions for cannabinoids (Zweigenbaum and Pierri 2020).

Another paper has proposed two different methods, one based on LC-MS/MS and the other based on GC-MS/MS, for the multiresidue quantitation of 367 pesticides in *Cannabis* flowers (Maguire et al. 2019). Analyte extraction was carried out by acetonitrile treatment, followed by partition with QuEChERS salts. After centrifugation, samples were diluted and directly injected into the LC-MS/MS apparatus; for GC-MS/MS analysis, a further purification step was needed, carried out by dispersive SPE (dSPE) using a mixture of magnesium sulphate and primary/secondary amine (PSA), C18 and graphitised carbon black (GCB) sorbents.

A different LC-MS/MS method has been proposed for the quantitation of 42 pesticides in marijuana samples after extraction and partition with QuEChERS salts (Daniel et al. 2019).

Three different methods, based on LC-MS/MS, GC-MS/MS and GC-MS, have been proposed for the determination of pesticides in medical *Cannabis* leaves, dried flowers and oils (Moulins et al. 2018). The three methods share the same extraction solvent, namely acetonitrile, and the following pre-treatment step, which is carried out by dSPE and SPE, albeit with different sorbent and procedures: for leaves, endcapped C18 (C18-E) followed by lipid removal (Lipid) sorbent, then graphitised non-porous carbon (Carb) and amino sorbents were used; for flowers, QuEChERS salts, C18-E, Lipid and Carb sorbent were used; for oils, Lipid sorbent followed by NaCl-MgSO$_4$ mixing was used. Up to 72 different pesticides could be determined with these methods.

Three different multiresidue extraction methods have been assessed for the analysis of pesticides in hemp by LC-MS/MS. Of the 61 tested pesticides, 37 were accurately determined using acetate buffered QuEChERS, 40 with modified citrate buffered QuEChERS and 46 with standard citrate buffered QuEChERS, with the last one providing best results for most method performance parameters (Pérez-Parada et al. 2016).

5.2.3.2 Heavy Metals

Heavy metals are among the most common contaminants in all products of plant origin, including, of course, *Cannabis*-related products. In this field, the different kinds of atomic spectrometry are undoubtedly the most suitable and most frequently exploited methods, although X-ray fluorescence (XRF) spectrometry is also represented.

A graphite furnace-atomic absorption spectrometry (GF-AAS) method has recently been published (Ribeiro Menezes et al. 2021) for the analysis of total Pb, Cd and As in different edible fibre hemp products: seeds, oil, butter and protein extracts. After method optimisation by ExDe (factorial design), its application revealed worrying levels of Pb (about five times the commonly accepted limit of 0.2 µg/g) and safe levels of Cd. Arsenic was always lower than the limit of quantitation (LOQ) of 0.6 µg/g, which is satisfactory for product safety, but less satisfactory as concerns method performance (also, the LOQ for Pb was 0.4 µg/g, which is higher than the common limit in food of 0.2 µg/g).

The same three heavy metals (Pd, Cd, As) have been determined by the same technique (GF-AAS) in CBD-rich products for medical applications after alkaline solubilisation (Nascimento et al. 2020). Limits of quantitation were similar to those of the previous method, but with higher sensitivity toward Pb (0.26 µg/g vs. 0.4 µg/g).

An innovative extraction method of As (V) from hemp oil includes the use of liquid ALIQUAT 336 (*N*-methyl-*N,N,N*-trioctylammonium) adsorbed on multiwalled carbon nanotubes: this procedure exploits the well-known metal-extraction properties of ALIQUAT 336 coupled to the large contact surface of carbon nanotubes to achieve high ratios of analyte concentration (Laza et al. 2020). Quantitation is then carried out by XRF directly on the solid.

5.3   CONCLUSION

Despite many years of relative neglect, scientific attention for *Cannabis* and its derived products is on the rise worldwide. As a consequence, new analytical methods are being published for the determination of cannabinoids, other specialised metabolites and contaminants of *Cannabis*.

As one would expect, also due to binding national and international regulations, most recent methods are based on extremely selective techniques such as high- or ultrahigh-performance chromatography (HPLC, UHPLC, GC) coupled to different "flavours" of MS or HRMS. The coupling of high separative power and extreme, certifiable specificity of detection makes these methods the gold standard for most applications, in particular, for forensic applications.

Less expensive, more readily available instrumentation, such as HPLC-UV, -DAD, -FL and GC-FID, is being used for less performance-intensive applications and less stringent requirements; for example, to evaluate analyte stability or for purely informative purposes.

Other techniques (HPTLC, NMR, electrochemistry, microelectronics) are also represented but limited to proof-of-concept or specific applications for now. More specialised techniques, such as AAS, are applied in their narrow field of excellence (heavy metal contamination in the case of *Cannabis*).

Regarding sample pre-treatment and purification, solvent extraction is still the most frequent approach, both due to widespread use, well-known principles and easy application. It is usually applied through some auxiliary instrumental procedure, such as UAE, VAE and MAE, to provide better performance and/or higher throughput. Higher performing procedures are being increasingly applied, such as SPE, dSPE and SPME, but they are still hindered by higher costs and more complicated procedure development. For some techniques (NIR, MS/MS), direct analysis on the solid sample is also possible but seldom applied due to the additional complications they present.

BIBLIOGRAPHY

Ahmed M, Ji M, Qin P, Gu Z, Liu Y, Sikandar A, Iqbal M, Javeed A. 2019. Phytochemical screening, total phenolic and flavonoids contents and antioxidant activities of Citrullus colocynthis L. and Cannabis sativa L. *Applied Ecology and Environmental Research* 17:6961–6979.

American Herbal Pharmacopoeia. 2013. Cannabis inflorescence. Cannabis spp. Standards of identity, analysis, and quality control. 65p. Available at; https://herbal-ahp.com/collect ions/frontpage/products/Cannabis-inflorescence-quality-control-monograph, accessed February 10, 2021.

Bakro F, Jedryczka M, Wielgusz K, Sgorbini B, Inchingolo R, Cardenia V. 2020. Simultaneous determination of terpenes and cannabidiol in hemp (Cannabis sativa L.) by fast gas chromatography with flame ionization detection. *Journal of Separation Science* 43:2817–2826.

Baratta F, Simiele M, Pignata I, Ravetto Enri L, Torta R, De Luca A, Collino M, D'Avolio A, Brusa P. 2019. Development of standard operating protocols for the optimization of cannabis-based formulations for medical purposes. *Frontiers in Pharmacology* 10:701.

Basas-Jaumandreu J, De Las Heras FXC. 2020. GC-MS metabolite profile and identification of unusual homologous cannabinoids in high potency *Cannabis* sativa. *Planta Medica* 86(5):338–347.

Brighenti V, Licata M, Pedrazzi T, Maran D, Bertelli D, Pellati F, Benvenuti S. 2019. Development of a new method for the analysis of cannabinoids in honey by means of high-performance liquid chromatography coupled with electrospray ionisation-tandem mass spectrometry detection. *Journal of Chromatography A* 1597:179–186.

Callado CS-C, Núñez-Sánchez N, Casano S, Ferreiro-Vera C. 2018. The potential of near infrared spectroscopy to estimate the content of cannabinoids in Cannabis sativa L.: a comparative study. *Talanta* 190:147–157.

Carcieri C, Tomasello C, Simiele M, De Nicolò A, Avataneo V, Canzoneri L, Cusato J, Di Perri G, D'Avolio A. 2018. Cannabinoids concentration variability in cannabis olive oil galenic preparations. *Journal of Pharmacy and Pharmacology* 70:143–149.

Cardenia V, Gallina Toschi T, Scappini S, Rubino RC, Rodriguez-Estrada MT. 2018. Development and validation of a fast gas chromatography/mass spectrometry method for the determination of cannabinoids in *Cannabis* sativa L. *Journal of Food and Drug Analysis* 26(4):1283–1292.

Ciolino LA, Ranieri TL, Taylor AM. 2018. Commercial cannabis consumer products part 2: HPLC-DAD quantitative analysis of cannabis cannabinoids. *Forensic Science International* 289:438–447.

Cirrincione M, Zanfrognini B, Pigani L, Protti M, Mercolini L, Zanardi C. 2021. Development of an electrochemical sensor based on carbon black for the detection of cannabidiol in vegetable extracts. *Analyst* 146:612–619.

Citti C, Ciccarella G, Braghiroli D, Parenti C, Vandelli MA, Cannazza G. 2016. Medicinal cannabis: principal cannabinoids concentration and their stability evaluated by a high performance liquid chromatography coupled to diode array and quadrupole time of flight mass spectrometry method. *Journal of Pharmaceutical and Biomedical Analysis* 128:201–209.

Citti C, Pacchetti B, Vandelli MA, Forni F, Cannazza G. 2018. Analysis of cannabinoids in commercial hemp seed oil and decarboxylation kinetics studies of cannabidiolic acid (CBDA). *Journal of Pharmaceutical and Biomedical Analysis* 149:532–540.

Citti C, Russo F, Sgrò S, Gallo A, Zanotto A, Forni F, Vandelli MA, Laganà A, Montone CM, Gigli G. 2020. Pitfalls in the analysis of phytocannabinoids in cannabis inflorescence. *Analytical and Bioanalytical Chemistry* 412:4009–4022.

Comeau ZJ, Boileau NT, Lee T, Melville OA, Rice NA, Troung Y, Harris CS, Lessard BH, Shuhendler AJ. 2019. On-the-Spot Detection and Speciation of Cannabinoids Using Organic Thin-Film Transistors. *ACS Sensors* 4:2706–2715.

Daniel D, Lopes FS, do Lago CL. 2019. A sensitive multiresidue method for the determination of pesticides in marijuana by liquid chromatography–tandem mass spectrometry. *Journal of Chromatography A* 1603:231–239.

Dei Cas M, Casagni E, Saccardo A, Arnoldi S, Young C, Scotti S, de Manicor EV, Gambaro V, Roda G. 2020. The Italian panorama of cannabis light preparation: determination of cannabinoids by LC-UV. *Forensic Science International* 307:110113.

del Mar Contreras M, Jurado-Campos N, Callado CS-C, Arroyo-Manzanares N, Fernandez L, Casano S, Marco S, Arce L, Ferreiro-Vera C. 2018. Thermal desorption-ion mobility spectrometry: a rapid sensor for the detection of cannabinoids and discrimination of Cannabis sativa L. chemotypes. *Sensors and Actuators B: Chemical* 273:1413–1424.

Di Marco Pisciottano I, Guadagnuolo G, Soprano V, De Crescenzo M, Gallo P. 2018. A rapid method to determine nine natural cannabinoids in beverages and food derived from Cannabis sativa by liquid chromatography coupled to tandem mass spectrometry on a QTRAP 4000. *Rapid Communications in Mass Spectrometry* 32:1728–1736.

Drugs UNOo. 2009. *Recommended Methods for the Identification and Analysis of Cannabis and Cannabis Products: Manual for Use by National Drug Testing Laboratories.* New York@ United Nations Publications.

Fu Q, Shu Z, Deng K, Luo X, Zeng C. 2016. Simultaneous determination of three kinds of effective constituents in cannabis plants by reversed-phase HPLC. *Fa yi xue za zhi* 32:261–263.

Gul W, Gul SW, Chandra S, Lata H, Ibrahim EA, ElSohly MA. 2018. Detection and quantification of cannabinoids in extracts of cannabis sativa roots using LC-MS/MS. *Planta Medica* 84(4):267–271.

Gür M, Verep D, Güney K, Güder A, Altuner EM. Determination of some flavonoids and antimicrobial behaviour of some plants' extracts. *Indian Journal of Pharmaceutical Education and Research* 51(3s):s225–s229.

Hädener M, König S, Weinmann W. 2019. Quantitative determination of CBD and THC and their acid precursors in confiscated cannabis samples by HPLC-DAD. *Forensic Science International* 299:142–150.

Ibrahim EA, Gul W, Gul SW, Stamper BJ, Hadad GM, Abdel Salam RA, Ibrahim AK, Ahmed SA, Chandra S, Lata H, Radwan MM, Elsohly MA. 2018. Determination of acid and neutral cannabinoids in extracts of different strains of *Cannabis* sativa using GC-FID. *Planta Medica* 84(4):250–259.

Ibrahim EA, Wang M, Radwan MM, Wanas AS, Majumdar CG, Avula B, Wang Y-H, Khan IA, Chandra S, Lata H. 2019. Analysis of terpenes in Cannabis sativa L. Using GC/MS: method development, validation, and application. *Planta Medica* 85:431–438.

Kleinhenz MD, Magnin G, Ensley SM, Griffin JJ, Goeser J, Lynch E, Coetzee JF. 2020. Nutrient concentrations, digestibility, and cannabinoid concentrations of industrial hemp plant components. *Applied Animal Science* 36:489–494.

Layton CE, Aubin AJ. 2018. Method validation for assay determination of cannabidiol isolates. *Journal of Liquid Chromatography & Related Technologies* 41:114–121.

Laza A, Orozco E, Baldo MF, Raba J, Aranda PR. 2020. Determination of arsenic (V) in cannabis oil by adsorption on multiwall carbon nanotubes thin film using XRF technique. *Microchemical Journal* 158:105265.

Leghissa A, Hildenbrand ZL, Schug KA. 2018. A review of methods for the chemical characterization of cannabis natural products. *Journal of Separation Science* 41:398–415.

Leiman K, Colomo L, Armenta S, de la Guardia M, Esteve-Turrillas FA. 2018. Fast extraction of cannabinoids in marijuana samples by using hard-cap espresso machines. *Talanta* 190:321–326.

Madej K, Kózka G, Winiarski M, Piekoszewski W. 2020. A simple, fast, and green oil sample preparation method for determination of cannabidioloic acid and cannabidiol by HPLC-DAD. *Separations* 7:60.

Maguire WJ, Call CW, Cerbu C, Jambor KL, Benavides-Montes VE. 2019. Comprehensive determination of unregulated pesticide residues in Oregon cannabis flower by liquid chromatography paired with triple quadrupole mass spectrometry and gas chromatography paired with triple quadrupole mass spectrometry. *Journal of Agricultural and Food Chemistry* 67:12670–12674.

Mandrioli M, Tura M, Scotti S, Gallina Toschi T. 2019. Fast detection of 10 Cannabinoids by RP-HPLC-UV method in Cannabis sativa L. *Molecules* 24:2113.

Marchei E, Tittarelli R, Pellegrini M, Rotolo MC, Pacifici R, Pichini S. 2020. Is "light *Cannabis*" really light? Determination of cannabinoids content in commercial products. *Clinical Chemistry and Laboratory Medicine* 58(9):E175–E177.

Marchetti L, Brighenti V, Rossi MC, Sperlea J, Pellati F, Bertelli D. 2019. Use of 13C-qNMR spectroscopy for the analysis of non-psychoactive cannabinoids in fibre-type Cannabis sativa L.(Hemp). *Molecules* 24:1138.

McRae G, Melanson JE. 2020. Quantitative determination and validation of 17 cannabinoids in cannabis and hemp using liquid chromatography-tandem mass spectrometry. *Analytical and Bioanalytical Chemistry* 412:7381–7393.

Meng Q, Buchanan B, Zuccolo J, Poulin M-M, Gabriele J, Baranowski DC. 2018. A reliable and validated LC-MS/MS method for the simultaneous quantification of 4 cannabinoids in 40 consumer products. *PLoS One* 13:e0196396.

Moulins JR, Blais M, Montsion K, Tully J, Mohan W, Gagnon M, McRitchie T, Kwong K, Snider N, Blais DR. 2018. Multiresidue method of analysis of pesticides in medical cannabis. *Journal of AOAC International* 101:1948–1960.

Mudge EM, Brown PN. 2020. Determination of Cannabinoids in Cannabis sativa Dried Flowers and Oils by LC-UV: Single-Laboratory Validation, First Action 2018.10. *Journal of AOAC International* 103:489–493.

Nascimento PA, Schultz J, Gonzalez MH, Oliveira A. 2020. Simple GFAAS method for determination of Pb, As, and Cd in cannabidiol extracts used for therapeutic purposes. *Journal of the Brazilian Chemical Society* 31:894–903.

Nemeškalová A, Hájková K, Mikulů L, Sýkora D, Kuchař M. 2020. Combination of UV and MS/MS detection for the LC analysis of cannabidiol-rich products. *Talanta* 219:121250.

O'Keefe SF, Ackman RG. 1986. Vitamins A, D_3 and E in Nova Scotian cod liver oils. *Proceedings of the Nova Scotian Institute of Science* 37:1–7.

Patel B, Wene D, Fan ZT. 2017. Qualitative and quantitative measurement of cannabinoids in cannabis using modified HPLC/DAD method. *Journal of Pharmaceutical and Biomedical Analysis* 146:15–23.

Pérez-Parada A, Alonso B, Rodríguez C, Besil N, Cesio V, Diana L, Burgueño A, Bazzurro P, Bojorge A, Gerez N. 2016. Evaluation of three multiresidue methods for the determination of pesticides in marijuana (Cannabis sativa L.) with liquid chromatography-tandem mass spectrometry. *Chromatographia* 79:1069–1083.

Ribeiro Menezes I, Nascimento PdA, Gonzalez MH, Oliveira A. 2021. Simple and Robust GFAAS methods for determination of As, Cd, and Pb in Hemp products using different sample preparation strategies. *Food Analytical Methods*14:1043–1053.

Rocha ED, Silva VE, Pereira F, Jean VM, Souza FLC, Baratto LC, Vieira A, Carvalho VM. 2020. Qualitative terpene profiling of Cannabis varieties cultivated for medical purposes. *Rodriguésia* 71:e01192019. https://doi.org/10.1590/2175-7860202071040.

Saingam W, Sakunpak A. 2018. Development and validation of reverse phase high performance liquid chromatography method for the determination of delta-9-tetrahydrocannabinol and cannabidiol in oromucosal spray from cannabis extract. *Revista Brasileira de Farmacognosia* 28:669–672.

Schmidt T, Kramell AE, Oehler F, Kluge R, Demske D, Tarasov PE, Csuk R. 2020. Identification and quantification of cannabinol as a biomarker for local hemp retting in an ancient sedimentary record by HPTLC-ESI-MS. *Analytical and Bioanalytical Chemistry* 412:1–12.

Smeriglio A, Galati EM, Monforte MT, Lanuzza F, D'Angelo V, Circosta C. 2016. Polyphenolic compounds and antioxidant activity of cold-pressed seed oil from Finola Cultivar of Cannabis sativa L. *Phytotherapy Research* 30:1298–1307.

Thalhamer B, Himmelsbach M, Buchberger W. 2017. Trace level determination of Δ^9-tetrahydrocannabinol in a perfume using liquid chromatography high resolution tandem mass spectrometry and gas chromatography mass spectrometry. *Flavour and Fragrance Journal* 32:46–53.

Tyśkiewicz K, Gieysztor R, Maziarczyk I, Hodurek P, Rój E, Skalicka-Woźniak K. 2018. Supercritical fluid chromatography with photodiode array detection in the determination of fat-soluble vitamins in hemp seed oil and waste fish oil. *Molecules* 23:1131.

Tzimas PS, Petrakis EA, Halabalaki M, Skaltsounis LA. 2021. Effective determination of the principal non-psychoactive cannabinoids in fiber-type Cannabis sativa L. by UPLC-PDA following a comprehensive design and optimization of extraction methodology. *Analytica Chimica Acta* 1150:338200.

Wang M, Wang YH, Avula B, Radwan MM, Wanas AS, Mehmedic Z, van Antwerp J, ElSohly MA, Khan IA. 2017. Quantitative determination of cannabinoids in cannabis and cannabis products using ultra-high-performance supercritical fluid chromatography and diode array/mass spectrometric detection. *Journal of Forensic Sciences* 62:602–611.

Wang Y-H, Avula B, ElSohly MA, Radwan MM, Wang M, Wanas AS, Mehmedic Z, Khan IA. 2018. Quantitative determination of Δ^9-THC, CBG, CBD, their acid precursors and five other neutral cannabinoids by UHPLC-UV-MS. *Planta Medica* 84:260–266.

Zhang X, Danaceau JP, Chambers EE, Quantitative analysis of THC and its metabolites in plasma using Oasis PRiME HLB for Toxicology and Forensic Laboratories. Available from https://www.waters.com/waters/library.htm?locale=en_US&lid=13491677, accessed on February 10, 2021

Zekič J, Križman M. 2020. Development of gas-chromatographic method for simultaneous determination of cannabinoids and terpenes in hemp. *Molecules* 25(24):Article no. 5872.

Zivovinovic S, Alder R, Allenspach MD, Steuer C. 2018. Determination of cannabinoids in Cannabis sativa L. samples for recreational, medical, and forensic purposes by reversed-phase liquid chromatography-ultraviolet detection. *Journal of Analytical Science and Technology* 9:1–10.

Zweigenbaum J, Pierri A. 2020. Marihuana safety: potency of cannabinoids, pesticide residues, and mycotoxin in one analysis by LC/MS/MS. *Analysis of Cannabis* 90:339.

6 Cannabis Microbial Testing
Methodologies and Considerations

Kyle Boyar

CONTENTS

DOI: 10.1201/9780429274893-6

6.1   INTRODUCTION

The microbial testing of cannabis and cannabis products presents a unique set of challenges. Unlike food testing, cannabis testing has various routes of administration to consider. Cannabis flowers express high levels of antimicrobial cannabinoids and terpenoids and thus represent a different matrix from traditional foods (Appendino et al. 2008). It is currently estimated that 70% of cannabis is consumed via vaporizing or smoking oils and flowers while the remaining 30% is consumed in marijuana-infused products or MIPs, which can encompass a variety of matrices (LeafLink 2020).

In a testing landscape that consistently focuses heavily on chemical analysis, the microbiological testing of cannabis is often overlooked. However, it is truly one of the most important analyses in the context of product safety because the accidental ingestion or inhalation of these contaminants can cause severe illnesses, infections, or worse, death. These contaminants are especially of concern for those with compromised immune function but are not limited to these populations.

The present chapter explores the microbial contaminants of interest in cannabis, current testing methodologies, and the challenges that testing laboratories face in this continuously evolving domain. Different perspectives for ensuring product safety are presented in the context of current regulations and their varying approaches. Tactics for the remediation of contaminated products and preventative strategies used by cultivators are also discussed in the context of the existing incongruent patchwork of regulatory framework. Microbial testing acceptance criteria, methods, and recommendations from various standards organizations are presented and efforts toward the standardization and development of reference methods are highlighted.

6.2 TYPES OF CANNABIS MICROBIOLOGICAL TESTING: TOTAL COUNTS AND PATHOGENS

Microbial testing for cannabis entails two different primary types of tests: total count tests and pathogen tests. Total count tests are broad tests that quantify specific classes of microorganisms while pathogen tests are targeted toward microorganisms that are known to cause illness in humans. Both types of testing arguably have their place, total count tests serve as a general reference point for how clean a cannabis sample is and can indicate the cleanliness of an operation. However, these tests cannot discern between what is harmful and what is not, therefore, solely utilizing these as a measure for product safety is inadequate. Species-specific testing for pathogens on the other hand can definitively determine whether a contaminant that is harmful to human health is present. Using a combination of these two test types, one can assess a product's safety.

Microbial testing for foods differs from cannabis in that the test masses utilized in these sectors are significantly greater. Typically, food testing employs 25-, 50-, and 100-gram sample sizes with established sampling protocols to produce a statistically relevant sample (Andrews and Hammack 2003). Cannabis, on the other hand, often only utilizes a single gram for analysis and sampling methods widely vary depending on the jurisdiction. This significant difference in test mass is largely due to the cost of the material being tested, which in the case of some kinds of cannabis extracts, can be upwards of US$100 per gram retail. Additionally, unlike food, cannabis has few reference methods to draw upon. Sampling practices vary widely from state to state, which also contributes to interlaboratory variation in results.

6.3 THE ROLE OF WATER ACTIVITY IN MICROBIAL GROWTH

The water activity (A_w) of a product is the ratio between the vapor pressure of the product itself, when in a headspace with the surrounding air media, and the vapor pressure of distilled water under identical conditions. An A_w value of 0.80 means the vapor pressure is 80% of that of pure water. The water activity increases with temperature. The moisture condition of a product can be expressed in a percentage as equilibrium relative humidity (ERH) or as the water activity that is expressed as a decimal. Water activity is not to be confused with general moisture content, which determines the amount of water by mass while water activity measures how much water is available for microbial growth. Water activity is considered a critical control point for preventing microbial contamination. Controlling water activity is a key component of a product's shelf life and stability (Roggen 2019).

Water activity is measured by equilibrating the liquid phase water in the sample with the vapor phase water in the headspace of a closed chamber and measuring the equilibrium relative humidity (ERH) in the headspace using a sensor. The relative humidity can be determined using a resistive electrolytic sensor, a chilled mirror sensor, or a capacitive hygroscopic polymer sensor.

Each microorganism has an ideal water activity maintaining the level that is essential for its reproduction. Any time water activity levels drop lower than this value, it dehydrates the microorganism and creates a state of osmotic pressure. This causes the organism to use energy to maintain desirable water activity and ultimately leads to its demise.

Dried biomass will typically have a water activity in the 0.50 to 0.70 A_w range. While the growth of pathogenic bacteria would pose the greatest risk at the typical water activity of biomass, the more likely contamination source is molds. All molds, except a few rare xerophilic species, stop growing at water activities less than 0.70 (Cannabis Science Tech). While molds are not particularly dangerous if consumed, some can produce mycotoxins as part of their metabolism, and these can cause severe reactions depending on the level of exposure. In addition, the presence of actively growing mold also means the presence of mold spores. This can be particularly dangerous for a product that is inhaled, resulting in mold spores in the respiratory tract, which can lead to wheezing and other asthmatic symptoms. Consequently, the water activity of any harvested biomass being stored or transported needs to be below 0.70 A_w. This means that water activity testing should begin with cultivators and processors.

6.4   STATE REGULATIONS FOR WATER ACTIVITY

Currently, governmental oversight of the production and selling of cannabis is handled at the state level with the actual state department varying by state. Consequently, regulations vary extensively between states. Water activity currently only appears in the regulations or guidance documents for a few states, and these tend to be the states that have had some form of legalized cannabis for the longest time, and therefore, have the most mature regulations. It is expected that additional states will add water activity testing requirements to their regulations as markets mature, and if regulations move to the federal level, water activity will likely be included in any national regulations or guidelines.

States that currently include water activity in their cannabis regulations include (Cannabis Science Tech):

- Nevada-NAC 453A.654: Required quality assurance tests; submission of wet marijuana for testing. NAC 453A.550: "Potentially hazardous marijuana products and ingredients" defined.
- California-CA Section 19344–5322: Water activity and moisture content.
- Oregon-OAR 333-007-0300 to 333-007-0500 and OAR 333-064-0100 to 333-064-0130: Must test water activity on usable marijuana for sales or further processing.
- Washington-WAC 314-55-102: Quality assurance testing Part (i) Moisture analysis. Must test water activity on usable marijuana intended for retail sale or further processing.

In addition to the inclusion of water activity in state cannabis regulations, ASTM standards have been established for water activity in cannabis. These include:

- ASTM D8916-18: Standard practice for determining water activity.
- ASTM D8197-18: Standard for maintaining water activity.

6.5 TOTAL COUNT TESTS AND THEIR THRESHOLDS

6.5.1 TOTAL YEAST AND MOLD

TYM, or total yeast and mold count, is the number of colony-forming units present per gram of product (CFU/g). A colony-forming unit is the measurement of counting and reporting the population of live bacteria or yeast and mold in a product. To determine the count, the cannabis sample is plated on a petri dish at different dilutions which are then incubated at 25–28°C for 48–60 hours (rapid methods) or three to five days using traditional media (Cannabis Science Tech). During this time, the yeast and mold present will grow and reproduce. Each colony is a type of yeast or mold in present in the sample and produces on spot on the dish which can vary in size. Each isolated growth is considered a colony-forming unit which is then multiplied by the appropriate dilution factor to get a total CFU/g count. Depending on the jurisdiction, this value can change, but typically a threshold of 10,000 CFU/g signifies a failure for TYM (Upton et al. 2014). As we will discuss later in the chapter, TYM methodology for cannabis and cannabis products is an ongoing discussion and there are a number of factors that should be considered.

6.5.2 TOTAL AEROBIC COUNT

Total aerobic count (TAC) tests are used as an indication of bacterial contamination on a cannabis sample. In the food industry, testing labs use TAC tests to gauge a manufacturer's sanitary quality and adherence to good manufacturing practices. However, TAC tests are unable to differentiate between pathogenic, beneficial, and benign bacteria, making them poor indicators of safety. A low TAC result does not mean a cannabis sample is free of pathogens. Similarly, a high TAC result does not mean a sample is harmful to consumers. This is especially true in cannabis, which has a diverse microbiome of beneficial microbes that are not harmful to humans. For example, many organic cannabis growers utilize the aerobic bacteria *Bacillus* as a fungicide which will trigger these tests. Depending on the jurisdiction, this value can change, but typically a threshold of 100,000 CFU/g signifies a failure for TAC.

6.5.3 TOTAL COLIFORMS

Coliform bacteria are defined as rod-shaped gram-negative, non-spore forming, motile or non-motile bacteria, which can ferment lactose with the production of acid and gas when incubated at 35–37°C. These organisms are naturally found in the digestive tracts of humans, however, there are some species that can cause illness. Depending on the jurisdiction, this value can change, but typically a threshold of 1000 CFU/g signifies a failure for total coliforms (TC) (Upton et al. 2014).

6.5.4 BILE TOLERANT GRAM-NEGATIVE

Bile-tolerant gram-negative (BTGN) bacteria can survive in the human stomach (bile-tolerant) and they have a protective cell wall that causes them to turn red when subjected to the gram staining process (gram-negative). This combination of characteristics makes BTGN bacteria potentially harmful to humans.

Gram-negative bacteria thrive in virtually all environments that support life. They are an important medical challenge because the outer membrane that protects them from gram staining also protects them from many antibiotics, detergents, and antimicrobial enzymes produced by the immune system. In fact, when immune cells lyse gram-negative bacteria cells, it can cause a toxic reaction that can include an increased respiratory rate and low blood pressure—a life-threatening condition known as septic shock. Depending on the jurisdiction, this value can change, but typically, a threshold of 1000 CFU/g signifies a failure for BTGN (Upton et al. 2014).

Interestingly, recent studies have demonstrated that cannabidiol is effective against this particular class of bacteria including those that are notoriously resistant to traditional antibiotics such as *Neisseria gonorrhoeae* and MRSA. Cannabidiol derivatives are being further investigated for their antimicrobial potential (Blaskovich et al. 2021).

6.6 PATHOGENS OF INTEREST IN CANNABIS AND CANNABIS PRODUCTS

The detection of pathogenic fungi and bacteria is of the utmost importance in cannabis products as many users are immunocompromised and are at risk of contracting opportunistic infections. The primary pathogens that are tested in cannabis include *Aspergillus* spp., *Salmonella*, and Shiga-toxin producing *Escherichia coli* (STEC). Some states like California only test for pathogens while other states have opted to include total count tests in their mandated microbial analysis.

6.6.1 *ASPERGILLUS*

Aspergillus spp. are by far the most common pathogen found in cannabis, and interestingly, some species are also endophytes of the cannabis plant. *Aspergillus* spp. are by far the number one consideration for inhalable cannabis products. However, many of the Aspergilli found in cannabis are not pathogenic, and therefore, it is important to be able to distinguish between those that produce mycotoxins as opposed to the less harmful and non-toxigenic species.

Aspergillus spp. are widespread and exposure to hyphal fragments and airborne conidia is universal. However, in those who are immunocompromised, exposure can cause aspergillosis, a lung infection where the pathogen colonizes the lungs, which, in some cases, can be fatal. These lung infections are not limited to the immunocompromised and have been well documented in the literature in even immunocompetent cannabis users (Upton et al. 2014; Blaskovich et al. 2021; Thompson et al. 2017; Sutton et al. 1986; Verweij et al. 2000; Ruchlemer et al. 2015; Gargani et al. 2011; Bal et al. 2010; Szyper-Kravitz et al. 2001; Marks et al. 1996; Llamas et al. 1978; Hamadeh et al. 1988; CHUSID et al. 1975; Cescon et al. 2008; Remington et al. 2015). Specifically, four pathogenic species of *Aspergillus* are tested for in Alaska, California, Colorado, Nevada, and others, and have been routinely found to represent the vast majority of failures for microbial testing at least in the state of California (*A. flavus*, *A. fumigatus*, *A. niger*, *A. terreus*) (Table 6.1). It is important to note that the numbers in the table only represent compliance testing batches and are therefore a low representation of the overall failures within the state.

While states cannot mandate the type of methodology used, the case for molecular methods in the context of *Aspergillus* is quite strong. The first reason behind this thinking is *Aspergillus* species are very difficult to discern with the naked eye and even highly trained mycologists can mistake the non-pathogenic forms for the pathogenic ones. This is exemplified in a case from Alaska where the state lab had to referee a dispute between two testing labs (Boyar 2019; Maguire 2018). Lab A using molecular methods passed the particular sample while Lab B failed it using culture-based methods. Sequencing of the sample in question revealed that Lab B

TABLE 6.1
Current Microbial Failure Rate in the State of California

Certificates of analysis received	Tested batches	Failed batches
153,000	153,000	7,535

Tested batches by category	Tested batches	Failed batches by category
Flower	71,733	3176
Inhalable (Cartridges, waxes, etc.)	57,857	2702
Other (Edibles, tinctures, topicals, etc.)	23,410	1657
Total	153,000	7535

Reasons for failure*	Failed batches by category
Label claims	2379
Pesticides	2303
Microbial impurities	1316
Residual solvents	399
Homogeneity	36
Foreign material	38
Moisture	71
Heavy metals	883
Water activity	120
Cannabinoids	116
Mycotoxins	12
Injurious to human health	2
Total:	7675

*Batches can fail for multiple categories

Cannabis Batch Testing Certificates of Analysis as of October 23, 2020. Source: Bureau of Cannabis Control.

had mistakenly identified *A. niger* as non-pathogenic *A. brasiliensis*. These kinds of mistakes can easily be remedied by the use of targeted PCR primer sets that are specific to the species of interest. Second, plating is limited by its unit of quantification, the colony-forming unit (CFU). *Aspergillus* tends to exhibit the formation of heterogeneous macrocolonies making accurate CFU per gram quantitation a very difficult proposition (Figure 6.1). Third, some studies have suggested that molecular methods exhibit much better detection than traditional plating methods, however,

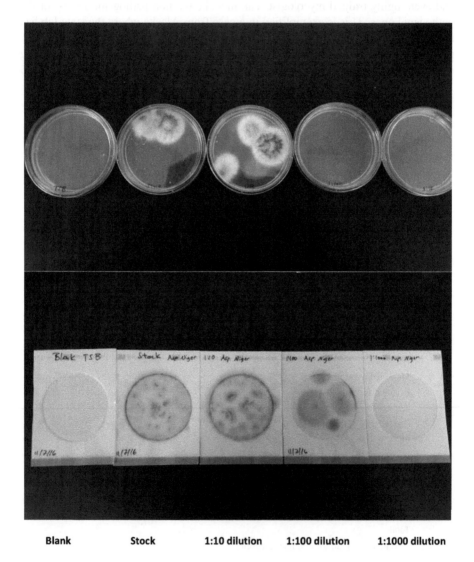

| Blank | Stock | 1:10 dilution | 1:100 dilution | 1:1000 dilution |

FIGURE 6.1   *Aspergillus* heterogeneous macrocolonies plated on SabDex agar (top) and rapid total yeast and mold 3M Petrifilm, which demonstrate why plating and the CFU/g unit is limiting when detecting and quantifying *Aspergillus* (Boyar, 2019).

this is currently under debate within the scientific community (Boyar 2019; Esposito or MC Labs 2021; McKernan et al. 2016).

6.6.2 *SALMONELLA* SPP.

Salmonella spp. are a group of gram-negative, rod-shaped bacteria that cause typhoid fever, gastroenteritis, and other illnesses. While the occurrence of *Salmonella* spp. is rare in cannabis, it cannot be ruled out as many organic farmers do utilize materials such as chicken feces as fertilizers for their soil. In January and February of 1981, 85 cases of enteritis caused by *Salmonella muenchen* were reported in the *New England Journal of Medicine* in Ohio, Michigan, Georgia, and Alabama. Initial investigation failed to implicate a food source as a common vehicle, but in Michigan, 76% of the patients, in contrast to 21% of the control subjects, admitted personal or household exposure to marijuana (P<0.001). Marijuana samples obtained from patients' households contained as many as 10^7 CFUs of *S. muenchen* per gram (Taylor et al. 1982).

6.6.3 SHIGA-TOXIN PRODUCING *E. COLI*

STEC is a group of *E. coli* that produce a Shiga toxin, which can induce stomach cramps and diarrhea that is often bloody. The most common of these STECs is the O157:H7 serovar. The presence of this group of *E. coli* is tested for on a qualitative presence/absence basis for ingestible products in most states with legal cannabis.

6.7 OTHER POTENTIAL ORGANISMS OF CONCERN

With people's cannabis use in the dark for so many years, and recently coming out of the shadows, cases of illness due to cannabis consumption are becoming more openly reported. Specifically, there have been instances of other molds such as *Rhizopus* (*Mucor*) leading to fatalities in cannabis users (Stone et al. 2019). Additionally, there are documented cases of immunocompetent users contracting meningitis derived from *Cryptococcus neoformans* contaminated cannabis (Shapiro et al. 2018). These organisms should be monitored to keep the public safe, however, proficiency testing for these microorganisms is lacking, which makes it difficult to mandate testing for these pathogens.

6.7.1 *BOTRYTIS CINEREA*

Botrytis cinerea is a necrotrophic fungus that affects many plant species, although its most notable hosts may be wine grapes. In viticulture, it is commonly known as "botrytis bunch rot"; in horticulture, it is usually called gray mold. It is a systemic infection and can remain dormant for long periods of time before sporulating. Botrytis often expresses itself from the inside out of a plant, which is why it is not readily apparent that infection has taken place until post-harvest when one breaks open a larger cola of cannabis only to find cobweb-like structures hidden.

6.7.2 *FUSARIUM* SPP.

Fusarium is a large genus of soil-borne filamentous fungi, part of a group often referred to as hyphomycetes that infects the root systems of plants and travels through the plant's vascular system to produce what is known as Fusarium wilt. An analogy to *Fusarium* infection would be that of arterial plaques whereby the circulatory system becomes clogged and the flow of blood containing nutrients is restricted. The fungus causes necrotic lesions throughout the xylem that causes various branches of the plant to become wilted as the disease progresses.

Interestingly, the US government investigated and genetically modified *F. oxysporum* as a cannabis eradication tool in the 1990s against the concerns of David Struhs, the Secretary of the Florida Department of Environmental Protection, who spelled out the dangers in a letter to Mr. McDonough (Head of Florida's Office of Drug Control) dated April 6, 1999. "Fusarium species are capable of evolving rapidly. Mutagenicity is by far the most disturbing factor in attempting to use a Fusarium species as a bioherbicide. It is difficult, if not impossible, to control the spread of Fusarium species" (Bragg 1999).

Some species of *Fusarium* produce mycotoxins themselves, for example, fumonisins, zearalenone, and trichothecenes. In a survey of mycotoxin residues in cannabis products by LC-MS/MS in Oregon conducted by Maguire et al. (2018), one in a hundred samples contained mycotoxin residues. Personal correspondence with Maguire indicated that this number may actually be much higher than initially estimated in his work:

> However, since that time we've been testing a lot more flower and extracts, and the frequency of samples positive for mycotoxins is much higher, closer to 1:15 or 1:20. In the majority of cases, these residues are fusarium toxins (nivalenol and its derivatives, zearalenone, or fumonisins) and found in extracts rather than flowers. Fusarium toxins are far more prevalent than Aspergillus in cannabis.
>
> **(Maguire 2018)**

The extent to which these *Fusarium* mycotoxins are of concern for human health is unclear as there have not been thorough investigations conducted on their inhalation in the context of cannabis use. More work is needed to determine the risk they pose to human health.

6.7.3 *LISTERIA* SPP.

Listeria is a gram-positive, rod-shaped bacterium that is found in contaminated foods. Listeria is typically soil-borne, which can lead to plant contamination. Animals that eat contaminated vegetation can become carriers. Therefore, it should come as no surprise the bacterium has been found on and in a variety of food types including meats, dairy products, fruits, and vegetables. To date, there have been no documented cases of listeria due to cannabis, however, due to the wide variety of matrices involved in cannabis products, this pathogen is something that regulators are keeping a close eye on.

6.7.4 *LEGIONELLA*

Legionella is a genus of gram-negative bacteria that includes the species *P. pneumophila*, the causal agent of a pneumonia-like illness called Legionnaires' disease. *Legionella* is found naturally in bodies of water where it typically takes residence in various types of amoebas.

Advanced age, diabetes, chronic immunosuppressive conditions, and tobacco use are risk factors for Legionnaires' disease and the literature suggests that cannabis users are at increased risk for the development of this condition due to THC's ability to lower immunity and this risk may be additive to that of tobacco use (Nguyen et al. 2010). In 2019, the Canadian licensed producer Organigram was linked to an outbreak of Legionnaires' disease that led to the hospitalization of 16 consumers. The source was found to be the cooling towers atop its production facility that had previously been cited as a potential source of such outbreaks (Magee 2020).

6.7.5 *RHIZOPUS, MUCOR, AND RHIZOMUCOR*

Mucormycosis is an angioinvasive disease caused by species of the order Mucorales, most commonly of the genera *Rhizopus*, *Mucor*, and *Rhizomucor*. Mucormycosis most commonly manifests as rhino-orbital-cerebral infection but may also present as pulmonary, cutaneous, gastrointestinal, central nervous system, or disseminated infection. Disease is typically seen in immunocompromised patients, including those with diabetes mellitus, particularly in the setting of diabetic ketoacidosis (Spellberg et al. 2005). There has been at least one documented fatality of pulmonary mucormycosis from the inhalation of contaminated cannabis (Stone et al. 2019).

6.7.6 POWDERY MILDEW

While not necessarily a concern for human health, powdery mildew is an obligate biotroph that can vascularize into the plant tissue and remain invisible to cultivators. It tends to emerge and sporulate two weeks into flowering thus destroying very mature crops with severe economic consequences. It is believed to travel in clones, and it is not known if it travels in seeds. It is interesting to note that the powdery mildew found on cannabis is not the same powdery mildew observed to infect other species.

It is important to note that there are numerous varieties of powdery mildew that infect different types of plants. Whole genome shotgun sequencing of a variety of cannabis-derived powdery mildew samples from across North America suggests that the type of powdery mildew that infects cannabis is a novel species showing greatest similarity in its internal transcribed spacer region (ITS) to *Golovinomyces ambrosiae* and *Golovinomyces orontii* (McKernan 2017).

6.8 METHODOLOGY: CULTURE-BASED VS. MOLECULAR

There is currently much debate among the cannabis-testing community about which methodologies are most appropriate for the microbial testing of cannabis. Frankly, they all have their own merits depending on the context in which they are used (Beadle 2021).

Culture-based techniques have represented the standard for some time, however, when one looks at the core of the concept, these are simply growth mediums that are meant to be selective based on the various ingredients and antibiotics used. The advantage of these methods is that they are much cheaper than molecular methods and typically cost between $1 and $3 per plate. However, plating techniques are not always as selective as they are often touted to be, especially when dealing with the cannabis matrix. A peer-reviewed study from McKernan et al. published in 2016 highlights this lack of selectivity via metagenomic analysis of the plates used to test cannabis. Specifically, total yeast and molds (TYM) counts are most affected by this lack of selectivity—in some cases, the reads from the plates surveyed displayed up to 60% bacterial growth (McKernan et al. 2016). Figure 6.2 provides an example of 16S ITS rDNA (bacterial) sequencing data performed on a total yeast and mold culture system highlighting the lack of specificity seen in these systems. This lack of specificity puts cultivators in a difficult spot as many of their crops will fail for what are often completely benign bacterial communities that can be beneficial for staving off more harmful microbial contaminants, which will be discussed further in a later section of this chapter.

In the context of yeasts and molds, molecular methods such as qPCR can provide much greater selectivity via amplification of internal transcribed spacer (ITS) regions. These are evolutionarily conserved regions of DNA associated with different classes of microbial contaminants. However, there are caveats to this, and certain types of fungi can have multiple copies of these ITS regions that could lead to

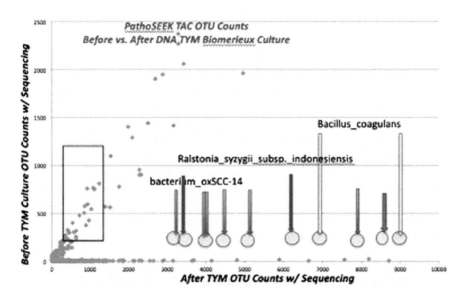

FIGURE 6.2 Metagenomic data that highlights a lack of specificity with culture-based TYM methods (McKernan, 2017).

higher counts depending on their composition. Additionally, those who are in favor of culture-based techniques often cite the lack of selectivity for live vs. dead DNA, however, there are economical methods available on the market for selective removal of dead DNA during sample preparation (Medical Genomics; Bio-Rad).

Another area where molecular methods have an advantage over plating techniques is their ability to detect endofungal pathogens such as *Ralstonia*, which acts as both a plant and human pathogen causing wilting in the former and potential lung infections in the latter (Coenye et al. 2002; Peeters et al. 2013; Boyar 2019). Plating techniques are unable to detect these pathogens as they reside intracellularly and infect many endophytic fungi found in cannabis such as *Aspergillus* and *Penicillium* (Boyar 2019).

However, there is controversy regarding the use of qPCR for total count tests that survey broad classes of microorganisms. Critics cite the ITS copy number variation mentioned previously as a challenge for developing equations that accurately convert Cq values produced by qPCR into the CFU/g values that are required by regulation. Concerns about the efficiency of lysis between different fungi and qPCR reaction kinetics have also been expressed as reasoning for not utilizing qPCR for the quantification of yeasts and molds in cannabis and cannabis products (MCR Labs 2021).

Matrix-specific suppression effects can also be seen in both molecular and plating methods. For the former, typical sources of such suppression are PCR inhibitors such as humic acid found in soil (Sidstedt et al. 2015). For the latter, this is demonstrated via spike-in experiments in Figure 6.3 where cannabis-infused candies were plated on Petrifilm for TC and total aerobic counts. The counts are completely suppressed showing little to no growth in the presence of the cannabis-infused candy when read at the appropriate time points per the manufacturer's recommendations (Boyar 2019). It is speculated that this is due to citrate content that is often utilized in the manufacturing of MIPs and can alter the readout chemistry of these plates.

6.9 CONTAMINANT CONFIRMATION USING MALDI-TOF-MS

Cannabis labs currently typically rely on only one screening method to obtain results for pathogen testing and often do not test in replicates or perform any kind of confirmatory step. For certain pathogens of interest in cannabis, like *Aspergillus*, plating as a method of confirmation is plausible but as mentioned previously, also highly prone to error, which makes confirmation via newer alternative methods like MALDI-TOF-MS an attractive option.

In the clinical world, matrix-assisted laser desorption ionization-time of flight-mass spectrometry (MALDI-TOF-MS) is regularly used to confirm the presence of microbial contaminants in human samples using the protein fragmentation patterns that are characteristic of a given organism. This still involves the act of culturing and once colonies begin to grow, a small sample of the growth is placed on a slide for screening on the MS. This process generates a spectral profile of the proteins in the sample that can then be used as a confirmatory step in screening for pathogens (Singhal et al. 2015).

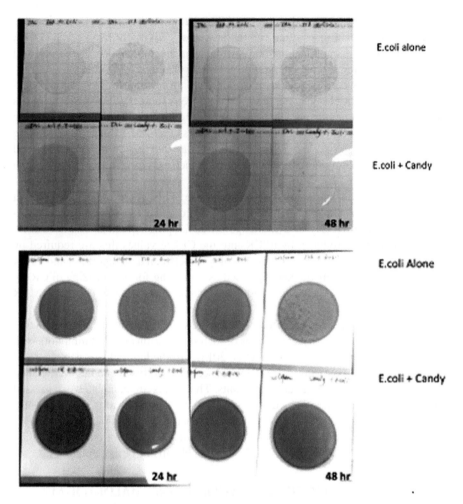

FIGURE 6.3   TC and TAC plates exhibiting matrix suppression in MIPs that utilize citric acid as a preservative. Alternative strategies for such matrices must be considered (Boyar 2019).

The benefits of running such a method are numerous, however, these instruments come at a hefty price tag and can cost up to half a million dollars. The high upfront cost of such an instrument can result in savings in the long term as using an alternative confirmatory method can be more costly than running a screen via MALDI-TOF-MS.

6.10   INSIGHTS FROM THE CANNABIS MICROBIOME

There have been a number of surveys of the microbiome of cannabis conducted by both the public and private sector that have provided considerable insights into the prevalence of certain types of microbial contaminants in cannabis and hemp (Thompson et al. 2017; McKernan Kevin et al. 2015; Vujanovic et al. 2020; Taghinasab and Jabaji 2020). These surveys have informed us that some of the pathogens of concern in cannabis are actually endophytes of the cannabis plant, some of which are capable of producing mycotoxins. Some of these are an innate component of the microbial communities found within cannabis while others are invasive and may actually be deleterious to overall plant health. Figure 6.4 highlights the different microbial communities that reside within the cannabis plant (Taghinasab and Jabaji 2020).

Most of the documented phytopathogens broadly include the fungal genera *Alternaria, Ascochyta/Phoma, Botrytis, Oidium, Sclerotinia, Septoria, Thanatephorus/Rhizoctonia, Verticillium, Pythium,* and *Phytophthora.* Host-specific pathogens, such as *Cercospora cannabina,* have also been reported in agricultural regions worldwide, including Eurasia (e.g., Cambodia, China, India, Pakistan, and Russia), Africa (e.g., Uganda), and North America (e.g., Mississippi and Wisconsin).

Moreover, the occurrence of fungal pathobiota, such as *Fusarium* on the *Cannabis sativa* host, shows certain site-specificity, as noted in the United States: California—*F. brachygibbosum, F. equiseti, F. radicicola, F. oxysporum,* and *F. solani;* Illinois—*F. oxysporum* f. sp. *cannabis, F. solani;* and Virginia—*F. sulphureum* (Vujanovic et al. 2020).

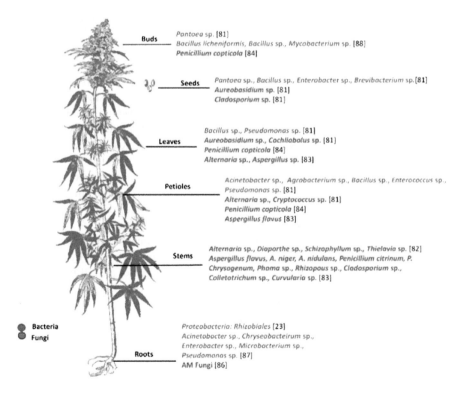

FIGURE 6.4 The most common endophytes harbored in different tissues of *Cannabis sativa* plants obtained from different geographical locations (Taghinasab and Jabaji 2020).

Investigations by Punja et al. examined the different pathogens found in cannabis by utilizing PCR assays that targeted the ITS region of ribosomal DNA. On inflorescences, they found *Penicillium* bud rot (caused by *Penicillium olsonii* and *Penicillium copticola*), *Botrytis* bud rot (*Botrytis cinerea*), and *Fusarium* bud rot (*F. solani*, *F. oxysporum*) were present to varying extents. Endophytic fungi present in crown, stem, and petiole tissues included soil-colonizing and cellulolytic fungi, such as species of *Chaetomium*, *Trametes*, *Trichoderma*, *Penicillium*, and *Fusarium*. Analysis of air samples in indoor growing environments revealed that species of *Penicillium*, *Cladosporium*, *Aspergillus*, *Fusarium*, *Beauveria*, and *Trichoderma* were present. The latter two species were the result of the application of biocontrol products for the control of insects and diseases, respectively, which will be discussed in more detail in the next section of this chapter (Punja et al. 2019).

6.11 CULTIVATION PRACTICES THAT REDUCE HARMFUL CONTAMINANTS: THE PLIGHT OF ORGANIC GROWERS

Many of the integrated pest management (IPM) techniques employed by organic cannabis growers involve utilizing probiotics such as *Trichoderma* spp., *Bacillus* spp., and other microorganisms. These organisms can trigger many total count tests, leading cultivators who utilize such practices to be often penalized in the form of failing products when adhering to protocols that mandate tight limits of total yeast and mold and total aerobic counts such as United States Pharmacopeia (USP), European Pharmacopoeia (Ph. Eur), and American Herbal Pharmacopeia (AHP).

This is one reason that many progressive jurisdictions such as California opt for species-specific testing for cannabis products. There is evidence to suggest that lactic acid-producing bacteria that are applied to cannabis as preventative measures are benign and often aid the plant due to their ability to increase levels of hexanoic acid. In essence, as these bacteria digest sugars, they produce hexanoate, which is a direct precursor to hexanoic acid, that feeds directly into the cannabinoid and terpene production pathways, which, in theory, would boost levels of these compounds. Hexanoic acid application also primes plant defense pathways that are triggered in response to *Botrytis* (Vujanovic et al. 2020; Taghinasab and Jabaji 2020). Furthermore, studies have demonstrated that some of the fungal endophytes (Figure 6.4) of cannabis inhibit the growth of various fungal pathogens found in cannabis (Kusari et al. 2013).

Beauveria bassiana is another type of preventative commonly used by cultivators to kill off any insects that would trigger TYM tests (Punja et al. 2019). Naturally found in soil, these fungi act as parasites to invading pests entering their circulatory system and harvesting nutrients from the blood.

Additionally, some of these probiotic microbes harbor chitinases, enzymes that degrade chitin, a polysaccharide that is an integral component of the cell wall of various fungi. *Bacillus* and *Pseudomonas*, which are both prevalent in the cannabis microbiome, express chitinases, and their presence has been demonstrated to provide antagonistic effects on the growth of aflatoxin-producing *A. flavus*, altering its morphological structure during spore germination and mycelial growth. Additionally, there is some anecdotal evidence to suggest that these microorganisms can aid in botrytis prevention, but the existing data does not support this assertion (Stout et al. 2012; Balthazar et al. 2020).

6.12 THE IMPORTANCE OF REPRESENTATIVE SAMPLING

As a natural product, cannabis is hardly homogenous. Microbial contamination may surface itself in some areas of the plant while other areas of the plant are largely unaffected. Therefore, obtaining a representative sample that accurately reflects a whole production batch of product is essential for ensuring consumer safety. Unfortunately, this is also another area of cannabis testing that is lacking in standardization.

Collecting a sample that is truly representative of a batch product can be challenging in many jurisdictions, especially those that do have regulations in place to ensure unbiased sampling methods are used. California serves as a good example as a state with regulations that ensure a representative sample is taken. In California, a minimum of 0.35% of the total batch of product is sampled at increasing amounts of random increments (different areas of the batch) with increased batch size (Bureau of Cannabis Control 2019).

Furthermore, the typical sample size for analysis in cannabis is significantly smaller than other industries due to its high value as a commodity. Using the California example, a five-pound batch of flowers would require a sample size of 18 g taken at eight random increments. After the sample is homogenized, typically only one of those 18 grams is utilized for microbial testing, which illustrates the case for enrichment, and is described in the next section.

6.13 TO ENRICH OR NOT TO ENRICH?

Enrichment is a technique used to increase the number of cells in a given sample prior to subsampling. This ensures that the target being screened for can be accurately detected within a small aliquot taken from the larger sample as a whole. Enrichment involves taking a homogenized sample and incubating it in enrichment media such as tryptic soy broth (TSB) or potato dextrose broth (PDB). Enrichment times and temperatures can vary depending on the pathogen of interest. An analogy would be if one were searching for a needle in a haystack, would it not be a lot easier to find a needle if there were numerous needles scattered throughout that haystack?

While this concept seems straightforward, depending on the microbial composition of the sample, out competition can occur from other microbial species present, which could in essence result in a false negative. When validating, it is critical to experiment with different incubation times with samples of varying microbial backgrounds to ensure that such out competition does not occur in real-world samples.

6.14 MICROBIAL REMEDIATION TECHNIQUES

In consideration of the fact that cannabis is a natural product and endogenous microbial communities exist within the plant, one may consider various techniques to render these microbes non-viable and hence greatly reduce the risk of opportunistic infection to the end-user. One such technique for rendering microbes non-viable is gamma irradiation.

Gamma radiation is generated by the decay of the radioisotope cobalt-60, with the resultant high-energy photons being an effective sterilant. A key characteristic of gamma irradiation is the high penetration capability, which allows for delivery of a target radiation dose to areas of products that may be higher in density. Hazekamp investigated the effects of gamma irradiation on the overall quality of cannabis and found that this technique does have drawbacks, especially in the context of terpene content, which is of utmost importance for the therapeutic properties of cannabis. Figure 6.5 from his work demonstrates up to a 38% reduction in the monoterpene terpinolene and conversion of the sesquiterpene β-caryophyllene into its oxidized counterpart caryophyllene oxide increasing its concentration by 75% (Hazekamp 2016). However, in the case of terpinolene it is important to note that a similar level of reduction would be seen if stored in a plastic bag.

Another methodology that can be utilized to effectively kill microbial contaminants is ultraviolet germicidal irradiation (UVGI). The UVGI disinfection method uses short-wavelength ultraviolet (ultraviolet C or UV-C) light to kill or inactivate microorganisms by destroying nucleic acids and disrupting their DNA, leaving them unable to perform vital cellular functions. Like gamma irradiation, UV is not without potential drawbacks as it has been demonstrated that UV light can convert and isomerize terpenes. One example of this is β-myrcene, which can be converted by UV light into hashishene (Figure 6.6), which is not naturally produced by the cannabis plant (Marchini et al. 2014). More work is needed to determine if specific wavelengths of UV light favor this reaction as this has not been studied in the context of remediation.

6.15 MICROBIAL CONSIDERATIONS FOR CANNABIS EXTRACTS

Cannabis extraction is a straightforward way to achieve higher concentrations of active components of the plant such as the cannabinoids and terpenes. The resulting extractions can be used as inhaled products or can be infused into oils and other carriers to produce ingestible products. Oftentimes, many cultivators that have moldy products will simply send them off for extraction as many assume that treatment with solvent will remove any viable microbial hazards from the contaminated raw material. However, this is far from the truth as other undesirable residual products are often left behind. There are a variety of methods that can be used to achieve these elevated concentrations but there are several factors to consider when examining what the microbial outcome might be.

6.16 SOLVENT POLARITY: WHY IT MATTERS

Because different solvents will capture different components at different efficiencies—the choice of solvent is critical for understanding whether it will impact the results of your microbial testing. In particular, knowing the polarity of the solvent and how it behaves under extraction conditions will determine whether the microbial contents of the extraction material will survive.

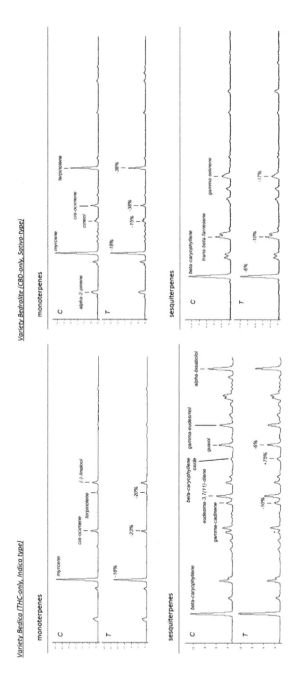

FIGURE 6.5 GC profiles of two studied varieties showing monoterpenes, sesquiterpenes, and cannabinoids in separate sections. C, control (non-irradiated); T, treated (irradiated); *, artifact. Numbers indicate the percentage of change in treated samples compared to non-treated controls (Hazekamp 2016).

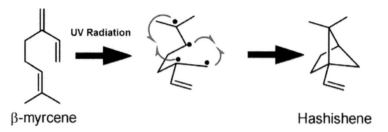

β-myrcene   Hashishene

FIGURE 6.6   UV light-induced rearrangement of beta myrcene into hashishene (Marchini et al. 2014). Further research is needed to determine if UV-based remediation techniques can result in chemical transformations that significantly alter the overall terpene profile.

TABLE 6.2
Anonymized qPCR Data of Various Butane Extracts That Illustrate That Although the Microbial Contaminants Present May Be Dead Their DNA Can Linger in the Final Product

Extract	Total aerobic count	Total yeast and mold
BHO 1	1876	363
BHO 2	252	0
BHO 3	61	0
BHO 4	11	0
BHO 5	35	0

Source: Boyar 2019.

Furthermore, DNA is negatively charged due to the sugar-phosphate backbone on the molecule. This negative charge means that it will not be soluble in non-polar solvents. In line with this, the data in Table 6.2 highlights that microbial DNA is much less likely to be present in extractions produced with non-polar solvents.

6.17   EXTRACTION SOLVENTS

6.17.1   ICE AND COLD WATER

When employing water or ice as your solvent there is a much greater likelihood of elevated microbial load because while the solvent is at a low temperature, it does not mean that the solvent will kill the microbes present. Additionally, because water is a polar solvent, it will simply carry the microbes from the extraction material into the resulting extract and concentrate them as well. This is often why bubble hash and ice hash produce elevated total aerobic and total yeast and mold counts.

6.17.2 HYDROCARBONS

Hydrocarbons, like butane and propane, are non-polar solvents and are commonly used for cannabis extraction. When in liquid form these exist at very cold temperatures under normal atmospheric conditions. Due to these properties, the microbes present in the extraction material are essentially frozen alive and rendered unviable. However, this does not mean the resulting extract is void of any microbial DNA or other microbial hazards as exemplified in Table 6.2, which shows the resulting CFU/g produced by an assay from a leading cannabis microbial testing vendor.

6.17.3 CO$_2$

CO_2 is also a commonly used technique in cannabis extraction in which this compound that normally exists as a gas at room temperature is subjected to extremely cold temperatures and high pressure to produce what is called a supercritical fluid. This high pressure coupled with extremely low temperatures will effectively kill microbial contaminants but the DNA from these contaminants can remain.

6.17.4 ETHANOL

Ethanol is also a very popular solvent for cannabis extraction. It is sometimes used as the primary solvent for extraction, while at other times, it is used as a refining agent for removing inactive lipid constituents. Ethanol as a solvent is amphiphilic and in higher concentration will render the vast majority of microbial contaminants unviable. However, due to its polarity, the DNA from microbial contaminants can carry over into the resulting extract.

6.18 ADDITIONAL CONCERNS FOR CANNABIS EXTRACTION: MYCOTOXINS AND OTHER CONTAMINANTS

While most of the commercially used extraction techniques available effectively kill any microbes present, there are other components from these contaminants that can be left behind. One of these components of concern is a class of compounds called mycotoxins. Mycotoxins are thermally resistant compounds that exhibit carcinogenic, nephrotoxic, and neurotoxic properties that can remain in the resulting extract as they are extremely stable (Daley et al. 2013; McPartland and McKernan 2017). For example, aflatoxins—AFBs (AFB1 and AFB2s)—and fumonisins—FUMs (FB1 and FB2)—are all very highly soluble in the same solvents that are used to concentrate cannabinoids from cannabis plant material (Bennett and Klich 2003). More research is needed to determine this potential risk as only a handful of mycotoxins are tested for in legal markets.

Furthermore, once cannabis material has been processed into an extract, proper storage of the resulting material is still paramount for ensuring consumer safety. One microorganism of particular concern when dealing with cannabis extracts is *Clostridium botulinum*, which is an anaerobic, spore-forming bacterium that produces botulinum toxin under ideal conditions. This compound is neurotoxic and causes muscular paralysis which can be fatal in even healthy individuals. McKernan et al. detected *C. botulinum* in their surveys of the cannabis microbiome and this microbial threat has been acknowledged by the Denver Department of Environmental Health and is continually being monitored (McKernan et al. 2016; https://www.medicinalgenomics.com/wp-content/uploads/2016/08/Special-concerns-with-marijuana-extractions-and-infusions_Denver_Botulism_160824.pdf).

6.19 DISTILLATION: A WORK AROUND

If contaminant DNA remains in many solvent extractions, then how does one deal with it? Distillation is often employed to further concentrate and refine extracts in which the starting material is heated to the point at which the various components vaporize. These components are then separated based on boiling point. The raffinate or undesirable fractions with a lower boiling point are typically discarded and the fraction with a higher boiling point containing the cannabinoids, or the distillate, is retained. By capturing the cannabinoid fraction and removing the other components, the vast majority of any contaminant DNA that may have been present in the crude extract will be successfully removed (Table 6.3). Mycotoxins, however, are a bit trickier. Since cannabinoid distillation is performed under vacuum, this effectively lowers the boiling point of the mycotoxins, which leaves room for the possibility of these compounds co-distilling with the cannabinoids. It is in the best interest of the operator to determine the optimal conditions for capturing the majority of the cannabinoids while excluding mycotoxins from the fraction (Boyar 2019).

6.20 REFERENCE METHODS AND STANDARDIZATION

6.20.1 AMERICAN HERBAL PHARMACOPEIA

The AHP monograph was one of the earliest monographs to establish microbial limits for cannabis and cannabis products. The thresholds provided by AHP by matrix are outlined in Table 6.4 (Upton et al. 2014). While these limits appear to be

TABLE 6.3

Anonymized PathoSEEK qPCR Data of Cannabis Distillates That Demonstrate the Vast Majority of Microbial Contaminant DNA Can Be Removed by Distillation

Extract	Total aerobic count	Total yeast and mold
Distillate 1	27	0
Distillate 2	27	0
Distillate 3	106	0
Distillate 4	87	0
Distillate 5	67	0

Source: Boyar 2019.

TABLE 6.4

Microbial and Fungal Limits for Orally Consumed Botanical Products in the US (CFU/g)

	TAC	TYM	TC	BEGIN	Pathogenic *E. coli* and *Salmonella* spp.
Unprocessed materials*	10^5	10^4	10^3	10^3	Not detected in 1 g
Processed materials*	10^5	10^4	10^3	10^3	Not detected in 1 g
CO_2 and solvent-based extracts	10^4	10^3	10^2	10^2	Not detected in 1 g

Source: Adapted from the American Herbal Pharmacopeia (AHP) Monograph Revision 2014 (Upton et al. 2014).

*Unprocessed materials include minimally processed crude cannabis preparations such as inflorescences, accumulated resin glands (kief), and compressed resin glands (hashish). Processed materials include various solid or liquid infused edible preparation, oils topical preparations, and water-processed resin glands ("bubble hash"). Significant microbial contamination can occur during post-harvest handling.

reasonable, it is also very important to recognize that when dealing with a natural product, endogenous microorganisms are inevitable and one needs to understand if elevated counts indeed pose a risk to the end consumer. As mentioned earlier in the chapter, many of the microorganisms that can trigger these tests are utilized as biocontrol agents in organic farming practices. Such probiotic and preventative microorganisms have shown efficacy against fungal pathogens such as *Aspergillus* spp. and other undesirable molds like *Botrytis cinerea* (Lamont et al. 2017; Akocak et al. 2015; Balthazar et al. 2020).

6.20.2 ASSOCIATION OF OFFICIAL AGRICULTURAL CHEMISTS

In 2019, the Association of Official Agricultural Chemists (AOAC) launched the Cannabis Analytical Sciences Program (CASP). CASP has been working with industry stakeholders on the development of various standard method performance requirements (SMPRs) for the cannabis industry.

AOAC SMPRs describe the minimum recommended performance characteristics to be used during the evaluation of a method. The evaluation may be an on-site verification, a single laboratory validation, or a multi-site collaborative study. SMPRs are written and adopted by AOAC stakeholder panels composed of representatives from industry, regulatory organizations, contract laboratories, test kit manufacturers, and academic institutions. AOAC SMPRs are used by AOAC expert review panels in their evaluation of validation study data for methods being considered for performance tested methods or for AOAC official methods of analysis and can be used as acceptance criteria for verification at user laboratories.

To date, CASP's Microbial Contaminants Working Group has worked with industry stakeholders to approve three SMPRs. SMPRs for the detection of *Aspergillus*, STEC, and *Salmonella* in cannabis and cannabis products have been completed and work is currently underway on a fourth SMPR for the quantification of total yeasts and molds in cannabis and cannabis products (AOAC 2019-2020). An important distinction in the testing marketplace is given to methods that have achieved AOAC validation as this is an extensive and peer-reviewed process.

6.20.3   EUROPEAN PHARMACOPOEIA

In European and Canadian jurisdictions, some have opted to employ the action limits put forth by Ph. Eur 5.1.4.-1, which gives different tolerances for TAC and TYM as well as specific microorganisms depending on their route of administration. Table 6.5 outlines the allowances based on the product's route of administration. These limits are very stringent in some cases and may not be feasible especially in the context of inhalation as some genera such as *Pseudomonas* are commonly found in the microbiome of hemp (Punja et al. 2019; Taghinasab and Jabaji 2020).

6.20.4   UNITED STATES PHARMACOPEIA

USP published a stimulus article entitled "The Advisability and Feasibility of Developing USP Standards for Medical Cannabis." The author cited the US Food and Drug Administration (FDA) *Bacteriological Analytical Manual* as a source of appropriate methods. Another source that is suggested is USP *<2021> Microbial Enumeration Tests-Nutritional and Dietary Supplements* and USP *<2022> Microbiological Procedures for Absence of Specified Microorganisms—Nutritional and Dietary Supplements* (Giancaspro et al. 2016).

Laboratories may opt to utilize USP methods to test for microbial contaminants. USP chapter "<1111> USP: Microbiological Examination of Nonsterile Products: Acceptance Criteria for Pharmaceutical Preparations and Substances for Pharmaceutical Use" provides two acceptance criteria tables for USP <61> and USP <62> methods. USP "<61> Microbiological Examination of Nonsterile Products: Microbial Enumeration Tests" includes methods for enumerating total aerobic bacterial count and the total yeasts and molds count. USP "<62> Microbiological Examination of Nonsterile Products: Tests for Specified Microorganisms" includes methods and specifications for the absence of *Salmonella* species and *Escherichia coli* and the enumeration of total bile-tolerant gram-negative bacteria.

This discussion was expanded upon recently with the publication of "Cannabis Inflorescence for Medical Purposes: USP Considerations for Quality Attributes" by the USP Cannabis Expert Panel. In line with previous publications such as the AHP Monograph—the panel recommended the following specifications for the microbial quality of cannabis inflorescence:

USP <61>:
- The total aerobic bacterial count—not more than 10^5 CFU/g
- The total combined molds and yeast count—not more than 10^4 CFU/g

USP <62>:
- The total bile-tolerant gram-negative bacteria—not more than 10^3 CFU/g
- Meets the requirements of the tests for the absence of *Salmonella* species and *Escherichia coli*

TABLE 6.5

The European Pharmacopoeia (Ph. Eur) Acceptance Criteria for Microbiological Quality of Non-Sterile Dosage Forms

Route of administration	TAC (CFU/g or CFU/mL)	TYM (CFU/g or CFU/mL)	Specified microorganisms
Non-aqueous preparations for oral use	10^3	10^2	Absence of *E. coli* (1 g or 1 mL)
Aqueous preparations for oral use	10^2	10^1	Absence of *E. coli* (1 g or 1 mL)
Rectal use	10^3	10^2	
Oromucosal use Gingival use Cutaneous use Nasal use Auricular use	10^2	10^1	Absence of *P. aeruginosa* (1 g or 1 mL) Absence of *S. aureus* (1 g or 1 mL)
Vaginal use	10^2	10^1	Absence of *P. aeruginosa* (1 g or 1 mL) Absence of *S. aureus* (1 g or 1 mL) Absence of *C. albicans* (1 g or 1 mL)
Transdermal patches (limits for one patch including adhesive layer and backing)	10^2	10^1	Absence of *P. aeruginosa* (1 patch) Absence of *S. aureus* (1 patch)
Inhalation use (special requirements apply to liquid preparations for nebulization)	10^2	10^1	Absence of *P. aeruginosa* (1 g or 1 mL) Absence of *S. aureus* (1 g or 1 mL) Absence of bile-tolerant gram-negative bacteria (1 g or 1 mL)
Special Ph. Eur provision for oral dosage forms containing raw materials of natural (animal, vegetal, or mineral) origin for which antimicrobial pretreatment is not feasible and for which the competent authority accepts TAC of the raw material exceeding 10^3 CFU/g or 10^3 CFU/mL	10^4	10^2	Not more than 10^2 CFU of bile-tolerant gram-negative bacteria (1 g or 1 mL) Absence of *Salmonella* (10 g or 10 mL) Absence of *E. coli* (1 g or 1 mL)

The authors also discuss *Aspergillus* extensively and note that molecular techniques like qPCR should be utilized to detect microbial contaminants (i.e., powdery mildew) that are not amenable to culture-based techniques. The expert panel also addresses water activity for the control of microbial growth and suggested the adoption of ASTM guidelines that limit the content to Aw values between 0.55 and 0.65. Reduced water activity greatly assists in the prevention of microbial proliferation and spoilage (Sarma et al. 2020).

6.21 CONCLUDING STATEMENTS

While different microbial testing methods have their own merits, certain scenarios require a critical eye in their application. Plating/culture-based techniques are the traditionally used methods that are most economical and widely accepted while molecular techniques are the most specific and sensitive. Some but not all molecular methods on the market can discern between live and dead DNA, which will be essential in medical markets where remediation techniques are likely to be used. There is a need for rapid secondary screening methods, which methods like MALDI-TOF-MS are well equipped to address.

Some of the testing costs for producers can potentially be mitigated by taking a risk/benefit approach where certain pathogens are only tested when elevated counts of the greater classes of organisms are detected. We are still learning a lot about what additional contaminants might be of concern to the public and these organisms of potential concern should be continually monitored to ensure public safety.

REFERENCES

Akocak PB, Churey JJ, Worobo RW. 2015. Antagonistic effect of chitinolytic Pseudomonas and Bacillus on growth of fungal hyphae and spores of aflatoxigenic Aspergillus flavus. *Food Bioscience* 10:48–58.

Andrews WH, Hammack TS. 2003. Food sampling/preparation of sample homogenate. *Bacteriological Analytical Manual* online, 8th edn. Center for Food Safety & Applied Nutrition, US Food and Drug Administration. http://www.cfsan.fda.gov/~ebam/bam-1 .html.

Appendino G, Gibbons S, Giana A, Pagani A, Grassi G, Stavri M, Smith E, Rahman MM. 2008. Antibacterial cannabinoids from Cannabis sativa: a structure–activity study. *Journal of Natural Products* 71:1427–1430.

Babu T, Griswold MK, Urban MA, Babu KM. 2017. Aspergillosis presenting as multiple pulmonary nodules in an immunocompetent Cannabis user. *Journal of Toxicology and Pharmacology* 1:004.

Bal A, Agarwal AN, Das A, Suri V, Varma S. 2010. Chronic necrotising pulmonary Aspergillosis in a marijuana addict: a new cause of amyloidosis. *Pathology* 42:197–200.

Balthazar C, Cantin G, Novinscak A, Joly DL, Filion M. 2020. Expression of putative defense responses in Cannabis primed by Pseudomonas and/or Bacillus strains and infected by Botrytis cinerea. *Frontiers in Plant Science* 11:1873.

Beadle, A. 2021. Techniques and technologies for microbiological contamination testing. *Analytical Cannabis*. https://www.analyticalcannabis.com/articles/techniques-and-t echnologies-for-microbiological-contamination-testing-307113. Accessed April 24, 2021.

Bennett J, Klich M. 2003. Mycotoxins. *Clinical Microbiological Reviews* 16:497–516.

Bio-Rad. Microbial solutions for cannabis testing. https://www.bio-rad.com/en-us/applicatio ns-technologies/microbial-detection-solutions-for-cannabis-testing. Accessed March, 2021.

Blaskovich MA, Kavanagh AM, Elliott AG, Zhang B, Ramu S, Amado M, Lowe GJ, Hinton AO, Zuegg J, Beare N. 2021. The antimicrobial potential of cannabidiol. *Communications Biology* 4:1–18. https://doi.org/10.1038/s42003-020-01530-y.

Boyar K. 2019. Cannabis microbiome sequencing and its implications for cannabis safety testing. *Abstracts of Papers of the American Chemical Society: Amer Chemical Soc*, Washington, DC.

Bragg, R. 1999. A fungus to kill marijuana has environmentalists wary. *The New York Times*, July 27, 1999, sec. U.S. https://www.nytimes.com/1999/07/27/us/a-fungus-to-kill-marij uana-has-environmentalists-wary.html.

Bureau of Cannabis Control. 2019. Text of Regulations (Order of Adoption) "Laws & Regulations - BCC." https://www.bcc.ca.gov/law_regs/. Accessed March 7, 2021.

Cannabis Science Tech. The what, how, and why of water activity in cannabis. https://www .cannabissciencetech.com/view/temperature-comparison-of-3m-rapid-yeast-and-mold -petrifilm-utilizing-manufacturers-suggested-temperatures-on-dried-cannabis-flower -cannabis-spp. Accessed April 19, 2021.

Cescon DW, Page AV, Richardson S, Moore MJ, Boerner S. 2008. Invasive pulmonary aspergillosis associated with marijuana use in a man with colorectal cancer. *Journal of Clinical Oncology* 26:2214–2215.

Chusid MJ, Gelfand JA, Nutter C, Fauci AS. 1975. Pulmonary aspergillosis, inhalation of contaminated marijuana smoke, chronic granulomatous disease. *Annals of Internal Medicine* 82:682–683.

Coenye T, Vandamme P, LiPuma JJ. 2002. Infection by Ralstonia species in cystic fibrosis patients: identification of R. pickettii and R. mannitolilytica by polymerase chain reaction. *Emerging Infectious Diseases* 8:692.

Daley P, Lampach D, Sguerra S. 2013. *Testing Cannabis for Contaminants.* BOTEC Analysis Corp. Retrieved from Steep Hill http://steephill.com/pdf/uploads/whitepapers/5c5be0 247e264b5020a99b669a936362.pdf (Archived by WebCite1 at http://www.webcitation .org/6bBnLWPed).

Gargani Y, Bishop P, Denning DW. 2011. Too many mouldy joints—marijuana and chronic pulmonary aspergillosis. *Mediterranean Journal of Hematology and Infectious Diseases* 3:e2011005.

Giancaspro GI, Kim N-C, Venema J, de Mars S, Devine J, Celestino C, Feaster CE, Firschein BA, Waddell MS, Gardner SM. 2016. The advisability and feasibility of developing USP standards for medical Cannabis. *Pharmacopeial Forum.* http://www.uspnf.com/ sites/default/files/usp_pdf/EN/USPNF/usp-nf-notices/usp_stim_article_medical_can- nabis.pdf

Hamadeh R, Ardehali A, Locksley RM, York MK. 1988. Fatal aspergillosis associated with smoking contaminated marijuana, in a marrow transplant recipient. *Chest* 94:432–433.

Hazekamp A. 2016. Evaluating the effects of gamma-irradiation for decontamination of medicinal cannabis. *Frontiers in Pharmacology* 7:108.

Kagen S. 1981. Aspergillus: an inhalable contaminant of marihuana. *The New England Journal of Medicine* 304:483–484.

Kusari P, Kusari S, Spiteller M, Kayser O. 2013. Endophytic fungi harbored in Cannabis sativa L.: diversity and potential as biocontrol agents against host plant-specific phyto- pathogens. *Fungal Diversity* 60:137–151.

Lamont JR, Wilkins O, Bywater-Ekegärd M, Smith DL. 2017. From yogurt to yield: potential applications of lactic acid bacteria in plant production. *Soil Biology and Biochemistry* 111:1–9.

LeafLink. 2020. January insights flash | LeafLink. *Resources.* https://www.resources.leaflink .com/insights-flash-january. Accessed April 5, 2021.

Llamas R, Hart DR, Schneider NS. 1978. Allergic bronchopulmonary aspergillosis associ- ated with smoking moldy marihuana. *Chest* 73:871–872.

Magee, S. 2020. Organigram admits role in moncton legionnaires' disease outbreak. *CBC News.* December 4, 2020.

Maguire, S. 2018. Disagreement between Laboratories as Steep Hill Alaska Considers Legal Options. https://www.alaskasnewssource.com/content/news/Auditing-marijuana-labs- -472254833.html. Accessed March 8, 2021.

Maguire W, et al. 2018. Survey of mycotoxin residues in Oregon cannabis crops by LC-MS/ MS [Conference Poster]. *Cannabis Science Conference*, Portland, OR, 2018.

Marchini M, Charvoz C, Dujourdy L, Baldovini N, Filippi J-J. 2014. Multidimensional analy- sis of cannabis volatile constituents: identification of 5, 5-dimethyl-1-vinylbicyclo [2.1. 1] hexane as a volatile marker of hashish, the resin of Cannabis sativa L. *Journal of Chromatography A* 1370:200–215. https://doi.org/10.1016/j.chroma.2014.10.045.

Marks WH, Florence L, Lieberman J, Chapman P, Howard D, Roberts P, Perkinson D. 1996. Successfully treated invasive pulmonary aspergillosis associated with smoking mari- juana in a renal transplant recipient. *Transplantation* 61:1771–1774.

McKernan K. 2017. Whole genome sequencing of several cannabis derived powdery mildew samples and the development of field portable colorimetric detection tools for infecting fungi. *ICRS* 2017. https://slideplayer.com/slide/12890792/

McKernan K, Spangler J, Helbert Y, Lynch RC, Devitt-Lee A, Zhang L, Orphe W, Warner J, Foss T, Hudalla CJ. 2016. Metagenomic analysis of medicinal Cannabis samples; pathogenic bacteria, toxigenic fungi, and beneficial microbes grow in culture-based yeast and mold tests. *F1000Research* 5:2471.

McKernan K, Spangler J, Zhang L, Tadigotla V, Helbert Y, Foss T, Smith D. 2015. Cannabis microbiome sequencing reveals several mycotoxic fungi native to dispensary grade Cannabis flowers. *F1000Research* 4:1422.

McPartland JM, McKernan KJ. 2017. Contaminants of concern in cannabis: microbes, heavy metals and pesticides. Pages 457–474. In: Suman Chandra, Hemant Lata, Mahmoud A. ElSohly (eds), *Cannabis sativa L. – Botany and Biotechnology*, New York: Springer.

MCR Labs. 2021. Broad species qPCR found inappropriate for total yeast and mold counts. https://mcrlabs.com/wp-content/uploads/2021/03/Mike-E-qPCR-PDF.pdf. Accessed April 23, 2021.

Medicinal Genomics. Grim reefer free DNA removal kit. https://www.medicinalgenomics. com/free-dna-removal-kit/. Accessed March 8, 2021.

Nguyen LT, Picard-Bernard V, Perriot J. 2010. Legionnaires disease in cannabis smokers. *Chest* 138:989–991.

Peeters N, Guidot A, Vailleau F, Valls M. 2013. R alstonia solanacearum, a widespread bacte- rial plant pathogen in the post-genomic era. *Molecular Plant Pathology* 14:651–662.

Punja ZK, Collyer D, Scott C, Lung S, Holmes J, Sutton D. 2019. Pathogens and molds affect- ing production and quality of Cannabis sativa L. *Frontiers in Plant Science* 10:1120.

Remington TL, Fuller J, Chiu I. 2015. Chronic necrotizing pulmonary aspergillosis in a patient with diabetes and marijuana use. *CMAJ* 187:1305–1308.

Roggen M. 2019. Healthy and concentrated cannabis plants: how to use acronyms to optimize production. *Journal of AOAC International* 102:421–426.

Ruchlemer R, Amit-Kohn M, Raveh D, Hanuš L. 2015. Inhaled medicinal cannabis and the immunocompromised patient. *Supportive Care in Cancer* 23:819–822.

Sarma ND, Waye A, ElSohly MA, Brown PN, Elzinga S, Johnson HE, Marles RJ, Melanson JE, Russo E, Deyton L. 2020. Cannabis inflorescence for medical purposes: USP con- siderations for quality attributes. *Journal of Natural Products* 83:1334–1351.

Shapiro BB, Hedrick R, Vanle BC, Becker CA, Nguyen C, Underhill DM, Morgan MA, Kopple JD, Danovitch I, IsHak WW. 2018. Cryptococcal meningitis in a daily cannabis smoker without evidence of immunodeficiency. *BMJ Case Reports* 2018 (January 26, 2018).

Sidstedt M, Jansson L, Nilsson E, Noppa L, Forsman M, Rådström P, Hedman J. 2015. Humic substances cause fluorescence inhibition in real-time polymerase chain reaction. *Analytical Biochemistry* 487:30–37.

Singhal N, Kumar M, Kanaujia PK, Virdi JS. 2015. MALDI-TOF mass spectrometry: an emerging technology for microbial identification and diagnosis. *Frontiers in Microbiology* 6:791.

Spellberg B, Edwards J, Ibrahim A. 2005. Novel perspectives on mucormycosis: pathophysiology, presentation, and management. *Clinical Microbiology Reviews* 18:556–569.

Stone T, Henkle J, Prakash V. 2019. Pulmonary mucormycosis associated with medical marijuana use. *Respiratory Medicine Case Reports* 26:176–179. https://doi.org/10.1016/j.rmcr.2019.01.008.

Stout JM, Boubakir Z, Ambrose SJ, Purves RW, Page JE. 2012. The hexanoyl-CoA precursor for cannabinoid biosynthesis is formed by an acyl-activating enzyme in Cannabis sativa trichomes. *The Plant Journal* 71:353–365.

Sutton S, Lum BL, Torti FM. 1986. Possible risk of invasive pulmonary aspergillosis with marijuana use during chemotherapy for small cell lung cancer. *Drug Intelligence & Clinical Pharmacy* 20:289–291.

Szyper-Kravitz M, Lang R, Manor Y, Lahav M. 2001. Early invasive pulmonary aspergillosis in a leukemia patient linked to aspergillus contaminated marijuana smoking. *Leukemia & lymphoma* 42:1433–1437.

Taghinasab M, Jabaji S. 2020. Cannabis microbiome and the role of endophytes in modulating the production of secondary metabolites: an overview. *Microorganisms* 8:355.

Taylor DN, Wachsmuth IK, Shangkuan YH, Schmidt EV, Barrett TJ, Schrader JS, Scherach CS, McGee HB, Feldman RA, Brenner DJ. 1982. Salmonellosis associated with marijuana: A multistate outbreak traced by plasmid fingerprinting. *The New England Journal of Medicine* 306(21):1249–1253. doi:10.1056/NEJM198205273062101.

Thompson GR, Tuscano J, Dennis M, Singapuri A, Libertini S, Gaudino R, Torres A, Delisle A, Gillece J, Schupp J. 2017. A microbiome assessment of medical marijuana. *Clinical Microbiology and Infection* 23:269–270.

Upton R, Craker L, ElSohly M, Romm A, Russo E, Sexton M. 2014. *Cannabis Inflorescence: Cannabis spp.; Standards of Identity, Analysis, and Quality Control.* Scotts Valley, CA: American Herbal Pharmacopoeia.

Van Klingeren B, Ten Ham M. 1976. Antibacterial activity of Δ^9-tetrahydrocannabinol and cannabidiol. *Antonie van Leeuwenhoek* 42:9–12.

Verweij PE, Kerremans JJ, Voss A, Meis JF. 2000. Fungal contamination of tobacco and marijuana. *Jama* 284:2875–2875.

Vujanovic V, Korber DR, Vujanovic S, Vujanovic J, Jabaji S. 2020. Scientific prospects for cannabis-microbiome research to ensure quality and safety of products. *Microorganisms* 8:290.

7 Cannabis Extract Formulations and Devices

Brad Douglass and Robert M. Strongin

CONTENTS

7.1   SAFETY CONSIDERATIONS FOR CANNABIS CONCENTRATES MEANT FOR INHALATION

The layman typically thinks in terms of safety: is it safe to do something or not? In contrast, scientists tend to think in terms of risk and hazard. The difference is subtle but meaningful. The concept of safety implies that something is either risk-full or risk-free: all or nothing. In reality, risk-free situations and substances are exceedingly rare. Take molecular oxygen and water as examples. Both are necessary for human life—water is even partly composed of oxygen. However, both water and oxygen can cause injury or death when misused.

Hazard and risk are continuous variables, which can be quantified. As such, scientists and public health officials can distill useful information about the *degree* of hazard or risk. Understanding the degree of the issue at hand enables the proper emphasis to be placed upon mitigation measures. This applies to such disparate applications as the tone of public service educational messages and the sensitivity of product quality testing standards.

Another important concept for understanding hazard determination is *relative risk*. Risk is always relative to something else. For example, if one were to compare the risk of inhaling ambient air in Beijing relative to inhaling pure oxygen or the exhaust stream from an automobile tailpipe, one would end up with a different conception of how "safe" it is to inhale Beijing air. It is critical to understand that risk

DOI: 10.1201/9780429274893-7

161

is inevitably present and must be compared with something else to imbue it with meaning. As such, when care is taken to evaluate a hazard in the context of a relevant alternative situation, the severity—or even preferability—of the hazard can be kept in context. The concept of relative risk allows us to make pragmatic judgments about the acceptability of solutions to perceived problems. If the hazard associated with A has been deemed acceptable, and B is less risky than A, then it logically follows that B also possesses an acceptable level of hazard.

A classic example of relative risk at work is cigarettes versus e-cigarettes. E-cigarettes possess inherent risks. This is an undisputed fact. Yet relative to normal cigarettes, a properly formulated and standardized e-cigarette is designed to present fewer toxicological risks. In addition, if the e-cigarette is properly engineered and used appropriately by the end-user, it may also have the potential to present a lesser overall hazard than a traditional cigarette. This understanding has led to the approval of electronic nicotine delivery systems (ENDS) by global regulatory bodies as a therapeutic treatment for smoking cessation. A similar relative risk calculation undergirds the acceptability of using methadone to treat opioid addiction. For manufactured cannabis products, it is often appropriate to compare the risk versus smoked cannabis—the traditional form of cannabis utilization.

7.2   MOLECULES FOUND NATURALLY OCCURRING IN CANNABIS

Cannabis produces an astonishing array of chemical compounds. These include the primary molecules of life on Earth: nucleic acids, proteins, fats, and carbohydrates. Yet there is also a plethora of secondary molecules manufactured by cannabis that are non-essential for basic life-sustaining biochemical functions, such as reproduction, repair, energy generation, and energy storage.

These secondary compounds include classes of molecules that a chemist would categorize as alcohols, aldehydes, alkaloids, cannabinoids, esters, ethers, fatty acids, flavonoids, hydrocarbons, ketones, lactones, spirans, steroids, and terpenoids amongst others, as detailed non-exhaustively in Table 7.1. The primary distinguishing characteristic of *Cannabis sativa* L. from other plant species is the cannabinoids. Very few plants on earth produce anything similar to the phytocannabinoids. They are the *sine qua non* of cannabis.

Aside from cannabinoids, there are very few compounds found in cannabis that are not also produced by other plants. Good examples are terpenes and terpenoids. Terpenoids have captured the collective imagination of cannabis culture yet are produced ubiquitously throughout the natural world. In fact, there are almost zero terpenoids that are uniquely produced by cannabis. Instead, what makes cannabis remarkable is the sheer variety of terpenoids it can express. For example, limonene typically composes greater than 90% of the terpene fraction of oranges (Coleman 1969; Vora 1983; Pino 1992). Whereas just two terpenoids—linalool and linalyl acetate—dominate the essential oil of lavender (Shellie 2002).

Cannabis stands out as a prolific producer of many terpenoids such that most cannabis varieties do not have one or even two compounds that compose a majority of the terpene fraction. Typically, the predominant terpenoid in cannabis only

TABLE 7.1
Molecules Found in Cannabis by Functional Group

Chemical class	Prefix	Name	Alternative ID(s)
Alcohol		Benzyl Alcohol	Benzyl alcohol
Alcohol	*cis-*	Hex-3-en-1-ol	(Z)-3-hexen-1-ol, (3Z)-hexenol
Aldehyde		Hexanal	
Aldehyde		Nonanal	
Alkaloid		Cannabisativine	
Cannabinoid		Cannabichromanon	CBCN
Cannabinoid		Cannabichromene	CBC, cannabichromen
Cannabinoid		Cannabichromenic acid	CBCA
Cannabinoid		Cannabicitran	CBT
Cannabinoid		Cannabicyclol	CBL
Cannabinoid		Cannabidiol	CBD
Cannabinoid		Cannabidiolic acid	CBDA
Cannabinoid		Cannabidivarin	CBDV
Cannabinoid		Cannabidivarinic acid	CBDVA
Cannabinoid		Cannabielsoic acid B	CBEA-B
Cannabinoid		Cannabielsoin	CBE
Cannabinoid		Cannabielsoin-C3	CBE
Cannabinoid		Cannabifuran	CBF
Cannabinoid		Cannabigerol	CBG
Cannabinoid		Cannabigerol monomethyl ether	CBGM, CBG-MME
Cannabinoid		Cannabigerolic acid	CBGA
Cannabinoid		Cannabinol	CBN
Cannabinoid		Cannabivarin	CBNV
Cannabinoid		Dehydrocannabifuran	DCBF
Cannabinoid	$(-)$-*trans*-Δ^9-	tetrahydrocannabinol	d9THC, Δ1-tetrahydrocannabinol (old nomenclature)
Cannabinoid	$(-)$-*trans*-Δ^8-	tetrahydrocannabinol	d8THC, Δ1,6-tetrahydrocannabinol (old nomenclature)
Cannabinoid	$(-)$-*trans*-Δ^9-	tetrahydrocannabinol-C4	d9THC-C4
Cannabinoid	$(-)$-*trans*-Δ^9-	tetrahydrocannabinolic acid A	THCA-A
Cannabinoid	$(-)$-*trans*-Δ^9-	tetrahydrocannabiorcol	d9THC-C1
Cannabinoid	$(-)$-*trans*-Δ^9-	tetrahydrocannabivarin	THCV
Cannabinoid	$(-)$-*trans*-Δ^9-	tetrahydrocannabivarinic acid A	THCVA-A
Ester		Hexyl butyrate	Hexyl butanoate, butanoic acid hexyl ester
Ester		Methyl acetate	Acetic acid methyl ester, methyl ethanoate

(Continued)

TABLE 7.1 (CONTINUED)
Molecules Found in Cannabis by Functional Group

Chemical class	Prefix	Name	Alternative ID(s)
Ester		Methyl palmitate	Methyl hexadecanoate, Hexanoic acid methyl ester, Methyl caproate
Fatty acids		Docosanoic acid	Behenic acid
Fatty acids		Hexadecanoic acid	Palmitic acid, C16:0
Fatty acids	α-	Linoleic acid	
Fatty acids	α-	Linolenic acid	C18:3ω6
Fatty acids		Octadecanoic acid	Stearic acid, C18:0
Fatty acids		Oleic acid	(9Z)-Octadec-9-enoic acid, *cis*-9-Octadecenoic acid, 18:1 *cis*-9
Flavonoid		Cannflavin A	Canniflavanone-2
Flavonoid		Cannflavin B	Canniflavone-1
Hydrocarbon		Dodecane	n-dodecane
Hydrocarbon		Hexadecane	
Hydrocarbon		Pentadecane	
Ketone	2-	Heptanone	Heptan-2-one, methyl n-amyl-ketone
Lactone	5,5-	dimethyl-2(5H)-furanone	
Phenylpropene	*cis*-	Anethole	Anise Camphor
Phenylpropene		Estragole	p-allylanisole, methyl chavicol
Spirans		Cannabispiradienone	
Spirans	α-	Cannabispiranol	
Spirans	β-	Cannabispiranol	Cannabispirol
Spirans		Cannabispirenone-A	
Spirans		Cannabispirenone-B	
Spirans		Cannabispirone	Cannabispiran
Spirans		Dehydrocannabispiran	Cannabispirenone
Steroids		Campesterol	
Steroids	β-	Sitosterol	
Steroids		Stigmasterol	
Stilbenoid		Canniprene	
Terpenoid		Alloaromadendrene	
Terpenoid		Aromadendrene	
Terpenoid	*trans*-α-	Bergamotene	
Terpenoid	*cis*-α-	Bergamotene	
Terpenoid	β-	Bisabolene	
Terpenoid	epi-α-	Bisabolol	
Terpenoid	α-	Bisabolol	
Terpenoid		Borneol	Camphol
Terpenoid	α-	Bulnescene	
Terpenoid	α-	Cadinene	

(Continued)

TABLE 7.1 (CONTINUED)
Molecules Found in Cannabis by Functional Group

Chemical class	Prefix	Name	Alternative ID(s)
Terpenoid		Camphene	
Terpenoid		Camphor	
Terpenoid	σ-	Cadinene	
Terpenoid	3-	Carene	
Terpenoid		Carvone	
Terpenoid	β-	Caryophyllene	(E)-Caryophyllene
Terpenoid	cis-	Caryophyllene	
Terpenoid		Caryophyllene oxide	
Terpenoid	1,8-	Cineol	Eucalyptol
Terpenoid		Citral B	Neral
Terpenoid	α-	Copaene	Aglaiene
Terpenoid	α-	Cubebene	
Terpenoid	α-	Curcumene	
Terpenoid	γ-	Curcumene	
Terpenoid	p-	Cymene	Dolcymen, Camphogen, P-Cymol
Terpenoid	p-	Cymene-8-ol	p-cymen-8-ol
Terpenoid	γ-	Elemene	
Terpenoid	α-	Eudesmol	
Terpenoid	β-	Eudesmol	
Terpenoid	γ-	Eudesmol	
Terpenoid	cis-β-	Farnesene	(Z)-β-Farnesene
Terpenoid	trans-β-	Farnesene	(E)-β-Farnesene
Terpenoid	β-	Farnesene	
Terpenoid		Farnesol	
Terpenoid	β-	Fenchol	Endo-Fenchol, Fenchyl alcohol
Terpenoid		Fenchone	
Terpenoid		Geranyl acetone	Geranylacetone
Terpenoid		Germacrene B	
Terpenoid	α-	Guaiene	
Terpenoid		Guaiol	Champacol, Guaiac alcohol
Terpenoid	(−)-α-	Gurjunene	
Terpenoid	β-	Humulene	
Terpenoid	α-	Humulene	α-Caryophyllene
Terpenoid		Ipsdienol	
Terpenoid		Limonene	p-Menth-1,8-diene, 1-methyl-4-(1-methylethenyl)cyclohexene, 1-methyl-4-(prop-1-en-2-yl)cyclohex-1-ene
Terpenoid		Linalool	β-linalool, 3,7-dimethyl-1,6-octadien-3-ol

(Continued)

TABLE 7.1 (CONTINUED)
Molecules Found in Cannabis by Functional Group

Chemical class	Prefix	Name	Alternative ID(s)
Terpenoid	*cis-*	Linalool oxide	(Z)-linalool oxide (furanoid)
Terpenoid	*trans-*	Linalool oxide	*trans*-linalool 3,6-oxide, *trans*-2-methyl-2-vinyl-5-(1-hydroxy-1-methylethyl) tetrahydrofuran
Terpenoid		Longifolene	
Terpenoid		Menthol	
Terpenoid	α-	Muurolene	Cadinene (group of isomers)
Terpenoid	γ-	Muurolene	Cadinene (group of isomers), murolene
Terpenoid	β-	Myrcene	
Terpenoid	(+)-	Nerolidol	
Terpenoid	*cis-*β-	Ocimene	(Z)-Ocimene
Terpenoid	*trans-*β-	Ocimene	(E)-Ocimene
Terpenoid	α-	Phellandrene	
Terpenoid	β-	Phellandrene	
Terpenoid		Phytol	
Terpenoid	α-	Pinene	
Terpenoid	β-	Pinene	
Terpenoid	*trans-*	Pinocarveol	Pinocarveol, 10-pinen-3-ol
Terpenoid		Sabinene	4[10]-Thujene
Terpenoid	*cis-*	Sabinene hydrate	4-Thujanol
Terpenoid	*trans-*	Sabinene hydrate	
Terpenoid	(+)-	Sativene	
Terpenoid		Selina-3,7(11)-diene	
Terpenoid	α-	Selinene	eudesma-3,11-diene
Terpenoid	β-	Selinene	eudesma-(4(14),11-diene
Terpenoid	α-	Terpinene	
Terpenoid	γ-	Terpinene	
Terpenoid	α-	Terpinene-4-ol	Terpinen-4-ol
Terpenoid	α-	Terpineol	Terpineol
Terpenoid		Terpinolene	σ-Terpinene, α-Terpinolene
Terpenoid	α-	Thujene	
Terpenoid	(+)-	Valencene	
Terpenoid		Verbenone	2-Pinen-4-one
Terpenoid	α-	Ylangene	

This is a non-exhaustive list of compounds found naturally occurring in cannabis. Only compounds reported by at least four peer-reviewed publications have been included in the table. Data provided by the Werc Shop Laboratory, LLC., Monrovia, CA.

represents a lesser minority, usually below 30%, of the total terpene fraction. This means that one singular compound is not responsible for the characterizing aroma of cannabis as is common for fruits and herbs. Furthermore, due to the promiscuity of terpenoid production by cannabis, the resulting essential oils and terpene-fractions are rich mixtures of compounds that vary greatly in concentration and composition. And therein, perhaps, lies the magic of cannabis polypharmacy.

The interplay of multiple compounds, including additive or antagonistic effects, represents a frontier for biochemistry and pharmacy. This is not just so for cannabis, but for many substances. How does the average human body respond to a mixture of Δ^9-tetrahydrocannabinol (THC) and ethanol, for example? This is not well understood. Without that knowledge, it is even harder to understand how those two molecules interact with the variety of individual physiologies that compose the human landscape.

Although it may not yet be clear to science and medicine what interaction effects mixtures of molecules instigate upon living organisms, one thing is clear: the source of the specific molecules is immaterial. Whether (–)-limonene is derived from oranges, cannabis, or a genetically engineered yeast strain, we can convincingly assert that (–)-limonene will have the same physical, chemical, and physiological properties.

Although the source of molecules does not impact how molecules function, their concentration assuredly does. An old real estate saying succinctly holds that "location, location, location" is what is important for the value and desirability of land or buildings. Similarly, "concentration, concentration, concentration" is critical to the effects of molecules—any molecule—on living organisms. Often, we think about concentration in terms of "dose" when speaking about physiology and therapeutics. This is a hallmark of Western medicine. Paracelsus, the father of Western medicine, is often attributed the paraphrased concept "only the dose separates the medicine from the poison" that undergirds the dose-response paradigm. Physiological response aside, concentration is a critical parameter for understanding how groups of molecules act (and react) together, including how easily they degrade into something else. Concentration plays an integral role in the remaining sections of this chapter and is a fundamental concept that demands inclusion in any serious hazard assessment of additives for cannabis vapor products.

7.3 FLAVOR ADDITIVES

There is more data available on the additives used in cigarettes and e-cigarettes than in cannabis vapor products. This is partly due to e-nicotine products having a longer commercial tenure. But it also reflects the historical use of additives in cigarettes and the more robust regulatory standards that have been recently adopted for e-cigarettes around the globe. In this vein, R.J. Reynolds now regularly publishes a list of all of the additives that they use in their collective products as shown in Table 7.2 for 2019.

The U.S. Food and Drug Administration (FDA) has also published a list of harmful and potentially harmful constituents (HPHCs) found in tobacco products and

TABLE 7.2
R.J. Reynolds Ingredient List (2019 Disclosure)

Chemical class	Prefix	Name	Single-substance (SS) or mixture (X)
Ketone		Acetanisole	SS
Carboxylic acid		Acetic acid	SS
Ketone		Acetoin	SS
Ketone		Acetophenone	SS
Nitrogen-containing		Acetylpyrazine	SS
Nitrogen-containing	2-	Acetylpyridine	SS
Nitrogen-containing	3-	Acetylpyridine	SS
Amino acid	DL-	Alanine	SS
Polysaccharide		Alginate, ammonium	SS
Base		Ammonium hydroxide	SS
Base		Ammonium phosphate, dibasic	SS
Ester		Amyl butyrate	SS
		Amyris oil	X
Phenyl propene	*trans-*	Anethole	SS
Ester		Anisyl acetate	SS
		Apple juice concentrate	X
Amino acid	L-	Arginine	SS
		Ascorbic acid	SS
Amino acid	L-	Aspartic acid	SS
		Balsam tolu	X
		Beeswax absolute	X
Aldehyde		Benzaldehyde	SS
Carboxylic acid		Benzoic acid	SS
Alcohol		Benzyl alcohol	SS
Ester		Benzyl benzoate	SS
Ester		Benzyl cinnamate	SS
		Brown sugar	X
Ketone	4-(2-Furyl)-3-	Buten-2-one	SS
		Butter starter distillate	X
Ester		Butyl isovalerate	SS
Carboxylic acid		Butyric acid	SS
		Caramel color	X
		Carbon	SS
		Carbon dioxide	SS
		Cardamom oil	X
		Cardamom powder	X
		Carob (extract and powder)	X
		Carob bean extract	X
		Carrot seed oil	X
Terpenoid	L-	Carvone	SS

(Continued)

TABLE 7.2 (CONTINUED)
R.J. Reynolds Ingredient List (2019 Disclosure)

Chemical class	Prefix	Name	Single-substance (SS) or mixture (X)
Terpenoid	β-	Caryophyllene oxide	SS
Terpenoid	β-	Caryophyllene	SS
		Castoreum extract	X
Polysaccharide		Cellulose	SS
		Chicory extract	X
		Chocolate liquor	X
Aldehyde		Cinnamaldehyde	SS
Carboxylic acid		Cinnamic acid	SS
		Cinnamon bark oil	X
Ester		Cinnamyl acetate	SS
Alcohol		Cinnamyl alcohol	SS
Acid		Citric acid	SS
		Citronella oil	X
		Clary oil	X
		Cocoa (extract, powder and extractive)	X
		Coffee beans, ground and extract	X
		Cognac, green, oil	X
		Coriander oil	X
		Corn mint oil	X
		Corn syrup	X
Ester	p-	Cresyl acetate	SS
Ester	p-	Cresyl isovalerate	SS
Ketone	β-	Damascenone	SS
Ketone	β-	Damascone	SS
Ketone	cis-β-	Damascone	SS
		Davana oil	X
Lactone	Δ-	Decalactone	SS
Lactone	γ-	Decalactone	SS
Carboxylic acid		Decanoic acid	SS
Ester		Decanoic acid, ester with 1,2,3-propanetriol octanoate	SS
Monosaccharide		Dextrose	SS
Nitrogen-containing	2,3-	Diethylpyrazine	SS
Alcohol	2,6-	Dimethoxyphenol	SS
Lactone	4,5-	Dimethyl-3-hydroxy-2,5-dihydro furan-2-one	SS
Nitrogen-containing	2,5-	Dimethylpyrazine	SS
Lactone	Δ-	Dodecalactone	SS
Ester		Ethyl 2-methylbutyrate	SS

(*Continued*)

TABLE 7.2 (CONTINUED)
R.J. Reynolds Ingredient List (2019 Disclosure)

Chemical class	Prefix	Name	Single-substance (SS) or mixture (X)
Ester		Ethyl acetate	SS
Alcohol		Ethyl alcohol	SS
Ester		Ethyl benzoate	SS
Ester		Ethyl butyrate	SS
Ester		Ethyl caproate	SS
Ester		Ethyl cinnamate	SS
Ketone		Ethyl cyclotene	SS
Ester		Ethyl heptanoate	SS
Ester		Ethyl isovalerate	SS
Ester		Ethyl lactate	SS
Ester		Ethyl levulinate	SS
Ketone		Ethyl maltol	SS
Ester		Ethyl myristate	SS
Ester		Ethyl pentanoate	SS
Ester		Ethyl phenylacetate	SS
Aldehyde		Ethyl vanillin	SS
Nitrogen-containing	3-	Ethyl-2,6-dimethylpyrazine	SS
Nitrogen-containing	3-	Ethyl-2-methylpyrazine	SS
Nitrogen-containing	2-	Ethyl-3,(5 or 6)-dimethylpyrazine	SS
Lactone	5-	Ethyl-3-hydroxy-4-methyl-2(5h)-furanone	SS
Terpenoid	4-	Ethylguaiacol	SS
Terpenoid		Eucalyptol	SS
		Fenugreek extract	X
		Fenugreek seed and absolute	X
		Fig extract	X
		Fig juice concentrate	X
Ketone		Furaneol	SS
Terpenoid		Geraniol	SS
		Geranium oil	X
Ketone		Geranyl acetone	SS
		Ginger extract	X
Glyceride		Glycerides, mixed decanoyl and octanoyl	
Alcohol		Glycerin	SS
		Graphite	SS
Terpenoid		Guaiacol	SS
		Guar gum	X
		Gum benzoin, sumatra	X
Lactone	γ-	Heptalactone	SS
Carboxylic acid		Heptanoic acid	SS

(*Continued*)

TABLE 7.2 (CONTINUED)
R.J. Reynolds Ingredient List (2019 Disclosure)

Chemical class	Prefix	Name	Single-substance (SS) or mixture (X)
Lactone	γ-	Hexalactone	SS
Carboxylic acid		Hexanoic acid	SS
Alcohol	1-	Hexanol	SS
Alcohol	cis-3-	Hexen-1-ol	SS
Ester	cis-3-	Hexen-1-yl acetate	SS
Ester		Hexyl acetate	SS
Ester		Hexyl phenylacetate	SS
		High fructose corn syrup	X
		Honey	X
		Hydrogenated glucose syrup	X
Ketone	4-p-	Hydroxyphenyl-2-butanone	SS
		Immortelle (absolute and extract)	X
Monosaccharide		Invert sugar	SS
Ketone	β-	Ionone	SS
Ester		Isoamyl acetate	SS
Ester		Isoamyl benzoate	SS
Ester		Isoamyl butyrate	SS
Ester		Isoamyl isovalerate	SS
Ester		Isoamyl phenylacetate	SS
Ester		Isobutyl cinnamate	SS
Ester		Isobutyl phenylacetate	SS
Nitrogen-containing		Isobutyl-3-methoxypyrazine, 2-	SS
Alcohol	α-	Isobutylphenethyl alcohol	SS
Aldehyde		Isobutyraldehyde	SS
Carboxylic acid		Isobutyric acid	SS
Ketone		Isophorone	SS
Carboxylic acid		Isovaleric acid	SS
		Jasmine, oil	X
		Labdanum absolute	X
		Labdanum oil	X
Carboxylic acid		Lactic acid	SS
Fatty acid		Lauric acid	SS
Carboxylic acid		Levulinic acid	SS
		Licorice (extract and powder)	X
Terpenoid		Linalool	SS
Ester		Linalyl acetate	SS
		Lovage (extract, root and oil)	X
Amino acid	L-	Lysine	SS
Carboxylic acid		Malic acid	SS
		Malt extract	X

(Continued)

TABLE 7.2 (CONTINUED)
R.J. Reynolds Ingredient List (2019 Disclosure)

Chemical class	Prefix	Name	Single-substance (SS) or mixture (X)
Polysaccharide		Maltodextrin	SS
Ketone		Maltol	SS
		Mate absolute	X
Terpenoid		Menthol	SS
Nitrogen-containing	2-	Methoxy-3-methylpyrazine	SS
Alcohol	2-	Methoxy-4-methylphenol	SS
Aldehyde	p-	Methoxybenzaldehyde	SS
Ketone		Methyl acetophenone	SS
Fatty ester		Methyl linoleate	SS
Fatty ester		Methyl linolenate	SS
Ketone	6-	Methyl-3,5-heptadien-2-one	SS
Ketone	6-	Methyl-5-hepten-2-one	SS
Aldehyde	3-	Methylbutyraldehyde	SS
Carboxylic acid	2-	Methylbutyric acid	SS
Ketone		Methylcyclopentenolone	SS
Nitrogen-containing	2-	Methylpyrazine	SS
Carboxylic acid	2-	Methylvaleric acid	SS
Carboxylic acid	3-	Methylvaleric acid	SS
		Molasses	X
		Myrrh absolute	X
		Myrrh extract and oil	X
Ether	Dodecahydro-3A,6,6,9A-Tetramethyl	Naphtho[2,1-B]furan	SS
		Neroli, bigarade oil	X
Terpenoid		Nerolidol	SS
Lactone	γ-	Nonalactone	SS
Carboxylic acid		Nonanoic acid	SS
		Nutmeg oil	X
Lactone	γ-	Octalactone	SS
Carboxylic acid		Octanoic acid	SS
Alcohol	1-	Octen-3-ol	SS
Aldehyde	(2e)-2-	Octenal	SS
		Orange oil sweet terpeneless	X
		Orris root extract	X
Ketone		Oxacycloheptadec-10-en-2-one	
Lactone		Pentadecalactone	SS
Ketone	2,3-	Pentanedione	SS
Ketone	2-	Pentanone	SS
		Pepper, black, oil	X

(Continued)

TABLE 7.2 (CONTINUED)
R.J. Reynolds Ingredient List (2019 Disclosure)

Chemical class	Prefix	Name	Single-substance (SS) or mixture (X)
		Peppermint oil, terpeneless	X
		Peru balsam oil	X
Ester		Phenethyl acetate	SS
Aldehyde		Phenylacetaldehyde	SS
Carboxylic acid		Phenylacetic acid	SS
Alcohol		Phenylethyl alcohol	SS
Acid		Phosphoric acid	SS
		Pineapple juice concentrate	X
Terpenoid	α-	Pinene	SS
Terpenoid	β-	Pinene	SS
Aldehyde		Piperonal	SS
		Pipsissewa Leaf extract	X
		Plum extract	X
Polyol		Polyethylene glycol	SS
Base		Potassium carbonate	SS
Salt		Potassium sorbate	SS
Carboxylic acid		Propionic acid	SS
Ester		Propyl acetate	SS
Alcohol		Propylene glycol	SS
Lactone	3-	Propylidenephthalide	SS
		Prune juice concentrate	X
		Pulp, cellulose	X
		Pyroligneous acids, hickory	X
		Rose oil turkish	X
		Rosemary oil	X
		Rum ether	X
		Sage oil	X
Aldehyde		Salicylaldehyde	SS
		Sandalwood, yellow, oil	X
Base		Sodium bicarbonate	SS
Base		Sodium carbonate	SS
Salt		Sodium citrate	SS
		Spearmint oil	X
		Specially denatured alcohol #4	X
		Specially denatured rum #4	X
		Styrax	X
Monosaccharide		Sucrose	SS
		Sugar beet juice concentrate	X
Carboxylic acid		Tartaric acid (d-, l-, dl-, meso-)	SS
Terpenoid	α-	Terpineol	SS

(Continued)

TABLE 7.2 (CONTINUED)
R.J. Reynolds Ingredient List (2019 Disclosure)

Chemical class	Prefix	Name	Single-substance (SS) or mixture (X)
Ester		Terpinyl acetate	SS
Nitrogen-containing	5,6,7,8-	Tetrahydroquinoxaline	SS
Nitrogen-containing	2,3,5,6-	Tetramethylpyrazine	SS
Ester		Tolyl isobutyrate	SS
Ester	p-	Tolyl phenylacetate	SS
Ester		Triacetin	SS
Ester		Triethyl citrate	SS
Ketone	2,6,6-	Trimethylcyclohex-2-ene-1,4-dione	SS
Nitrogen-containing	2,3,5-	Trimethylpyrazine	SS
Lactone	Δ-	Undecalactone	SS
Lactone	γ-	Undecalactone	SS
Nitrogen-containing		Urea	SS
		Valerian root oil	X
Lactone	γ-	Valerolactone	SS
		Vanilla extract	X
Aldehyde		Vanillin	SS
Phenylpropene		Vanitrope (propenyl guaethol)	SS
Aldehyde		Veratraldehyde	SS
		Water	SS
		Wheat absolute	X

A reportedly exhaustive list of chemicals, including flavor additives, deployed in R.J. Reynolds' suite of products in 2019. These are organized by chemical class and whether the ingredient is a single molecule (M) or a complex mixture (X).

tobacco smoke, which is shown in Table 7.3 (Center for Tobacco Products 2019). This list includes 93 entries consisting of very few flavor additives. Many components are the result of unintentional contamination of the base materials (e.g., metals). Others are mainly combustion or thermal degradation byproducts of other ingredients found in manufactured tobacco and nicotine products.

Similarly, in Europe, the list of substances prohibited as ingredients in e-cigarettes is lengthy. But only two are flavor additives as can be seen in Table 7.3. Although flavor additives have the potential to cause harm, very few present *known* acute, toxicological risk when consumed in *low* concentrations. Diacetyl (butane-2,3-dione) and pentane-2,3-dione, which impart buttery flavors, are exceptions. Initially investigated due to worker exposure incidents that occurred in microwaveable popcorn manufacturing facilities that led to a condition dubbed "popcorn lung," it is now understood that even at low concentrations, these compounds can downregulate multiple genes involved in the biogenesis of cilia that line human airways (Brass 2017, Park 2019).

TABLE 7.3

Harmful and Potentially Harmful Constituents (HPHC) in Tobacco Products and Tobacco Smoke

Chemical class	Prefix	Name	Toxicological Class
Aldehyde		Acetaldehyde	CA, RT, AD
Amide		Acetamide	CA
Ketone		Acetone	RT
Aldehyde		Acrolein	RT, CT
Amide		Acrylamide	CA
Nitrogen-containing		Acrylonitrile	CA, RT
Polycyclic chromene		Aflatoxin B1	CA
Nitrogen-containing	4-	Aminobiphenyl	CA
Nitrogen-containing	1-	Aminonaphthalene	CA
Nitrogen-containing	2-	Aminonaphthalene	CA
Nitrogen-containing		Ammonia	RT
Nitrogen-containing		Anabasine	AD
Nitrogen-containing	o-	Anisidine	CA
Metal		Arsenic	CA, CT, RDT
Nitrogen-containing		A-α-C (2-Amino-9$\underline{H}$-pyrido[2,3-$\underline{b}$] indole)	CA
Polycyclic aromatic hydrocarbon (PAH)		Benz[$\underline{a}$]anthracene	CA, CT
Polycyclic aromatic hydrocarbon (PAH)		Benz[$\underline{j}$]aceanthrylene	CA
Aromatic hydrocarbon		Benzene	CA, CT, RDT
Polycyclic aromatic hydrocarbon (PAH)		Benzo[$\underline{b}$]fluoranthene	CA, CT
Polycyclic aromatic hydrocarbon (PAH)		Benzo[$\underline{k}$]fluoranthene	CA, CT
Polycyclic aromatic hydrocarbon (PAH)		Benzo[$\underline{b}$]furan	CA
Polycyclic aromatic hydrocarbon (PAH)		Benzo[$\underline{a}$]pyrene	CA
Polycyclic aromatic hydrocarbon (PAH)		Benzo[$\underline{c}$]phenanthrene	CA
Metal		Beryllium	CA
Unsaturated hydrocarbon	1,3-	Butadiene	CA, RT, RDT
Metal		Cadmium	CA, RT, RDT
Carboxylic acid		Caffeic acid	CA
Gas		Carbon monoxide	RDT
Benzene-like		Catechol	CA
Polyhalogenated aromatic hydrocarbon		Chlorinated dioxins/furans	CA, RDT
Metal		Chromium	CA, RT, RDT
Polycyclic aromatic hydrocarbon (PAH)		Chrysene	CA, CT
Metal		Cobalt	CA, CT
Benzene-like		Coumarin	Banned in food
Benzene-like	o-, m-, andp-	Cresols	CA, RT
Aldehyde		Crotonaldehyde	CA
Polycyclic aromatic hydrocarbon (PAH)		Cyclopenta[$\underline{c,d}$]pyrene	CA

(Continued)

TABLE 7.3 (CONTINUED)

Harmful and Potentially Harmful Constituents (HPHC) in Tobacco Products and Tobacco Smoke

Chemical class	Prefix	Name	Toxicological Class
Polycyclic aromatic hydrocarbon (PAH)		Dibenz[a,h]anthracene	CA
Polycyclic aromatic hydrocarbon (PAH)		Dibenzo[a,e]pyrene	CA
Polycyclic aromatic hydrocarbon (PAH)		Dibenzo[a,h]pyrene	CA
Polycyclic aromatic hydrocarbon (PAH)		Dibenzo[a,i]pyrene	CA
Polycyclic aromatic hydrocarbon (PAH)		Dibenzo[a,l]pyrene	CA
Nitrogen-containing	2,6-	Dimethylaniline	CA
Nitrogen-containing		Ethyl carbamate (urethane)	CA, RDT
Benzene-like		Ethylbenzene	CA
Epoxide		Ethylene oxide	CA, RT, RDT
Aldehyde		Formaldehyde	CA, RT
Aromatic heterocycle		Furan	CA
Nitrogen-containing		Glu-P-1 (2-Amino-6-methyldipyrido[1,2-a:3',2'-d]imidazole)	CA
Nitrogen-containing		Glu-P-2 (2-Aminodipyrido[1,2-a:3',2'-d]imidazole)	CA
Nitrogen-containing		Hydrazine	CA, RT
Nitrogen-containing		Hydrogen cyanide	RT, CT
Polycyclic aromatic hydrocarbon (PAH)		Indeno[1,2,3-cd]pyrene	CA
Nitrogen-containing		IQ (2-Amino-3-methylimidazo[4,5-f]quinoline)	CA
Unsaturated hydrocarbon		Isoprene	CA
Metal		Lead	CA, CT, RDT
Nitrogen-containing		MeA-α-C (2-Amino-3-methyl)-9H-pyrido[2,3-b]indole)	CA
Metal		Mercury	CA, RDT
Ketone		Methyl ethyl ketone	RT
Polycyclic aromatic hydrocarbon (PAH)	5-	Methylchrysene	CA
Nitrogen-containing		4-(Methylnitrosamino)-1-(3-pyridyl)-1-butanone (NNK)	CA
Polycyclic aromatic hydrocarbon (PAH)		Naphthalene	CA, RT
Metal		Nickel	CA, RT
Nitrogen-containing		Nicotine	RDT, AD
Nitrogen-containing		Nitrobenzene	CA, RT, RDT
Nitrogen-containing		Nitromethane	CA
Nitrogen-containing	2-	Nitropropane	CA
Nitrogen-containing	N-	Nitrosodiethanolamine (NDELA)	CA
Nitrogen-containing	N-	Nitrosodiethylamine	CA
Nitrogen-containing	N-	Nitrosodimethylamine (NDMA)	CA

(Continued)

TABLE 7.3 (CONTINUED)

Harmful and Potentially Harmful Constituents (HPHC) in Tobacco Products and Tobacco Smoke

Chemical class	Prefix	Name	Toxicological Class
Nitrogen-containing	N-	Nitrosomethylethylamine	CA
Nitrogen-containing	N-	Nitrosomorpholine (NMOR)	CA
Nitrogen-containing	N-	Nitrosonornicotine (NNN)	CA
Nitrogen-containing	N-	Nitrosopiperidine (NPIP)	CA
Nitrogen-containing	N-	Nitrosopyrrolidine (NPYR)	CA
Nitrogen-containing	N-	Nitrososarcosine (NSAR)	CA
Nitrogen-containing		Nornicotine	AD
Alcohol		Phenol	RT, CT
Nitrogen-containing		PhIP (2-Amino-1-methyl-6-phenylimidazo[4,5-b]pyridine)	CA
Radioactive metal		Polonium-210	CA
Aldehyde		Propionaldehyde	RT, CT
Epoxide		Propylene oxide	CA, RT
Nitrogen-containing		Quinoline	CA
Metal		Selenium	RT
Benzene-like		Styrene	CA
Benzene-like	o-	Toluidine	CA
Benzene-like		Toluene	RT, RDT
Nitrogen-containing		Trp-P-1 (3-Amino-1,4-dimethyl-5H-pyrido[4,3-b]indole)	CA
Nitrogen-containing		Trp-P-2 (1-Methyl-3-amino-5H-pyrido[4,3-b]indole)	CA
Radioactive metal		Uranium-235	CA, RT
Radioactive metal		Uranium-238	CA, RT
Unsaturated ester		Vinyl acetate	CA, RT
Unsaturated chlorocarbon		Vinyl chloride	CA

All constituents identified by the US Food and Drug Administration (FDA) as harmful or potentially harmful, organized by chemical and toxicological classes. Carcinogen (CA), respiratory toxicant (RDT), addictive (AD). https://www.federalregister.gov/documents/2019/08/05/2019-16658/harmful-and-pote ntially-harmful-constituents-in-tobacco-products-established-list-proposed-additions

Substances that perhaps present a greater toxicological risk than low concentration flavor additives have been the focus in Europe. This includes anything that is carcinogenic, mutagenic, or a known reproductive toxin as well as many common metals (Table 7.4). Compounds that can alter user perception about the inherent risk of nicotine-containing products are also forbidden, such as vitamins and minerals. Vitamins may convey the false impression that e-cigarettes containing them are "healthy." In addition, substances that possess independent stimulant effects are prohibited. Caffeine and taurine, as examples, can lead to unexpected additive or

TABLE 7.4

Ingredients Prohibited as E-Cigarette Additives in the EU

Substance	CAS no.	Prohibition rationale	
		Substance class	Notes
Diacetyl (butane-2,3-dione)	431-03-8	Activated carbonyl	Known inhalation hazard. No intentional addition permitted.
Pentane-2,3-dione	600-14-6	Activated carbonyl	
Formaldehyde	50-00-0	Volatile carbonyl	Known inhalation hazard.
Acetaldehyde	75-07-0	Volatile carbonyl	No intentional addition permitted.
Acrolein	107-08-8	Volatile carbonyl	May unintentionally be present in aerosol stream due to thermal degradation of other ingredients.
Diethylene glycol	111-46-6	Polyol	Substance and metabolites have known
Ethylene glycol	107-21-1	Polyol	neuro-, renal-, and cardio-toxicology. Can be contaminants in propylene glycol and glycerin.
Cadmium (Cd)	7440-43-9	Metal	Exposure to metals presents risks via most
Chromium (Cr)	7440-47-3	Metal	routes of human exposure, but especially
Iron (Fe)	7439-89-6	Metal	for inhalation where metals can deposit on
Lead (Pb)	7439-92-1	Metal	delicate alveolar tissue and disrupt
Mercury (Hg)	7439-97-6	Metal	gas-exchange capacity.
Nickel (Ni)	7440-02-0	Metal	
Vitamins and minerals		Vitamins	Any ingredient that can create the impression that a vaping product has a health benefit or presents reduced health risks.
Caffeine	58-08-2	Stimulant	Avoid compounds that are associated with
Taurine	107-35-7	Stimulant	energy and vitality to avoid cross-psychoactivity and user expectations.
Emission colorants		Pigments	Unnecessary risk
Carcinogenic, mutagenic, and/or reproductive toxicants (CMRs)		CMRs	
Respiratory sensitizers		Respiratory sensitizers	A chemical that will lead to hypersensitivity of the airways following inhalation of the chemical. In contrast to respiratory irritation, respiratory sensitization is an immunological response to previous exposure to a chemical.

A composite list sourced from the European Tobacco Products Directive (2016) and the Vaping Products Manufacturing Guide from the British Standards Institute. It is important to note the differences between this table and Table 7.5 that detail the components that must be tested for and controlled in the aerosol streams of finished vaping products.

synergistic effects. In general, the focus in Europe has been on harm minimization by focusing on the greatest hazards and controlling those substances that have definitive harmful effects.

Since the goal of a harm minimization approach is to minimize the harm experienced by the user, it should not be surprising that Europe also focuses on testing the emissions from actual e-cigarettes *after* heating and aerosolization rather than simply testing the unheated vape fluid that a manufacturer adds to a cartridge. Table 7.5 lists the emission contaminants that are commonly assessed. Comparing this list to that in Table 7.4—the substances that are prohibited and/or tested provide a few key insights. The first and most important is that simply because a manufacturer does not intentionally add a substance to a vape formulation does not mean it will not be present in the aerosol stream that exits the device. Intentional ingredients, such as the diluent propylene glycol (PG), can have unintentional and harmful contaminants like ethylene glycol if not using United States Pharmacopeia (USP)

TABLE 7.5
Emission Contaminants Tested for in E-Cigarettes in the EU

		Limit value	
Chemical substance	CAS No.	BSI	AFNOR
Diacetyl (butane-2,3-dione)	431-03-8	Emission measured	490 µg/200 puffs
Formaldehyde	50-00-0	Emission measured	200 µg/200 puffs
Acetaldehyde	75-07-0	Emission measured	3200 µg/200 puffs
Acrolein	107-08-8	Emission measured	16 µg/200 puffs
Al		Emission measured	
Cd		Emission measured	2 µg/200 puffs
Cr		Emission measured	3 µg/200 puffs
Fe		Emission measured	
Pb		Emission measured	5 µg/200 puffs
Ni		Emission measured	5 µg/200 puffs
As		Emission measured	2 µg/200 puffs
Sb		Emission measured	20 µg/200 puffs
Sn		Emission measured	
Silica particles		Emission measured	
Solid particles			No emission
Carcinogenic substances			No emission
Toxic/dangerous substances in general		No substances must be emitted above the toxicological value as defined by toxicological risk assessment (TRA)	No emission beyond technical avoidable concentrations

Although EU member nations are bound to follow the EU Tobacco Products Directive, they have flexibility in how they enforce the provisions. For example, emission testing can differ depending on the jurisdiction. Shown here are the emission analytes and tolerances, if any, as recommended by the British Standards Institute and the French equivalent, Association Française de Normalisation (AFNOR).

grade PG. Testing for these contaminants ensures that manufacturers enforce acceptable standards of purity and impurities in their ingredients. Intentional and acceptable ingredients can also experience thermal degradation or pyrolysis upon vaping. For example, triacetin (a flavor and solubilization enhancer) can thermally degrade into acetic acid, which can increase the decomposition of PG and glycerin (VG) into acrolein, acetaldehyde, and formaldehyde—three substances found in Table 7.5 (Vreeke 2018). Since these reactions depend on reaching the necessary activation energy to occur, a higher temperature (i.e., more energy) leads to more degradation. Testing for these contaminants is therefore an indirect way to both assess the proper operation of the vapor device (does it heat the material to the intended temperature?) and the interaction between the vape device and the vape fluid (heat transfer). Lastly, the presence of metals in emission streams underscores the fact that the user is not simply inhaling the vapor. Rather, they are inhaling a complex mixture of vaporized components and nanosized particles (viz. liquid droplets). Testing for metals also helps provide insight about device quality (does the heating element sinter?) and formulation-device interactions (does the vape fluid leach lead from cheaply made glass cartridge housings?).

Flavor and aroma compounds have been largely untested for safety in vapor and aerosol products—whether nicotine- or cannabis-containing—for a variety of reasons. In the United States, tobacco companies have been reluctant to evaluate the potential hazards of flavor compounds without a clear mandate to do so, especially because these ingredients have a long-running history of use in traditional cigarettes. Flavoring nicotine products is also a contentious issue because it is posited that some flavored products can make products especially appealing to children, even if the flavored products can help adults quit smoking. Right or wrong, the debate has hampered investigations in the United States into if, and under what conditions, flavor additives can be harmful. Lastly, flavor compounds have been largely neglected in terms of toxicology in the face of other contaminants that present known hazards (e.g., heavy metals) or constituents utilized in higher concentrations than flavor compounds, such as diluents (e.g., propylene glycol). Other classes of compounds are strictly prohibited in nicotine products including carcinogens, mutagens, and reproductive toxins (CMR), as well as other psychoactive substances (e.g., caffeine, ethanol).

What we do know about the flavor additives used in cannabis vapor products is limited to mostly unpublished reports and inside information. Largely, it appears that many companies producing products specific for cannabis vapor products have sought to avoid some of the problem compounds traditionally used in e-cigarettes (e.g., diacetyl). Others have focused upon only using compounds found naturally occurring in cannabis irrespective of the source of those ingredients. On average, it appears that the nascent cannabis vapor industry is taking steps to responsibly address potentially hazardous compounds and act proactively to avoid them.

The differing polarities between e-cigarette and cannabis vapor formulations is another reason why the flavor compounds used in each do not exhibit perfect overlap. Some newer e-cigarette products utilize nicotine salts, which are more polar than free-base nicotine. They also serve to mask the harsh taste of neutral (free-base) nicotine. Even those e-cigarette solutions that merely use neutral nicotine (i.e., free-base nicotine) are more polar compared with cannabinoid-containing formulations. This is one reason why VG and PG are rarely used in cannabis vapor products—they are too polar to effectively dissolve cannabinoids. Table 7.6 shows a number of compounds believed to be in use for manufactured cannabis products that are not found to be naturally occurring in cannabis along with the characterizing flavor/aroma of each compound.

At the current time, a ready-made corpus of data does not exist that provides adequate insight into the potential hazards of inhaling flavor compounds at any temperature, let alone elevated temperatures, for short durations. The Flavor Extracts Manufacturers Association (FEMA) has rightly pointed out that lists of compounds generally recognized as safe (GRAS) for food flavor use and ingestion cannot be relied upon as an indication of acceptability for use in vapor and aerosol products. GRAS determinations are conducted for specific uses and functions of substances and not simply for the substance itself.

There are overlapping principles between the toxicology of ingestion and inhalation, however. For example, a carcinogenic or mutagenic substance will be carcinogenic or mutagenic irrespective of the route of exposure. The magnitude and hence the degree of risk imparted may change according to the route of exposure, but the qualitative hazard remains nonetheless. But the specifics of ingestion and inhalation toxicology vary considerably.

Two broad reasons can be identified for why flavor additives that are GRAS *for ingestion* may nevertheless present a hazard when inhaled in vape products. The first may be obvious. The types of tissues that compose the oral cavity and the alimentary

---

TABLE 7.6

Flavor Additives Utilized In Cannabis Vapor Products

Flavor molecules used in cannabis vapor products			
Chemical class	**Prefix**	**Name**	**Characterizing flavor**
Aldehyde		Benzaldehyde	Cherry, almond
Ester		Isoamylacetate	Banana
Ester		Ethylvalerate	Green apple
Aldehyde		Ethyl methylphenylglycidate	Strawberry
Ester		Methyl anthranilate	Grape
Ester		Octyl ethanoate	Orange
Terpenoid, aldehyde	(E- and Z-)	Citral	Lemon
Terpenoid	α-	Terpinene	Lime
Ester		Hexyl lactate	Pear
Lactone	γ-	Nonalactone	Coconut

A shortlist of flavor additives used in cannabis vapor products organized by chemical class and characterizing flavor/aroma. Not included in this table are the plethora of essential oils and other complex botanical mixtures that are utilized by some manufacturers.

---

canal differ significantly from those that line airways and lungs. Different tissues mean different cellular reactions can occur. Diacetyl (butane-2,3-dione) is a prime example. Diacetyl appears to downregulate the biogenesis of cilia in cells that line the human airway. These hair-like cell structures function to move contaminants and other unwanted matter up and out of the lungs by both producing mucus and rhythmically beating upward for ultimate excretion via the nose and mouth. The digestive tract does not contain respiratory cilia. As such, diacetyl presents little hazard when eaten even though it is hazardous to inhale.

The second reason may be less obvious to the non-scientist. Commercially available forms of vaporization devices involve a heating step that converts a liquid into a gaseous stream of vapors and liquid/solid particles, i.e., an aerosol, that a user then inhales. This heat is introduced quickly, resulting in high temperatures—sometimes exceedingly high. Other than causing matter to change state (e.g., liquid to gas), heat also catalyzes chemical reactions. This should be obvious to anyone who has grilled a filet mignon and watched it change from red, to pink, to brown (and hopefully no further).

Engineers often use a rule of thumb based upon the Arrhenius equation to estimate that each *10°C increase* in temperature leads to a doubling of reaction rate. This means that if molecule X changes into molecule Y, then approximately twice as much Y will form at 35°C than at 25°C during the same time period. With a 20°C increase, four times as much Y will form at 45°C than at 25°C. For the high temperatures inside of a vape-device atomizer, which are routinely greater than 200°C but can extend above and beyond 500°C, chemistry can be activated and accelerated in a manner that is vastly different from what happens at ambient temperature.

The thermal degradation of alpha-tocopherol acetate (also known as vitamin E acetate, VEA) to ketene is a relevant example. At room temperature, this degradation reaction does not proceed. Even at temperatures below 500°C, this reaction does not appreciably occur. But upwards of 600°C, ketene is calculated to form in quantities such that it could become concentrated enough to create chemical burns if inhaled (Wu and O'Shea 2020). Depending on the device, a formulation may be hazardous, or it may not be. This principle should be alarming. We delve further into this complexity in the following sections of this chapter where we discuss the interactions between the composition of vapor formulations, the design of vape devices, and the manner in which vapers use such devices. We raise the principle here because it sets the groundwork for predicting what substances could present likely hazards for vape applications. Chapter 9 additionally describes specific chemical reactions and aerosol products that have been identified upon vaping and dabbing cannabis concentrates.

Since a corpus of safety data for heated and inhaled substances does not yet exist, all determinations of safety (if done at all) for vapor devices are done on an *ad hoc* basis. One exposes the aerosols generated by the heating of complex formulations in complex devices to lung cells and tissue/animal models to see if there is a hazard. That is a top-down approach. If instead one wanted to take a bottom-up approach, one could individually evaluate the toxicology of the thousands of substances that may be used in vape devices at temperatures ranging from 100°C to 1000°C and also expose them to *in vitro* and *in vivo* tests of cardiopulmonary toxicology to understand the risks. The magnitude of such an undertaking in terms of time and resources is difficult to estimate but is likely to require decades and hundreds of billions of dollars. A relevant example is the Flavor Extracts Manufacturers Association (FEMA) undertaking over the past six decades to determine under what conditions roughly 4000 compounds can be safely used as flavor compounds for food at an estimated cost in USD billions or tens of billions. Even still such an exhaustive bottom-up approach is open to uncertainty surrounding mixture effects—how chemicals can interact in ways that are additive, synergistic, or antagonistic.

While it clearly makes sense to pursue both top-down and bottom-up approaches to inhalation toxicology, there remains a need for assessing the potential hazards of compounds now. Why sit on our hands and wait for data if we can deduce some cautionary insight now? In fact, this same principle was pursued for food flavor compounds while FEMA was conducting the time-consuming bottom-up work on individual compounds and developed into a "decision-tree" approach by Cramer, Ford, and Hall (1976; Schnabel and Taylor 2015). The clear benefit of such an approach is that decisions are based upon structural homology with the rationale being that similar molecular motifs lead to similar decomposition pathways, metabolic routes, and toxicological insults.

If a decision-tree approach were developed for substances meant to be heated and inhaled, current data suggests a few key chemical classes that may warrant caution. For example, the class of compounds that have similar aryl acetate moieties to alpha-tocopherol acetate and could either decompose to ketene with extreme heat or directly acetylate biological nucleophiles, such as amino acid side chains (e.g. lysine), may have sufficient cause to be avoided. Small chemical modifications of proteins can often lead to drastic changes in function that can be difficult for organisms to recognize and repair. Other classes of compounds that have similar reactivity in potentially "capping" biological nucleophiles may be used with caution or in limited concentration. This includes the so-called "activated carbonyls." Activated carbonyls possess electron-withdrawing characteristics that increase the electrophilic character of the carbonyl—making for more facile reactions with nucleophiles. Activated carbonyls include alpha-beta unsaturated carbonyls and alpha-diketones. In fact, 2,3-butanedione (diacetyl) is an alpha-diketone and instigates harmful effects on lung tissue through chemical modification of lung proteins in addition to its putative effects on cilia growth and function.

7.4 DILUENTS AND NON-FLAVOR ADDITIVES

The e-cigarette, or vaping, product use-associated lung injury (EVALI) outbreak of 2019 led to intensive scrutiny of manufactured cannabis concentrate products, and specifically ingredients such as the diluent vitamin E acetate (tocopheryl acetate, VEA). The CDC website notes that as of February 18, 2020, there had been 2807 hospitalized patients and 68 deaths attributed to EVALI. There has been a steady decline since August 2019, but new cases continue to be reported by states (CDC 2020).

Personal communications from clinicians in New York and California hospitals in December of 2020 revealed that they observe approximately two EVALI patients admitted per month. Although this information is anecdotal, it is in agreement with the CDC's report of a decline in cases, but also highlights a need for continued vigilance. Moreover, of concern is the fact that EVALI sufferers, COVID-19 patients, and patients with other respiratory issues present similar symptoms.

The rapidity of EVALI's harmful effects is one of its unique hallmarks and major challenges. For example, its rapid onset is in stark contrast to the deadly, chronic health effects of traditional smoking that take decades to appear. Currently, very little is known about the etiology of EVALI. A better understanding of the underlying causes of EVALI specifically, and lung injuries from vaping in general, is needed to address potential future related outbreaks, more chronic potential health problems, and guide the design of products affording harm reduction.

Although the focus on illicit THC products and VEA has led to public awareness and the targeting of related illegal operations by law enforcement, there have been peer-reviewed reports of EVALI patients having vaped nicotine, but not cannabis, products (Lozier 2019).

Clinicians have reported that EVALI symptoms resemble lipoid pneumonia. It is unclear, though, if the inhalation of exogenous lipids or the accumulation of endogenous lipids is involved. In addition, chemical burn-like symptoms have also been reported. For example, a detailed histopathological investigation led researchers to conclude that EVALI represents a form of airway-centered chemical pneumonitis from one or more inhaled toxic substances rather than exogenous lipoid pneumonia. Research into the causes of EVALI and the putative role of VEA is ongoing. Meantime, in responding to the EVALI outbreak, the CDC has stated that a primary proactive regulatory strategy is ensuring that chemicals of concern are not introduced into the supply chain. However, as noted earlier in this chapter, there is a dearth of knowledge about the inhalation toxicology of common vaping ingredients.

The high viscosity of THC and CBD can cause challenging processing and handling issues. Once cannabinoids are enriched via the distillation of manufactured extracts, the resultant high potency distillates are mixed with viscosity modifiers such as VEA and/or other thickening/thinning agents. Terpenes can also be used, and a variety of terpene formulations are sold for this purpose as well as to enhance flavor and aroma.

Although vitamin E and viscosity modifiers and additives are naturally occurring in the cannabis plant material, their levels are altered during post-distillation and related manufacturing processes. VEA, for example, has been found in cannabis vape samples at levels of up to approximately 70% v/v. As highlighted previously, significantly enhanced levels of molecular components where the inhalation toxicology is unknown can put consumers at risk. The chemical structures of some currently common cannabis oil additives are shown in Figure 7.1. These include medium-chain triglycerides (MCTs, coconut oil), triethyl citrate (TEC), alpha-(−)-bisabolol, phytol, and squalane (SQL). One investigation to date has found that additives sometimes found in vaping products, such as MCTs, TEC, and SQL can thermally degrade into chemical byproducts. Some of these byproducts are known respiratory toxins and

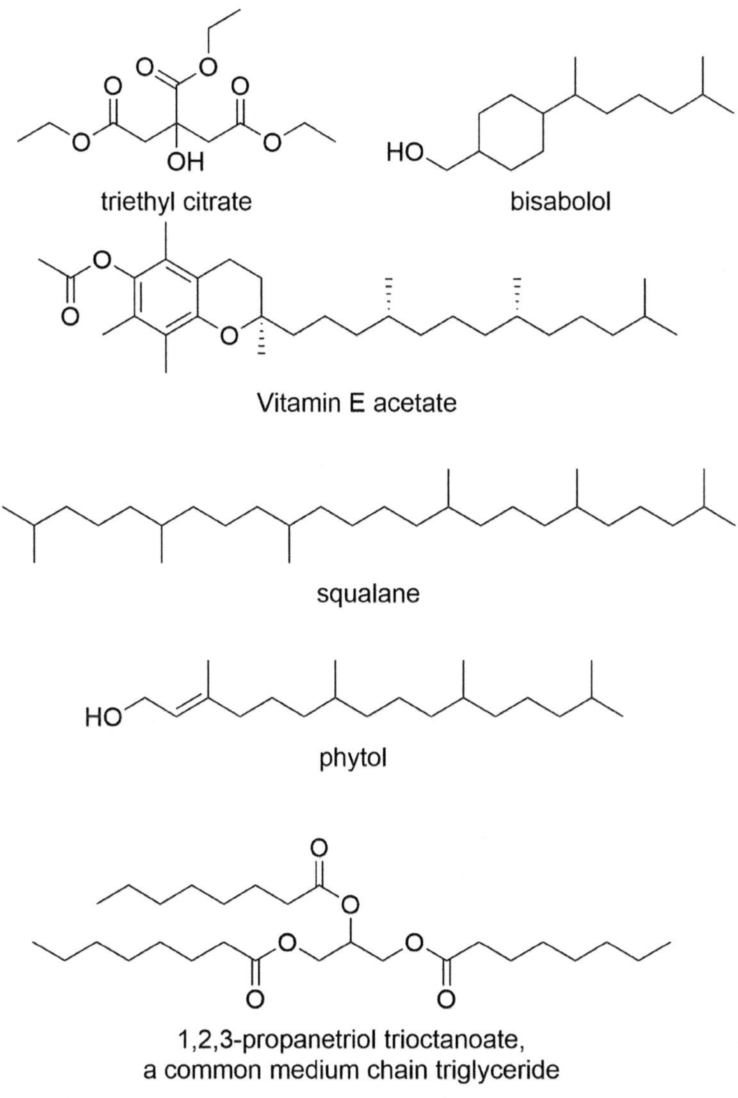

FIGURE 7.1 Structures of select non-flavor additives that have been used in cannabis concentrate formulations.

carcinogens, which can result in a reduction in human airway epithelial cell viability (Jiang 2020). More research is needed to validate and understand the molecular and biomolecular mechanisms related to these initial findings, as well as their relevance to real-world usage patterns and cannabis oil concentrate formulations.

In addition to cannabis product formulations and aerosol chemical components, another critical factor impacting human health is the aerosol particulate matter formed upon vaping cannabis products. E-cigarette aerosols consist of gaseous and particulate phases. The particulate phase actually consists of liquid droplets formed by aerosol components that partition preferentially into the liquid phase as opposed to the gas phase. Tobacco-derived e-cigarette products create particles in the nanometer size regime, which is concerning because small particles are deposited more deeply in the lungs. In addition, the high surface area to volume ratio of nanoparticles can render the particles highly reactive and/or catalytic. In general, smaller particles can more readily pass through and penetrate cell membranes.

A preliminary study was reported by Jaques (2018) showing that vaping and dabbing cannabis concentrates can produce potentially concerning concentrations of indoor PM2.5. The levels of PM2.5 in this study exceed US Environmental Protection Agency and World Health Organization thresholds. More recently, a study of VEA-derived aerosols showed that they contained extremely small (ca. 50 nanometers) particles (Mikheev 2020). It is important to note that, similar to flavor compounds, it is the *concentration* of the particles at these small size ranges that can have the most impact on toxicological properties. More research is needed in this area directed toward addressing the effects of various chemical formulations, user topography (puff behavior), and vaping devices on aerosol particle properties.

In addition to the GRAS for food-use diluents and additives described previously, there have been reports of cannabis vaping products adulterated with pine rosin, the primary toxic ingredient in solder fumes (Meehan-Atrash 2020). Pine rosin should not be confused with "rosin," which refers to a type of solventless cannabis concentrate. This finding demonstrates that consumers, regulators, and industry stakeholders should remain vigilant of illicit cannabis additives, even in the "post-EVALI" era.

7.5   VAPING DEVICES AND USER BEHAVIOR

Vaping is a popular route of administration for medical marijuana patients unable to smoke due to their condition. Unlike edible products that can take hours to afford pain relief or other intended results, the effects of vaping are felt immediately. Vaping cannabis has also gained popularity among recreational users, particularly young adults and teens, as a less detectable method of consuming cannabis compared with smoking.

Manufactured cannabis extracts (aka concentrates, oils) are the cannabis formulations most often used in the types of e-cigarettes that are marketed as vape pens. Cannabis extracts are highly enriched in THC (Δ^9-THC) or, alternatively, CBD. Two types of extracts are butane hash oil (BHO) and supercritical fluid extract (SFE). THC concentrations in commercial extracts are commonly in the range of 50–90% (w/w), while the THC range typically encountered in cannabis plant material for smoking is 10–25%. Vacuum distillation of BHO or SFE to manufacture an even purer cannabinoid product has become a prevalent industry practice. The second most abundant class of compounds in cannabis extracts is typically terpenes and terpenoids.

The distilled cannabinoids are then recombined with terpenes (and other additives, e.g., Section 7.4), affording the popular extract products termed "distillates," which are often marketed as having the highest, relative levels of THC enrichment.

In addition to vaping with a vape pen, dabbing is another common route of administration. Dabbing entails flash vaporizing cannabis extracts on a hot surface at typically ca. ~300–400°C (or higher). An analysis of >2.2 million posts on a cannabis-focused Reddit forum found that, from 2010–2016, "dabbing" and "BHO" showed the greatest relative increases in mentions about usage patterns (Meecham 2018). A national web survey of cannabis consumers found that nearly 60% of respondents had dabbed at least once and that 38% endorsed dabbing on a regular basis (Daniulaityte 2018).

There is a gap in our current understanding about how different vape pens and dab "rigs" produce specific aerosol chemical profiles. Physical variables such as specific device components and routes of administration can modulate levels of concerning aerosol chemical products. For example, wicking and heat transfer efficiency, which can vary due to heating element design, are the most critical factors in determining levels of aerosol toxicants at a given power setting in electronic cigarettes (Strongin 2019). An e-cigarette set to a power level of 60 W can counterintuitively produce lower levels of aerosol toxicants compared with a different device set at 8 W *so long as* the 60 W device has superior wicking properties and power distribution. In the latter e-cigarette example, the cotton wick and heating coils are likely more effectively immersed in e-liquid during the vaping process, avoiding "hot spots" that can lead to burnt e-liquid and excessive aerosol toxicant formation. In tobacco e-cigarettes, factors such as the number of heating coils and coil turns, as well as the total surface area and type of coil material, among others, modulate wicking efficiency and heat transfer (Strongin 2019).

Due to the general design similarities between tobacco and cannabis e-cigarettes, cannabis device heat transfer efficiency will also be a major determinant of aerosol toxicant production. However, heat transfer efficiency is more challenging to achieve with cannabis extracts compared with tobacco e-liquids due to the higher viscosity of cannabis extracts and the higher boiling points of cannabinoids. For example, the common cotton wicking material used in tobacco e-cigarettes burns when one uses it for vaping cannabis extracts, and cannabis vape pens thus use alternative materials, as described later.

The styles of devices used for vaping cannabis extracts (CEs) are numerous and continuously evolving. But for the sake of simplicity, one can divide them into two main classes: cartridge vaporizers (CVs) and top-loading vaporizers (TLVs). CVs are small electronic cigarette-like devices that use battery-powered, resistive heating to aerosolize cannabis extracts. A button-activated battery powers an atomizer in a cartridge pre-loaded with CE to generate aerosol when a user inhales. CVs include popular pre-filled cartomizers and necessitate using extracts that have relatively low viscosity, relying on wicking analogous to typical nicotine e-cigarettes. TLVs use a battery to power a resistively heated coil but differ from CVs in that users manually place the CE directly onto exposed heating coils in the atomizer. Most types of cannabis extracts can be used in TLVs without significant concern for viscosity.

Heating coil materials can include titanium and quartz, which have been replacing older stainless steel and ceramics. Heating elements can vary as having either a (i) wick (typically silica- or fiberglass-derived) or (ii) one to three ceramic or quartz heating rods. Some vape pen models avoid direct contact between the heating element and the extract via a quartz or ceramic dish positioned above the heating element to hold the sample during heating. Battery types include either 510 threaded or magnetic connections.

Dab platforms vary based on their specific components (Figure 7.2). Variables that can impact aerosolization efficiency and toxicant formation include the nail (heating element) as a function of material (quartz, titanium, glass, or ceramic) and method of heating (e-nail, electronically programmed) or via a torch. In addition, some dabbing platforms use a water "filter" (analogous to water pipes) and/or "carb caps." Carb caps are small plates used to "cap" the nail. After a dab is placed onto the nail, the user takes a long inhalation. Once the volatilization of the oil slows down due to the temperature drop, the user caps the nail to drop the pressure and increase volatilization while continuing inhalation. This enables larger inhalation duration and volume.

The study of user topography, which includes duration, volume, and intervals between puffs is an area of research currently lacking in the field of cannabis vaping. User topography can modulate dosing, the degree of thermal degradation products, and other aerosol properties along with potential health effects. To address this issue, researchers have implemented puffing regimens similar to those in e-cigarette research to date, such as vaping with smoking machines according to cannabis-adapted CORESTA protocols (Meehan-Atrash 2019). A variety of low, moderate, and high flow rates can be used to cover a range of potential vaping topographies and to mimic direct-to-lung (DTL) and mouth-to-lung (MTL) vaping inhalation practices (Korzun 2018). Since dabbing involves a distinct user topography compared with vaping, it is challenging to model dabbing in the laboratory using similar equipment and methods compared with those used with vape pens (Meehan-Atrash 2019).

7.6   QUALITY CONTROL AND TESTING

The primary testing focus to date of state regulatory agencies has been on the quality of concentrate products prior to vaping. Since the EVALI outbreak, this issue has received global attention. As of this writing, however, a major shift in priorities may have begun as the Colorado Marijuana Enforcement Division (CMED), commencing January 1, 2022, will begin requiring the testing of aerosols derived from vaping

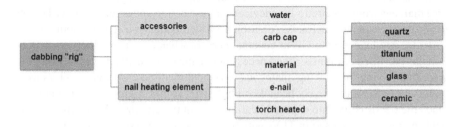

FIGURE 7.2   Dabbing devices (colloquially termed "rigs") enable more intense acute dosing compared with vape pens. They differ by the type of heating, heating mass ("nail") holding the sample, and accessories shown.

products for "metals contamination" at a "Regulated Marijuana Testing Facility." This will include determining arsenic, lead, cadmium, and mercury for every production batch of cannabis extracts in vaporized delivery devices.

This new requirement is widely viewed as the beginning of a trend by regulatory agencies to require aerosol testing. For instance, a recent article including an interview with the Chairman of the CMED sampling committee noted that CMED already plans to expand emissions testing protocols to also check for industrial pollutants, not long after the guidance on metals goes into effect, and to use tobacco e-cigarette regulations as a guide (Kaplan 2021).

Examining the chemical compounds in aerosols is more relevant to human exposure than testing products prior to vaping. It is well-known that, in both tobacco and cannabis vaping, constituent profiles can be altered during the heating and aerosolization process. Metals and plastics can leach from device components, and the cannabinoids, terpenes, and other starting ingredients can undergo thermal decomposition, to varying degrees, leading to a range of aerosol levels of compounds including some known HPHCs (Tables 7.3 and 7.6).

In theory, requiring aerosol testing as a method of quality control serves the consumer. However, aerosol testing is not straightforward. It is more technically challenging and time-consuming to analyze aerosols than it is to analyze CEs and vape formulations prior to vaping. Compliance with aerosol testing mandates will increase the expense and time to market for vaping products, possibly creating a relatively larger burden on smaller businesses.

ENDS regulations have varied by states and national guidance has been in flux for years. The current (6/11/19) recommended guidance by the FDA for PMTA (Premarket Tobacco Product Application for Electronic Nicotine Delivery Systems) approval describes reporting extensive details about product design and operation, e-liquid ingredient aerosol emissions and particle sizing, manufacturing, clinical and nonclinical studies, and human health risks. For example, the document instructs firms manufacturing ENDS products to

> provide aerosolization properties of each of the ingredients (e.g., constituents, humectants, metals, flavors included), particle size of these ingredients in the product, and deposition of these particles through inhalation. We also recommend that you discuss how these properties could affect the product's toxicity profile.

The FDA's PMTA guidance document is a rather comprehensive resource of recommended approaches to address and ensure quality control and regulatory compliance. The PMTA Guidance can be considered a window into FDA's thinking about cannabis vapor products, should they ever be called upon to promulgate regulations in the area.

The AOAC (Association of Official Analytical Collaboration International), established in 1884, sponsors a newsletter, various training programs, and working groups in cannabis analytical science. The AOAC website includes links to a number of publications (SMPRs, Standard Method Performance Requirements) for evaluating cannabis and cannabis products for pesticides, metals, microbes, solvents, and so on. Many of the methods encompass a variety of materials and products; however, some address specific product types such as cannabis concentrates. The AOAC supports the establishment and validation of standards, methods, and technologies to ensure the safety of food and other products impacting global health. It is an independent, non-profit organization. The AOAC also partners with the ISO (International Organization for Standardization) toward developing international standards.

The USP (United States Pharmacopeia) is another recognized non-profit organization that establishes reference standards for products such as pharmaceuticals, food ingredients, and dietary supplements. The USP is currently working with researchers, industry, regulators, and health care practitioners to create standards for the reliable characterization of cannabis for medical use.

The tobacco vaping field has well-documented instances of interlaboratory variability in the reporting of aerosol molecular components. For example, published reports of aerosol formaldehyde levels have varied, in the same device type, over five orders of magnitude (Chen 2018). Reported aerosol levels of other toxic electrophiles such as acrolein and acetaldehyde have been similarly inconsistent. Due to issues such as the generally higher viscosity of cannabis formulations for vaping and the challenges of modeling dabbing topography in the laboratory, issues of interlaboratory variability in reporting aerosol levels of specific molecules and metals can be expected to similarly challenge the cannabis industry. To help promote safety and public confidence for vape products, standardized and compendial methods should be developed to enable best practices in both industry and basic research.

7.7 CONCLUSION

It typically requires decades for the health effects of smoking to manifest. Vaping tobacco and cannabis products may thus also require a generation of usage for conclusive epidemiological evidence of harm reduction compared with their combustion analogs. Vaping cannabis products, however, has been associated with EVALI, a serious acute lung injury, though scientists have yet to establish a clear causative agent. A greater current understanding, prior to the manifestation of acute or chronic health effects, of the potential risks and benefits of these popular new products and routes of administration is clearly needed. More investigations that generate evidence-based chemical, biological, and clinical data are required. The degree of current health-related research and knowledge significantly lags in the prevalence of cannabis extract vaping and dabbing. To enable best practices in both industry and basic research, standard methods development is one established way to help promote safety and public confidence.

REFERENCES

Brass, D. M., and Palmer, S. M. 2017. Models of toxicity of diacetyl and alternative diones. *Toxicology* 388: 15–20.
CDC (Centers for Disease Control and Prevention). 2020. CDC, states update number of hospitalized EVALI cases and EVALI deaths. https://www.cdc.gov/media/releases/2020/s0225-EVALI-cases-deaths.html (accessed March 26, 2021).

Center for Tobacco Products. 2019. Established list of HPHCs in tobacco products and tobacco smoke. U.S. Food and Drug Administration. https://www.fda.gov/tobacco-pr oducts/rules-regulations-and-guidance/harmful-and-potentially-harmful-constituents -tobacco-products-and-tobacco-smoke-established-list (accessed October 12, 2020).

Chen, W. H., Wang, P., Ito, K., Fowles, J., Shusterman, D. et al. 2018. Measurement of heating coil temperature for e-cigarettes with a "top-coil" clearomizer. *PLOS ONE* 13: e0195925.

Coleman, R. L., Lund, E. D., and Moshonas, M. G. 1969. Composition of orange essence oil. *J. Food Sci.* 34: 610–11.

Cramer, G., Ford, R., and Hall, R. 1976. Estimation of toxic hazard—A decision tree approach. *Food Cosmet. Toxicol.* 16: 255–276.

Daniulaityte, R., Zatreh, M. Y., Lamy, F. R., Nahhas, R. W., Martins, S. S., Sheth, A., and Carlson, R. G. 2018. A Twitter-based survey on marijuana concentrate use. *Drug Alcohol Depen.* 187: 155–159.

Jaques, P., Zalay, M., Huang, A., Jee, K., and Schick, S. F. 2018. Measuring aerosol particle emissions from cannabis vaporization and dabbing. Proceedings of the 15th Meeting of the International Society for Indoor Air Quality and Climate. 22–27 July 2018.

Jiang, H., Ahmed, C. S., Martin, T. J., Canchola, A., Oswald, I. W., Garcia, J. A., Chen, J. Y., Koby, K. A., Buchanan, A. J., Zhao, Z., and Zhang, H. 2020. Chemical and toxicological characterization of vaping emission products from commonly used vape juice diluents. *Chem. Res. Toxicol.* 33: 2157–2163.

Kaplan, D. 2021. Everything you need to know about Colorado's Cannabis vape emissions testing. https://www.greentanktech.com/news/everything-you-need-to-know-about-c olorados-cannabis-vape-emissions-testing/ (accessed March 26, 2021).

Korzun, T., Lazurko, M., Munhenzva, I., Barsanti, K. C., Huang, Y., Jensen, R. P., Escobedo, J. O., Luo, W., Peyton, D. H., and Strongin, R. M. 2018. E-cigarette airflow rate modulates toxicant profiles and can lead to concerning levels of solvent consumption. *ACS Omega* 3: 30–36.

Lozier, M. J., Wallace, B., Anderson, K., Ellington, S., Jones, C. M., Rose, D., Baldwin, G., King, B. A., Briss, P., Mikosz, C. A., and Force, S. T. 2019. Update: demographic, product, and substance-use characteristics of hospitalized patients in a Nationwide outbreak of E-cigarette, or vaping, product use–associated lung injuries—United States, December 2019. *MMWR Morb. Mortal. Wkly. Rep.* 68: 1142.

Meacham, M. C., Paul, M. J., and Ramo, D. E. 2018. Understanding emerging forms of cannabis use through an online cannabis community: an analysis of relative post volume and subjective highness ratings. *Drug Alcohol Depen.* 188: 364–369.

Meehan-Atrash, J., Luo, W., McWhirter, K. J., and Strongin, R. M. 2019. Aerosol gas-phase components from cannabis e-cigarettes and dabbing: mechanistic insight and quantitative risk analysis. *ACS Omega* 4: 16111–16120.

Meehan-Atrash, J., and Strongin, R. M. 2020. Pine rosin identified as a toxic cannabis extract adulterant. *Forensic Sci. Int.* 312: 110301.

Mikheev, V. B., Klupinski, T. P., Ivanov, A., Lucas, E. A., Strozier, E. D., and Fix, C. 2020. Particle size distribution and chemical composition of aerosolized vitamin E acetate. *Aerosol Sci. Technol.* 54: 993–998.

Park, H. R., O'Sullivan, M., Vallarino, J., Shumyatcher, M., Himes, B. E., Park, J. A., Christiani, D. C., Allen, J., and Lu, Q. 2019. Transcriptomic response of primary human airway epithelial cells to flavoring chemicals in electronic cigarettes. *Sci. Rep.* 9: 1–11.

Pino, J., Sanchez, M., Sanchez, R., and Roncal, E. 1992. Chemical composition of orange oil concentrates. *Food/Nahrung* 36: 539–542.

Schnabel, J., and Taylor, S. 2015. Estimation of toxic hazard–A revised Cramer–Ford–Hall decision tree. *Toxicol. Lett.* 2: S7.

Shellie, R., Mondello, L., Marriott, P., and Dugo, G. 2002. Characterisation of lavender essential oils by using gas chromatography–mass spectrometry with correlation of linear retention indices and comparison with comprehensive two-dimensional gas chromatography. *J. Chromatogr. A* 970: 225–234.

Strongin, R. M. 2019. E-cigarette chemistry and analytical detection. *Annu. Rev. Anal. Chem.* 12: 23–29.

Vora, J. D., Matthews, R. F., Crandall, P. G., and Cook, R. 1983. Preparation and chemical composition of orange oil concentrates. *J. Food Sci.* 48: 1197–1199.

Vreeke, S., Peyton D. H., and Strongin, R. M. 2018. Triacetin enhances levels of acrolein, formaldehyde hemiacetals, and acetaldehyde in electronic cigarette aerosols. *ACS Omega* 3: 7165–7170.

Wu, D., and O'Shea, D. F. 2020. Potential for release of pulmonary toxic ketene from vaping pyrolysis of vitamin E acetate. *Proc. Natl. Acad. Sci. USA* 117: 6349–6355.

8 Transdermal Delivery

Jessica Painter, Carolyn Burek,
and Monica Vialpando

CONTENTS

DOI: 10.1201/9780429274893-8

8.1   INTRODUCTION

In the past five to ten years, product formulations have increasingly become more complex and sophisticated as both the hemp and regulated cannabis industries continue to evolve. The integration of cannabinoids from the *Cannabis* plant* into various product forms should involve a high level of scientific due diligence. Research, development, and testing of formulated cannabis products continue to advance and enable scientists and companies to create innovative products and technologies. Ultimately, with new products coming to market, it is even more imperative to manufacture products that are both efficacious and safe for administration.

In the realm of topical products, there is a wide degree of complexity and diversity in product types, ranging from medicinal to cosmetic. Advanced cannabis topical formulations, particularly those that enhance permeation of the cannabinoids, typically involve numerous ingredients and excipients, target enhanced dermal bioavailability, and/or can target a unique administration route with a highly specific epithelium. These components to topical formulation require a greater understanding of the technologies employed to improve the product's efficacy, consistency, and safety. This requires extensive knowledge of the structure and function of the skin in different locations on the body, the physicochemical properties of the active cannabinoids, and how and when it is appropriate to include technologies that can enhance the water solubility of the cannabinoids. In addition, it requires an understanding of the biochemical foundation for targeting specific cell types and associated receptors to activate the potential benefits of the cannabinoids and create a more effective topical product.

In regard to the advancement of cannabis drug delivery, research in vaginal administration of cannabinoids is increasing in popularity. Drugs applied to the vaginal mucosa in clinical studies have shown the systemic absorption capabilities that the female reproductive system has, which allows bypassing first-pass metabolism in the gastrointestinal tract. The delivery of cannabinoids vaginally is vastly different from topical and transdermal applications for local or systemic relief, respectively. There are notable differences in the permeation and bioavailability of the vaginal versus topical delivery that requires additional research and a physiological foundation with subject matter experts to ensure the product will not harm but help the consumer.

Therefore, this chapter will provide a greater understanding of the field of topical formulations and will lead into the advancements of vaginal delivery of cannabinoids. These routes of administration require an understanding of the structure and biochemistry of the epidermal layers, best practices for topical and vaginal formulation, and considerations to improve safety and efficacy to further advance the development of novel cannabis products and technologies.

---

* With respect to the hemp and regulated cannabis industries, it is important to note that cannabidiol (CBD), in particular, comes from the same *Cannabis* plant genus; however, CBD that is derived from hemp must have a concentration of Δ^9-tetrahydrocannabinol (Δ^9-THC) below 0.3% by mass.

8.2 OVERVIEW OF THE SKIN

8.2.1 STRUCTURE AND FUNCTION OF THE SKIN

The skin is the largest organ in the human body, comprising more than 10% of body mass and nearly 2 m² of the body surface area (Walters and Roberts, 2002; McGrath et al., 2004). Serving as a protectant and homeostatic regulator, the skin perceives and responds to different external stimuli. The skin is broadly composed of three main layers: epidermis, dermis, and hypodermis. The outermost layer of the epidermis is mainly composed of nonviable and viable keratinocytes, in which the nonviable keratinocytes make up the outermost stratum corneum (SC) layer. The dermis consists of connective tissue, sensory nerve endings, lymphatic vessels, blood capillaries, and various appendages (sweat glands, sebaceous glands, and hair follicles), with the sebaceous glands being the hardest to target (Yeoh and Modi, 2020). The deepest layer is the hypodermis, which is mostly subcutaneous tissue including adipose tissue, connective tissue, and larger lymphatic and blood vessels (Biga et al., 2019).

The epidermis can be further subdivided into four additional layers called, from external to internal, the stratum corneum, stratum granulosum, stratum spinosum, and stratum basale. The stratum corneum is the outermost layer of the skin and acts as the primary barrier (Ng and Lau, 2015). Therefore, the diffusion across the stratum corneum is the rate-limiting step surrounding effective transdermal permeation, and techniques to overcome this physical barrier have been widely studied in the field of transdermal products. Figure 8.1 shows all the layers and components of the skin.

8.2.2 EXISTENCE OF THE ENDOCANNABINOID SYSTEM IN THE SKIN

One of the skin's primary functions is to maintain homeostasis and modulate inflammatory immune responses (Tuting and Gaffal, 2017). Therefore, it is not surprising

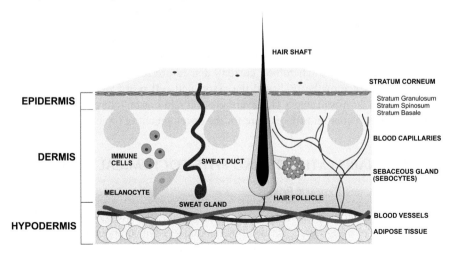

FIGURE 8.1 Dermal layers of the skin.

that the dermal layers of the skin involve functions and pathways associated with the endocannabinoid system (ECS). Studies have shown that endocannabinoid receptors largely exist within various cell types in the skin, including keratinocytes, melanocytes, sebocytes, sensory neurons, dermal immune cells, and cells in hair follicles (Toth et al., 2019). In these cell types, the ECS has been shown to regulate cell proliferation, differentiation, and apoptosis, as well as cytokine, endocannabinoid, and hormone expression (Caterina, 2014). Therefore, the existence of the ECS and associated receptors within the dermal layers and the homeostatic nature of the skin makes it an excellent target for the topical administration of cannabinoids.

Keratinocytes make up a large proportion of the cell types that exist within the epidermis, dermis, and hair follicles. Viable keratinocytes express cannabinoid receptors (CB1 and CB2) and transient receptor potential (TPR) channels, all of which have demonstrated binding to various endogenous and exogenous cannabinoids (Caterina, 2014). Binding to these receptors has been shown to regulate antigen-specific immune responses through the release of cytokines and chemokines (Albanesi, 2010). Numerous studies demonstrate that cannabinoids can down-regulate allergic inflammation and exhibit anti-inflammatory properties upon activation of the CB_1 and CB_2 receptor targets. In particular, keratinocytes containing CB_1 receptors alleviate inflammation and promote the homeostatic regeneration of epidermal integrity (Albanesi, 2010).

A study from 2009 (Biro et al., 2009) demonstrated the expression of both G-protein coupled receptors CB_1 and CB_2, and TRP ion channels in various cell types, including keratinocytes, melanocytes, sebocytes, sensory neurons, dermal immune cells, and cells in the hair follicle root sheath and bulge (Caterina, 2014). In these cell types, the ECS is shown to regulate cell proliferation, differentiation, and apoptosis, as well as cytokine, endocannabinoid, and hormone expression (Biro et al., 2009).

Cannabinoids are also found to bind to various TRP channels that are involved in cutaneous functions such as nociception, thermoception, homeostasis, and regulation of hair follicles and sebaceous glands (Caterina, 2014). Endocannabinoids (AEA, 2-AG, etc.), as well as phytocannabinoids, cannabidiol (CBD), and cannabigerol (CBG) have shown binding and activation of the transient receptor potential vanilloid 1 (TRPV1) cation channels, also known as the "capsaicin receptors" (De Petrocellis et al., 2011). Therefore, current, and future research is working to elucidate the presence of the ECS and the associated cell types and receptors in the epidermis and dermis (Table 8.1). Nevertheless, it remains an interesting therapeutic target and one to continuously explore for the development of topical formulations.

8.3   CANNABIS EXTRACTS AND PHYSICOCHEMICAL PROPERTIES

8.3.1   CANNABIS EXTRACT FORMS

As previously described in Chapter 1, the cannabis plant has over 85 cannabinoids and a variety of terpenoids, not to mention other common plant compounds such as flavonoids, alkaloids, fatty acids, polyphenols, and so on. The chemical composition of an extract is dependent on the extraction methodology used, and the current industry focus is to concentrate the cannabinoids and terpenoids using lipophilic solvents (Hazecamp

TABLE 8.1
Dermal Cell Types and ECS Receptors

Cell type	Receptors/channels
Keratinocytes	CB_1, CB_2, TRPV1, TRPV3, TRPV4, TRPA1
Sebocytes	CB_1, CB_2, $TRPV_1$
Langerhans cells	TRPV1, TRPV2, TRPV3
Melanocytes	CB_1, TRPV1, TRPA1
Hair follicle root sheath and bulge	CB_1, CB_2, TRPV1, TRPV3

et al., 2013). Despite the large diversity in cannabis extract types, three categories may be used to classify the majority of available products: full-spectrum, distillate, and isolate. Full-spectrum cannabis oil is intended to have a concentrated number of cannabinoids and terpenoids and will contain co-extracted plant compounds. Isolates are purified single cannabinoid substances and have the highest level of purity. Distillates contain full-spectrum cannabinoids, some fatty acids and vitamins, and limited terpenes as the majority evaporate throughout processing. Isolates are advantageous to formulators given their inherent consistency and purity. Full-spectrum extracts with minor cannabinoids present may offer additional advantages over single cannabinoid extracts in a phenomenon known as the "entourage effect" (Russo, 2011).

To stay true to the ethos of "cannabis as medicine," many companies prefer to use extract forms that promote the entourage effect. However, the type of extraction performed, and the parameters used, can impact the molecular profile of the end product. The profiles can even change from plant harvest to plant harvest, and therefore, from extraction run to extraction run. There are also additional post-refinement steps that could alter the molecular profile, resulting in various extracts and diminished product consistency. When formulating products that have numerous non-cannabis ingredients, it is important to understand all of the molecules that are present and if any could cause an unintended chemical reaction, promote degradation of the cannabinoids/terpenes, or cause adverse reactions upon administration in the user. Without adequate testing to confirm which compounds exist within various extract forms, it creates a challenge for formulators to develop products using full-spectrum cannabis oil with consistent effects.

To add additional complexity, some companies make skin or hair products using hemp seed oil, derived from *Cannabis sativa* seeds, that have a drastically different chemical profile than the previously mentioned extracts. Studies have shown that hemp seed oil contains around 30% fatty acids, 25% proteins, and dietary fiber, tocopherols, vitamins, and minerals. It is exceptionally abundant in two essential polyunsaturated fatty acids: linoleic acid (18:2 ω-6) and α-linolenic acid (18:3 ω-3) (Callaway, 2004). Hemp seed oil typically contains these fatty acids in a ratio that ranges between 1:2 and 1:3 ω-6:ω-3. As a dietary oral supplement, this has been shown to aid in the treatment of atopic dermatitis (Callaway, 2005). In addition, metabolites of these fatty acids are also found in hemp seed oil, mainly γ-linolenic acid (18:3 ω-6; GLA) and stearidonic acid (18:4 ω-3) (Callaway, 2004).

8.3.2   STABILITY CHALLENGES WITH CANNABIS EXTRACT

If *Cannabis sativa* is improperly stored, the compound profile can change, which may compromise the efficacy of the end product. The stability and shelf life of both the active and inactive ingredients in a product are critical factors in product development not only for efficacy but also for flavor and overall effect. There are over 100 terpenic phytochemicals known to exist from the *Cannabis sativa* plant. Specifically, these molecules are produced from the glandular trichomes and accumulated on the surface of a female *Cannabis sativa* plant.

There are multiple factors other than storage conditions that can degrade medically significant phytochemicals in *Cannabis sativa*, including but not limited to interactions between ingredients, homogeneity, the age of the active ingredient before infusion, packaging, and the product's stability in water (if applicable). To determine the long-term stability of a product infused with cannabis, conditions should ideally be at $25 \pm 2°C$, $60 \pm 5\%$ relative humidity (RH) for at least 12 months (FDA guidelines, 2003). The long-term stability of an infused product is critical for understanding how many units are produced at a time and how long the product is efficacious.

8.3.3   PHYSICOCHEMICAL PROPERTIES OF PHYTOCANNABINOIDS

The skin is a selective barrier that modulates the diffusion of compounds through the epidermis. The rate of diffusion is calculated as a function of permeation per unit area, per unit time, with units expressed as mg cm^{-2} h^{-1}. The two main variables that affect diffusion rate are the permeant's molecular mass and hydrophilicity, which is typically expressed as an octanol-water partition coefficient (log$P$). The skin's buffering capacity is optimal near its physiological pH of 4.6 (Ng et al., 2015). Hydrolyzable phenolic protons on cannabinoids such as tetrahydrocannabinol (THC) and CBD have pKa values of ~10.6 (PubChem: dronabinol) and ~9, respectively (ChEMBL), and will not be dissociated in a typical cannabis formulation. The major challenge for the primary phytocannabinoids, CBD and THC, is the high octanol-water partition coefficients of 5.8–6.3 and ~6.9, respectively (PubChem: dronabinol and cannabidiol, ChEMBL). This elevated hydrophobicity is above the desired range for effective penetration through the stratum corneum (Figure 8.2).

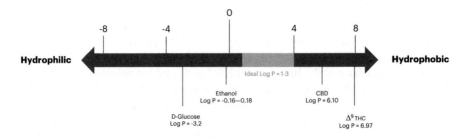

FIGURE 8.2   LogP of cannabinoids in relation to ideal permeation range.

Therefore, to promote the diffusion of cannabinoids through the epidermal layers to reach the blood capillaries within the dermis, transdermal formulations typically require specialized excipients, which is the topic for the next section of this chapter.

8.4 FUNDAMENTALS OF TOPICAL FORMULATION AND DEVELOPMENT

8.4.1 ADVANTAGES OF TOPICAL CANNABIS PRODUCTS

The bioavailability of the cannabinoids largely depends on their physicochemical properties, which will dictate their permeation efficiency through the dermis. Additionally, the efficacy of a topical product relies on the administered dose, frequency, and location of application (Yeoh and Modi, 2020). In developing a topical formulation, it is important to note that it may not be possible to deliver cannabinoids to the bloodstream. For some consumers, this is an advantage, particularly when the desire is to benefit from topical THC administration without experiencing psychotropic effects. Some topicals can be effective in providing localized relief to a specific area of the skin, such as a topical ointment for the treatment of fibromyalgia. One recent study suggests both THC and CBD are effective in treating various symptoms, with minimal side effects (Sagy et al., 2019). Transdermal patch application on the other hand utilizes permeation technology to house major benefits including potential cannabinoid delivery to the bloodstream bypassing the first-pass metabolism and the opportunity for a low dose to extended over a long period. Given the diversity of applications, determining an optimal route of topical administration is highly dependent on the intended application.

8.4.2 EMULSIONS AND EXCIPIENTS

Emulsions are composed of a stable mixture of oil and water and can be defined as water in oil (W/O) or oil in water (O/W), depending on the final volumes of each phase. The O/W emulsion has a smaller volume of oil that exists within a larger volume of water and a W/O emulsion is a smaller volume of water that exists within a larger volume of oil. For topical formulations, emulsions are common and either emulsion type can be used based on the goals of the final product. Emulsions can be formed by the addition of an amphiphilic molecule, commonly a surfactant or phospholipid emulsifying agent (i.e., emulsifiers), or using co-solvents that stabilize the formulation. Amphiphilic molecules contain a polar (hydrophilic) head group with a nonpolar (hydrophobic) tail that allow the formation of micelles, which are thermodynamically stable solution aggregates in oil-water suspensions. As with all formulations, it is important to pay attention to the toxicity limit and daily maximum level to ensure the safety of the final product, especially when formulating with surfactants. It is also crucial to verify that the combined excipients are compatible with each other and the intended packaging.

8.4.3 CHEMICAL PENETRATION ENHANCERS

Chemical penetration enhancers (CPEs) are commonly used in the pharmaceutical industry to promote permeation of compounds through the dermis either by disrupting the lipid barrier in the stratum corneum or by or acting as a carrier to facilitate uptake of the permeant. It is important to note that excessive disruption of the lipid barriers can cause skin irritation, and careful analysis of CPE concentration must be considered in any formulation. There are several CPEs in published research and can include water, sulfoxides (DMSO), or similar, less toxic aprotic solvents, pyrrolidones, fatty acids, alcohols, glycols, surfactants, and terpenes/terpenoids (Williams and Barry, 2012). In fact, natural terpenes found in the cannabis plant can effectively act as CPEs to promote penetration through the stratum corneum layer. Terpenes function by disrupting the intercellular lipids within the stratum corneum, either by fluidization, increasing the partitioning of active ingredients (i.e., cannabinoids) in the stratum corneum, or by modifying keratinized protein conformations (Chen et al., 2016). Although some terpenes can be irritating to the skin, they can enhance the permeation of both hydrophilic and lipophilic active ingredients and are considered a safe alternative to synthetic CPEs to promote permeation (Chen et al., 2016). Some common terpenes that are also found in cannabis are listed in Table 8.2.

To conclude this section, topicals and transdermal products can be highly effective and useful cannabis products and offer several ways to enhance the permeation, if desired. For transdermal products, such as patches or gels, systemic absorption through the dermis is an effective way to bypass first-pass metabolism. However, the active molecule must fall within the ideal range of properties (Figure 8.2), where the majority of molecules, including cannabinoids, do not and require penetration enhancers. But what about other forms of permeation in other areas of the body? Are there differences in biologically sexed male and female product permeation and physiological effects? Are there benefits to creating products that could be administered where the epithelial lining is easier to permeate or where the cannabinoids could offer a unique medicinal benefit?

TABLE 8.2
Natural Terpenes as Penetration Enhancers

Terpene/terpenoid	Type	Molecular weight (g/mol)	LogP
α-Bisabolol	Sesquiterpene	222.4	5.07
Borneol	Monoterpene	154.2	2.71
Geraniol	Monoterpene	154.2	3.28
Limonene	Monoterpene(s)	136.2	4.45
Linalool	Monoterpene	154.3	3.28
α-Pinene oxide	Monoterpene	152.3	2.11
α-Terpineol	Monoterpene(s)	154.3	2.79

Source: Chen et al. (2016).

The remainder of this chapter addresses these questions and will focus on the advancement of a new and innovative route of administration: vaginal delivery of cannabinoids. The benefits of vaginal delivery are similar to transdermal delivery in that the cannabinoids are intended to permeate through the epithelial layers. However, it is advised to formulate these products with careful consideration for various reasons mentioned herein. It is very important to note that while the aspects mentioned previously in this chapter may pertain to vaginal permeation, vaginal products must be regulated in a separate category of cannabis products from topicals or transdermals, with special consideration for specific safety standards.

8.5 DIFFERENCES IN SKIN AND CANNABIS USE AMONG BIOLOGICAL SEXES

8.5.1 BIOLOGICAL SEX SKIN DIFFERENCES

Biologically sexed males typically have higher levels of thickness, hydration, transepidermal water loss, microcirculation, pigmentation, sebum, and pore size than females. On the contrary, biologically sexed females have a higher pH level on their skin than their male counterparts (Rahrovan, 2018). Additionally, keratinocytes in biologically sexed females range from 34–44 µm, whereas biologically sexed male keratinocytes range from 37–46 µm, respectively. Even with these vast differences in skin structure, there are no differences when it comes to permeation. According to a recent study, a TEWL measurement was conducted on both male and female skin to objectively assess the barrier function in both *in vivo* and *in vitro* studies. They found that there were no significant permeation or barrier function differences found between biological sexes (Alexander, 2018).

8.5.2 BIOLOGICAL SEX DIFFERENCES OF CANNABIS INTAKE AND EFFECTS

When administering cannabis, it is important to remember that there are slight differences such as the effect of cannabinoid metabolism, use, regulation of energy homeostasis, and cannabis-induced antinociception (Wagner, 2016). Microsomes metabolizing THC in biologically sexed males are different from biologically sexed females. In an *in vivo* study, liver metabolism was observed after administering THC in both male and female rats. In male rats, THC transformed either by hydroxylation at 11-, 8-, and 3- carbon positions of the dibenzopyran backbone, respectively, whereas female rats followed by a lesser amount of THC-11-oic acid and 8α, 11-diOH-THC (Narimatsu et al., 1991). In addition to metabolism differences, biologically sexed men and women differ in consumption rate and physiological effects. Biologically sexed males typically consume cannabis at a faster rate with shorter intervals between inhalations and experience increased cardiac effects than biologically sexed female counterparts (Perez-Retes et al., 1988). Despite biologically sexed male increased consumption, it is currently exhibited that rapid progression from first cannabis use to cannabinoid use disorder is heightened in biologically sexed females (Cooper and Haney, 2014; Hernandez-Avila et al., 2004). Finally, the

FDA has reported studies of laboratory animals that demonstrated male reproductive toxicity using CBD. A decrease in testicular size, inhibition of sperm growth and development, and decreased circulating testosterone were observed, among other issues (FDA Website). In fact, not only did males using CBD experience these results but male offspring of CBD-treated pregnant females were affected as well (FDA Website). This can raise concerns that CBD can potentially negatively affect a biologically sexed man's fertility, however, further human-based clinical studies need to be performed to confirm this assumption.

8.6 VAGINAL DELIVERY AND CONSIDERATIONS

8.6.1 INTRODUCTION AND HISTORY

The earliest references to cannabis use for female gynecology dates back to the 7th century BCE in Ancient Mesopotamia. In these reports 4000 years ago, hemp seeds, also known as azallû, were mixed with other ingredients, such as saffron and mint, in fermented beverages for unspecified female-specific ailments such as difficulty during childbirth and painful menstrual cycles (Russo, 2002). In fact, the use of cannabis in gynecology steadily increased into the modern era until the prohibition of cannabis in the last century abruptly derailed the trend. Although there have been historical uses of topicals applied to female genitals, modern medicine still did not consider the capacity of vaginal drug absorption until Dr. David Macht investigated the vaginal absorption rate of morphine, atropine, and potassium, leading to a breakthrough in biologically sexed female health (Alexander, 2004). In his study, Macht observed that the vagina does in fact have the capability of absorbing drugs systemically, expanding opportunity for a variety of offerings and confirming ancient medicine suspicions. The basic understanding of this work led to the proliferation of female contraceptives such as NuvaRing and IUD, as well as a hormone treatment for a variety of ailments. Today, as both cannabis and hemp legalization proliferate nationwide, the popularity of cannabis products and the sophistication of the market have led to a diverse selection of available product offerings such as lubricants, suppositories, and massage oils.

The majority of cannabis-infused topical products on the market are oil-based formulations where the absorption site is local (e.g., muscle relief). As a result, topically applied products do not readily enter the bloodstream and therefore do not exhibit intoxicating effects like the inhalation of cannabis provides. On the other hand, transdermal products are specifically designed to deliver cannabinoids to the bloodstream. Most often presented in a transdermal patch, they are formulated with penetration enhancers, as discussed previously in Section 8.4.3, to facilitate absorption through the stratum corneum, the uppermost layer of the skin. Although these transdermal applications dissolute to the blood, the rate and extent of the dose are low. In contrast, products that are advertised to be applied vaginally, directly to the mucosa, have been shown to enable high bioavailability.

Regulatory requirements and pathways for the development of safe vaginal cannabinoid products are currently immature and unclear and there is a critical need for regulatory clarity to implement safe formulation parameters. In California, the Bureau of Cannabis Control (BCC, 2018) currently regulates sexual wellness products such as lubricants and salves under the same regulatory umbrella as topicals designed for dermal application (BCC, 2018). Surprisingly, vaginal suppositories are listed as a concentrate, in the same regulatory category as extracts, vape cartridges, capsules, and shatter (BCC, 2018). Furthermore, in the current FDA regulations for hemp (products containing *Cannabis sativa* with less than 0.3% THC), the FDA does not recognize CBD as an over-the-counter drug (FDA, 2020). Rather, it is categorized as a nutraceutical, which is not regulated with the same scrutiny as traditional FDA-regulated products (FDA, 2019). To add further complexity to the framework of regulating vaginal suppositories, there requires an understanding of the differences between the administration of isolate and full-spectrum extracts. Full-spectrum extracts would require further scrutiny of the individual components that are derived from the cannabis plant and how each would either facilitate a therapeutic effect or cause an adverse reaction. The next section discusses the complexities around vaginal drug delivery, potential benefits, and considerations in efficacious product design.

8.6.2 DRUG DELIVERY SYSTEM IN BIOLOGICALLY SEXED FEMALE REPRODUCTIVE ORGANS

Foundationally, a major advantage for the delivery of cannabinoids through the vagina is the high bioavailability that the female reproductive system possesses. When compared with oral administration, vaginal topicals can deliver cannabinoids more quickly and at a higher dose into the bloodstream. Drugs introduced to the vaginal tract are transported across the vaginal membrane by several routes such as transcellular (through the cell) and/or paracellular (in between the cell). The vaginal membrane consists of four major layers: epithelium, lamina propria, muscularis, and adventitia (Figure 8.3).

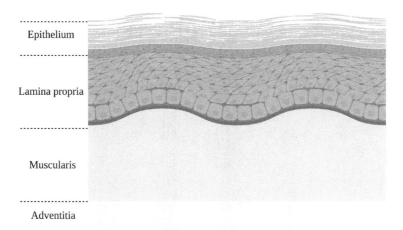

FIGURE 8.3 Layers of the vaginal wall.

In short, as cannabinoids are introduced to the vaginal mucosa, they permeate through the lamina propria layer that consists of connective tissues rich in blood and lymphatic vessels and capillaries. Once cannabinoids reach this layer, blood vessels and capillaries drain into the exterior iliac vein, where it unites with the common iliac vein (Figure 8.4).

Simultaneously, as drugs penetrate the common iliac vein, they bypass the first-pass metabolism, resulting in faster onset times. Most notably, drugs delivered to the vagina are found in large concentrations in the uterus. This is due to the high degree of direct vagina-to-uterus transport, also known as the "first uterine pass effect" (Bulletti, 2006). In a study that investigated the *ex vivo* uterine perfusion model of

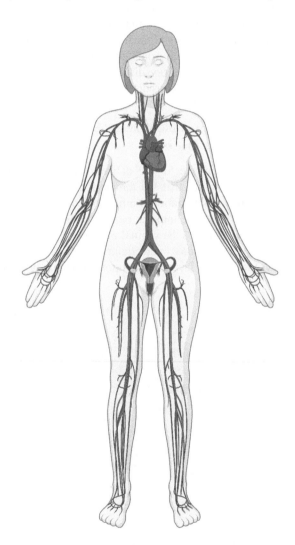

FIGURE 8.4   Reproductive organ reaching common iliac vein.

[3]H-progesterone, the authors demonstrated this first uterine pass effect. Here, the authors applied ^{3}H-progesterone on the rim of vaginal tissues in patients in both proliferative and secretory phases of the cycle. It was concluded that the migration of ^{3}H-progesterone was found in the uterus, with high concentrations in both the myometrium and endometrium, respectively (Bulletti et al., 1997). The first uterine pass effect is important to consider when selecting ingredients for products intended to be applied vaginally, as the bioavailability of these compounds proliferates in the uterus at a high concentration. Materials that are toxic to the uterus might cause a negative or hazardous effect on the end consumer. On the contrary, the first uterine pass effect can assist with a targeted approach to help treat ailments in the uterus such as uterine tract infections (UTIs) among others.

8.6.3 THE ENDOCANNABINOID SYSTEM IN BIOLOGICALLY SEXED FEMALE REPRODUCTIVE ORGANS

Following the administration of cannabis or hemp, phytocannabinoids are introduced into the body, activating endocannabinoid receptors. Our bodies produce endocannabinoids such as anandamide, known as the "bliss molecule" among others. CB_1 and CB_2, the most prevalent receptor binding sites, are continuously uncovered as scientists investigate the many factors that play a critical role in their function. Similar to the skin's primary function to maintain homeostasis and provide protection from foreign invaders (Tuting and Gaffal, 2017), the vaginal mucosa also works to maintain homeostasis by moderating physiological pH. Therefore, it is not surprising to find the receptors commonly associated with the ECS present within various cell types of the female reproductive system.

In biologically sexed female reproductive organs, CB_1 receptors proliferate around the ovaries and the central nervous system, while CB_2 receptors are found in the ovarian cortex, ovarian medulla, and ovarian follicles, respectively, among others (Walker et al., 2019; El-Talatini, 2009). Additionally, there are CB_1 and CB_2 receptors found outside female reproductive organs that have been found to impact functionality and operation. Interactions between the ECS and pain-associated mechanisms have been observed in both *in vitro* and *in vivo*. In one study, endometriosis patients treated with cannabis were observed at several levels: changes in the central and peripheral neural system; involvement of neuropathic and inflammatory pain; psychological interaction with the pain experience; hormonal variability of the pain; and the expression of cannabinoid receptors, enzymes, and ligands (Fine, 2013). Endometriosis is an extremely painful ailment that nearly six million women suffer from in the United States alone. Scientists have observed that phytocannabinoids do in fact have efficacy in the treatment of endometriosis as well as other chronic pain conditions. Furthermore, there is a great promise as a therapeutic supplement in treating peripheral and central neuropathic pain and inflammation-mediated chronic pain (Fine, 2013). The potential relief from biologically sexed female chronic pain should be further examined and researched to determine a targeted and consistent approach with more natural remedies such as phytocannabinoids.

8.6.3.1 ECS and Pregnancy

When a woman conceives a child, the ECS is hard at work, ensuring the embryo implants smoothly. The ECS in the uterus influences receptivity, placental remodeling, embryo implantation, and embryo-uterus cross talk (Ezechukwu Henry, 2020). Cross talk, an important function in early pregnancy, assists with the successful implantation and fertilization of an embryo. Adequate concentrations of anandamide-mediated through the CB_1 receptor are responsible for the early stages of pregnancy and endometrial thickness, which must be maintained throughout pregnancy (Ezechukwu Henry, 2020).

Furthermore, outside of female reproductive organs, endocannabinoid receptors are found to have an impact on functions in reproductive organs, and consequently, pregnancy. Specifically, CB_1 receptors found intracellularly on the mitochondrial membrane (energy regulator for cells) are affected by cannabis intake and can dysregulate energy metabolism. Foundationally, mitochondrial function regulates apoptosis, therefore, dysregulating the energy metabolism can subsequently impact the process of producing quality gametes. As a result, dysregulating the energy metabolism affects embryogenesis and can lead to the production of poor-quality embryonic stem cells (Walker et al., 2019; Ramalho-Santos, 2009). In brief, disrupting the ECS by introducing phytocannabinoids in the body may lead to problems with conception (Walker et al., 2019).

8.6.3.2 ECS and Cancer

Cervical cancers are the second leading cause of malignancy-related deaths in biologically sexed females worldwide, with over 250,000 deaths being reported each year. The role of the ECS in gynecological cancers has been a recent topic of research in the development, progression, and prognosis of these devastating diseases. This research is speculative and preliminary, and no evidentiary conclusions can be made at this time. Nevertheless, there are early observations of an association of the ECS and dysregulation of biologically sexed female gynecological cancers. Cannabinoids impact the eCB, a signals receptor target, that may potentially influence the functional dysregulation of some gynecological cancers. In an exploratory study with different cervical cancer lines with CBD, a decrease in cell proliferation and induced cell death by the accumulation of cells in the cell death phase (sub-G0) was observed (Taylor, 2020). This heeds the path of CBD potentially making a significant impact and therapeutic tool for the treatment of cervical cancer. Continued research on interactions between gynecological cancers and the endocannabinoid system is desperately needed to understand the intricate role and potential benefit of phytocannabinoids.

8.6.4 Safety: Ingredients and Dosage

In view of the variability in both the vaginal mucosa and epithelial thickness throughout a woman's cycle, the effectiveness and extent of a formulation reaching the lamina propria are difficult to predict. This is due to fluid volume, pH, viscosity, cell wall thickness, and hormones, which all play a role in vaginal composition, as decreasing estrogen leads to increased vaginal mucosa pH (Gorodeski, 2005). The fluctuation of hormones in the vaginal mucosa can potentially alter the chemical composition of the drug and inactive ingredients, influencing the safety and efficacy of the overall product. Furthermore, there is an overall discrepancy in female testing in clinical study settings. Women are often excluded from study designs due to unknown genotoxic, epigenetic, and reproductive side effects that may occur as a result of their participation. This is a positive practice to protect women, but unfortunately inhibits the research that would enable safer and more efficacious ingredients for vaginal permeability products for women.

In the vagina, there is a layer of mucosa that proliferates near the epithelium in the vaginal canal called mucosa flora. Lactobacilli, a compound found in this vaginal mucosa flora, produces hydrogen peroxide as a byproduct. The primary role of the hydrogen peroxide byproduct is to prevent overgrowth of other "bad" bacteria found in the mucosa such as *Gardnerella vaginalis* and even some sexually transmitted infections (STIs) (van de Wijgert, 2017). Hydrogen peroxide along with other symbiotic bacteria found in the mucosa flora accomplish this task by retaining an acidic environment in the vaginal canal that is unfavorable to many pathogenic microbes (Panda et al., 2014). The vaginal pH typically ranges from 3.8–4.2 in healthy reproductive-aged women and 6.5–7 in menopausal women, respectively (Panda et al., 2014). As biologically sexed females age, the pH of the vaginal mucosa changes as well. Any topicals inserted into and on biologically sexed female reproductive organs can vastly disrupt the pH of vaginal mucosa and therefore interfere with the body's natural protection against infection.

When creating an efficacious product, it is important to not only look at the safety of the product but if it is effective as well. As the bioavailability of vaginally applied products is significantly more permeable than traditional dermal application, it is recommended to evaluate the influence of the dose strength when compared with other routes of administration. Of the regulated vaginal products reviewed in the cannabis and hemp market, the majority claim a 100 mg dose per package, a similar package strength to that of THC-infused edibles. Nonetheless, the high absorption from a 10 mg THC suppository will yield a much higher psychotropic experience than ingesting a 10 mg THC edible. The California Bureau of Cannabis Control regulations currently states that cannabis topicals labeled for recreational use may not exceed 1000 milligrams (mg) per package. Products applied to biologically sexed female reproductive organs are much more permeable than other dermal application sites. Furthermore, the bioavailability of respected application sites is vastly different, which, in return, affects the overall potency and efficacy of the product.

8.6.5 DRUG PRODUCT DESIGN

Local and transmucosal administrations can be facilitated through self-administration and oftentimes with vaginal products, this is a messy, difficult, or inconvenient experience. Currently in the cannabis and hemp space, products are still immature and lack sophisticated application devices to ease the burden on the consumer. In addition to product application, product capacity carries its own unique challenges. Cannabis molecules are naturally hydrophobic, and therefore a simple approach would be to add other oils in the formulation. Unfortunately, this leads to a product that is not compatible with latex condoms. While there are latex-friendly and water-based formulations, these formulations may lack the traditional condom capacity testing as this is not required in the regulations. The next section focuses on the risks of incorporating nanoemulsions in sexual wellness products, as well as the obstacles with other applications like suppositories, creams, and salves face.

8.6.5.1   Oil-Based Suppositories

Suppositories bear their own challenges for consumers, as the internal temperatures of a vaginal canal interact with oil-based suppositories and often leave a mess. Inside the vaginal canal, the basal temperature ranges from 36.1°C–36.4°C (97°F–97.5°F) before ovulation to 36.4°C–37°C (98.6°F–98.6°F) after ovulation, respectively (University of Michigan). The majority of suppositories in the current cannabis and hemp spaces contain carrier oils that are either coconut oil or cocoa butter. Both of these oils have a melting point of around 25.5°C–34.1°C (78.0°F–93.4°F), respectively. The range of the basal temperature melts both oils in the suppositories, which eventually drips out of the vaginal canal, leaving an undesired feeling. Furthermore, the melting of the oil presents a challenge with the absorption of the drug as well, as the cannabinoids are likely to be attached to the said carrier oil, therefore, the consumer is not receiving the full dose advertised on the product's packaging.

8.6.5.2   Creams and Salves

Creams and salves can be extremely greasy, and the application of these products can often leave consumers frustrated. Often presented without a proper applicator, this product type can be hard to dose out properly and has a greater chance of incorrect dosage. Additionally, creams and salves are also more susceptible to product contamination. This can happen in a multitude of ways, but most often due to the introduction of a dirty finger to the product jar. In the same way, the use of your fingers for application thereafter may introduce bad bacteria to the vaginal canal, leaving more issues than benefits. There is a greater chance that these product types can cross contaminate if hands are not thoroughly cleaned after application, and currently in the cannabis industry, the majority of suppositories, creams, and salves on the market do not come with an applicator. As the sophistication of cannabis products grows, addressing these critical application parameters is key in the success of consumer enjoyment and product efficacy.

8.6.5.3   Oil vs. Water-Based Lubricants

Oil-based lubricants, often made with medium-chain triglyceride (MCT) oil are used in formulations to carry cannabinoids through the epithelial lining in the emergence of this niche market. These formulations have a great disadvantage to the product user, as the oils in the oil-based formulation will interact and deteriorate latex condoms—a warning that is not always indicated on the label.

Cannabis nanoemulsions are the most commonly applied water-based soluble enhancing technology. These more complex formulations are on the rise in a variety of products for a variety of application sites including oral applications. In traditional oral applications, nanotechnology solutions can reduce the onset time and create a consistent dose effect, which will be beneficial to the consumer. However, in the case of sexual wellness products, the main advantage of incorporating these technologies is to offer a formulation that is latex compatible.

In a formulation, the mixing of cannabis oil and water ingredients seems impossible to stabilize alone. This is where surfactants play a role. Surfactants stabilize the formulation by offering a hydrophilic head and hydrophobic tail. With the inclusion of surfactants and other emulsifiers like phospholipids, a micelle can be formed (Figure 8.5). To enhance the water solubility of a lubricant, a critical micelle concentration (CMC) must be achieved. In terms of vaginal applications, this can be a hindrance, as surfactants have been shown to negatively affect vaginal mucosa and the increase of these surfactants pose a greater risk to the consumer.

Physicochemical characterization of the finished formulation is critical in products with nanosolutions. Important characteristics to consider when verifying these products include, but are not limited to, the amount of oil encapsulated in the micelle if it remains in the micelle after infusion and if the micelles remain intact once introduced to vaginal mucosa. If the integrity of the nanoemulsion is compromised in any verification step, it can show that there are free-floating oils in the formulation, creating an environment that might lead to the compromise of latex condom protection. Finally, in addition to ingredient selection and internal verification of encapsulation, it is important to note that all products formulated for sexual pleasure or wellness should undergo the same process checks as commercialized FDA-regulated products. This is to ensure the compatibility and capacity with condoms, and if not capable, to clearly demonstrate that on the label.

8.6.6 Future of Vaginally Administered Products

The ideal vision for future vaginally administered products are hygienic, easy to use, and discrete methods that are currently practiced in pharmaceuticals and over-the-counter products. Most commercialized products utilize airless dispensers for

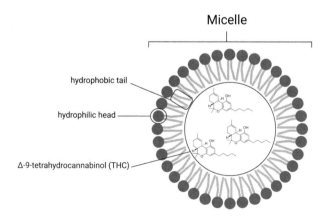

FIGURE 8.5 Illustration of a micelle encapsulating Δ^9-tetrahydrocannabinol (Δ^9-THC).

creams and salves and applicators for suppositories, creating a mess-free and easy application to consumers. Typically made from sterilized materials, commercialized product applicators create a more efficacious design as it greatly reduces the potential for bacteria to come into contact with both the formulation and the vaginal canal, and for the product to be accidentally dosed to others. Furthermore, the use of an applicator can also extend the storage capacity of the formulation and potency as there are fewer opportunities for contamination and light degradation. It is typical in commercialized products to stick an applicator in the formulation tube to extract the dose needed, preserving the formulation inside from air, light, bacteria contamination, and temperature variation. To conclude, the sophistication and improvement of suppositories, creams, and salves in cannabis and hemp spaces can subsequently lead to the empowerment of biologically sexed females and the management of their own pain in a discrete and mess-free manner.

8.7   CONCLUSION

Research in the cannabis space continues to advance, creating opportunities to alleviate specific ailments using a targeted cell approach and providing products with improved safety and efficacy. Topical, transdermal, and vaginal routes of administration require an understanding of the structure and biochemistry of the skin, the physicochemical properties of the cannabinoids, best practices for topical formulation, and consideration of the site of application. Advanced cannabis topical formulations, particularly those that enhance permeation of the cannabinoids, typically involve numerous ingredients and excipients, target enhanced bioavailability, and/or target a unique administration route with a highly specific epithelium. These components of topical formulation require a greater understanding of the technologies employed to improve the product's efficacy, consistency, and safety. In addition, it is important to understand how and when it is appropriate to include these technologies, particularly any that would enhance the water solubility of cannabinoids and cannabis extract.

For creating a product that will be applied in a more permeable area (e.g., vaginal mucosa), the considerations outlined in this chapter are especially important to consider during product development and formulation. The application of products vaginally is vastly different from dermal applications such as on arms and knees as there is increased permeability and bioavailability with vaginal applications. These differences alone require more stringent regulations on ingredient, manufacturing, and application safety (e.g., condom compatible). Regardless, as cannabis and hemp regulations continue to be refined, it is imperative to receive guidance from a subject matter expert for each application site, especially regarding biologically sexed female reproductive organs.

BIBLIOGRAPHY

360 Research Reports. 2020. Global CBD skin care sales market report 2020. https://www.360researchreports.com/global-cbd-skin-care-sales-market-16697271   (accessed January 21, 2021).

Albanesi, C. 2010. Keratinocytes in allergic skin diseases. *Current Opinion in Allergy and Clinical Immunology* 10: 452–456.

Alexander, H. 2018. Research techniques made simple: transepidermal water loss measurement as a research tool. *Journal of Investigative Dermatology*. 138: 2295–2300. doi:10.1016/j.jid.2018.09.001

Alexander, N.J., et al. 2004. Why consider vaginal drug administration? *Fertility and Sterility* 82, 1: 1–12.

Biga, L.M., et al. 2019. Anatomy and Physiology. Corvallis, OR: OpenStax Oregon State University, 221. https://open.oregonstate.education/aandp/

Biorender. 2020. Retrieved from https://app.biorender.com/biorender-templates (accessed January 29, 2021).

Biro, T., et al. 2009. The endocannabinoid system of the skin in health and disease: novel perspectives and therapeutic opportunities. *Trends in Pharmacological Sciences* 30, 8: 411–420.

Bulletti, C., et al. 1997. Vaginal drug delivery: the first uterine pass effect. *Annals of the New York Academy of Sciences* 828: 285–290. doi:10.1111/j.1749-6632.1997.tb48549.x

Bureau of Cannabis Control. 2018. California code of regulations title 16 division 42. https://bcc.ca.gov/law:regs/readopt_text_final.pdf (accessed February 2, 2021).

Callaway, J.C. 2004. Hempseed as a nutritional resource: an overview. *Euphytica* 140: 65–72.

Callaway, J.C., Pate, D.W. 2009. *5 – Hempseed Oil, Gourmet and Health-Promoting Specialty Oils*. AOCS Press, 185–213. doi:10.1016/B978-1-893997-97-4.50011-5

Callaway, J.C., et al. 2005. Efficacy of dietary hempseed oil in patients with atopic dermatitis. *Journal of Dermatological Treatment* 16: 87–94.

Calvi, L., et al. 2018. Comprehensive quality evaluation of medical Cannabis sativa L. inflorescence and macerated oils based on HS-SPME coupled to GC–MS and LC-HRMS (q-exactive orbitrap®) approach. *Journal of Pharmaceutical and Biomedical Analysis* 150: 208–219.

Caterina, M.J. 2014. TRP channel cannabinoid receptors in skin sensation, homeostasis, and inflammation. *ACS Chemical Neuroscience* 5: 1107–1116.

Chang, C., et al. 2010. Gamma-linolenic acid inhibits inflammatory responses by regulating NF-κB and AP-1 activation in lipopolysaccharide-induced RAW 264.7 macrophages. *Inflammation* 33, 1: 46–57.

Chen, J., et al. 2016. Natural terpenes as penetration enhancers for transdermal drug delivery. *Molecules* 21, 1709: 1–22.

Cooper, Z.D., Haney, M. 2014. Investigation of sex-dependent effects of cannabis in daily cannabis smokers. *Drug and Alcohol Dependence* 1, 136: 85–91. doi:10.1016/j.drugalcdep.2013.12.013

De Petrocellis, L., et al. 2011. Effects of cannabinoids and cannabinoid-enriched Cannabis extracts on TRP channels and endocannabinoid metabolic enzymes. *British Journal of Pharmacology* 163: 1479–1494.

De Petrocellis, L., et al. 2012. Cannabinoid actions at the TRPV channels: effects on TRPV3 and TRPV4 and their potential relevance to gastrointestinal inflammation. *Acta Physiologica* 204: 255–266.

El-Talatini, M.R., et al. 2009. Localisation and function of the endocannabinoid system in the human ovary. PLoS One 4, 2. doi: 10.1371/journal.pone.0004579.

European Bioinformatics Institute of the European Molecular Biology Laboratory (EMBL). 2018. ChEMBL Database. Cannabidiol, ID=CHEMBL190461. https://www.ebi.ac.uk/chembl/compound_report_card/CHEMBL190461/ (accessed June 9, 2020).

Ezechukwu, H., et al. 2020. Role for endocannabinoids in early pregnancy: recent advances and the effects of cannabis use. *American Journal of Physiology-Endocrinology and Metabolism* 319, 3: E557–E561.

Fine, P.G., Rosenfeld, M.J. 2013. The endocannabinoid system, cannabinoids, and pain. *Rambam Maimonides Medical Journal* 4, 4: E0022. doi:10.5041/RMMJ.10129

Gorodeski, G.I., et al. 2005. Estrogen acidifies vaginal pH by up-regulation of proton secretion via the apical membrane of vaginal-ectocervical epithelial cells. *Endocrinology* 146, 2: 816–824. doi:10.1210/en.2004-1153

Hazecamp, A., et al. 2013. Cannabis oil: chemical evaluation of an upcoming cannabis-based medicine. *Cannabinoids* 1, 1: 1–11.

Hernandez-Avila, C.A., et al. 2004. Opioid-, cannabis- and alcohol-dependent women show more rapid progression to substance abuse treatment. *Drug and Alcohol Dependence* 74, 3: 265–272. doi:10.1016/j.drugalcdep.2004.02.001

Kapoor, R., Huang, Y. 2006 Gamma-linolenic acid: an antiinflammatory omega-6 fatty acid. *Current Pharmaceutical Biotechnology* 7, 6: 531–534.

McGrath, J., et al. 2004. Anatomy and organization of human skin. In: *Rook's Textbook of Dermatology*, 7th ed., eds. Rook, A., Burns, T. Malden: Blackwell Science.

Method for labial, vaginal, transmucosal and transdermal metered dose dispensing. United States, US 2012/065619 A1, filed (September 14, 2011), and issued (March 15, 2012).

Narimatsu, S., et al. 1991. Sex difference in the oxidative metabolism of Δ^9-tetrahydrocannabinol in the rat. *Biochemical Pharmacology* 41, 8: 1187–1194. doi:10.1016/0006-2952(91)90657-Q

National Center for Biotechnology Information. PubChem Database. Dronabinol, CID=16078. https://pubchem.ncbi.nlm.nih.gov/compound/16078 (accessed June 9, 2020).

National Center for Biotechnology Information. PubChem Database. Cannabidiol, CID=644019. https://pubchem.ncbi.nlm.nih.gov/compound/644019 (accessed June 9, 2020).

Ng, K.W., Lau, W.M. 2015. Skin deep: the basics of human skin structure and drug penetration, In: *Percutaneous Penetration Enhancers Chemical Methods in Penetration Enhancement*, eds. Dragicevic, N., Maibach, H. Berlin, Heidelberg: Springer.

Panda, Subrat, et al. 2014. Vaginal pH: a marker for menopause. *Journal of Mid-Life Health* 5, 1: 34–37. doi:10.4103/0976-7800.127789

Perez-Reyes, M., et al. 1988. Interaction between marijuana and ethanol: effects on psychomotor performance. *Alc. Clinic Exp. Res.* 12: 268–276.

Rahrovan, S. et al. 2018. Male versus female skin: what dermatologists and cosmeticians should know. *International Journal of Women's Dermatology* 4, 3: 122–130. doi:10.1016/j.ijwd.2018.03.002

Revision 2. U.S. Department of Health and Human Services Food and Drug Administration, Guidance for Industry Q1A(R2) Stability Testing of New Drug Substances and Products. Office of Training and Communication Division of Drug Information. 2003. https://www.fda.gov/media/71707/download (accessed March 3, 2021).

Ramalho-Santos, J. et al. 2009. Mitochondrial functionality in reproduction: from gonads and gametes to embryos and embryonic stem cells. *Human Reproductive Update* 15: 553–572.

Russo, E. 2002. Cannabis treatments in obstetrics and gynecology: a historical review. *Journal of Cannabis Therapeutics* 2: 5–35. doi:10.1300/J175v02n03_02

Russo, E. 2011. Taming THC: potential cannabis synergy and phytocannabinoid-terpenoid entourage effects. *British Journal of Pharmacology* 163: 1344–1364.

Sagy, I., Schleider, L.B., Abu-Shakra, M., Novack, V. 2019. Safety and efficacy of medical cannabis in fibromyalgia. *Journal of Clinical Medicine* 8, 807: 1–12.

Taylor, A.H., et al. 2020. (Endo)Cannabinoids and gynaecological cancers. *Cancers (Basel)* 13, 1: 37. doi:10.3390/cancers13010037

Tóth, K.F., Ádám, D., Bíró, T., Oláh, A. 2019. Cannabinoid signaling in the skin: therapeutic potential of the "c(ut)annabinoid" system. *Molecules* 24, 5: 918.

Tuting, T., Gaffal, E. 2017. Regulatory role of cannabinoids for skin barrier functions and cutaneous inflammation. Handbook of Cannabis and Related Pathologies 57: 543–549.

U.S. Food & Drug Administration. 2019. LRB QBR for rectal and vaginal products. fda.g ov/drugs/how-drugs-are-developed-andapproved/lrb-qbr-rectal-and-vaginal-products (accessed February 10, 2021).

U.S. Food & Drug Administration. 2020. What to know about products containing Cannabis and CBD. fda.gov/consumers/consumer-updates/what-you-need-know-and-what -wereworking-find-out-about-products-containing-cannabis-or-cannabis (accessed February 10, 2021).

University of Michigan Medicine. 2020. Charting Michigan medicine basal body temperature (BBT) charting. uofmhealth.org/health-library/hw202058 (accessed January 22, 2021).

van de Wijgert, J.H.M. 2017. The vaginal microbiome and sexually transmitted infections are interlinked: consequences for treatment and prevention. *PLoS Medicine* 14, 12: 27. doi:10.1371/journal.pmed.1002478

Wagner, E. 2016. Sex differences in cannabinoid-regulated biology: a focus on energy homeostasis. *Frontiers in Neuroendocrinology* 40: 101–109. doi:10.1016/j.yfrne.2016.01.003

Walker, O.S., et al., 2019. The role of the endocannabinoid system in female reproductive tissues. *Journal of Ovarian Research* 12: 3. doi:10.1186/s13048-018-0478-9

Walters, K., Roberts, M. 2002. Dermatological and transdermal formulations. In: Drugs and Pharmaceutical Sciences, ed. Walters, K. Volume 119. New York: Informa Healthcare USA, Inc.

Williams, A. 2003. *Transdermal Drug Delivery: From Theory to Clinical Practice.* Pharmaceutical Press. ISBN 10: 0853694893.

Williams, A., Barry, B.W. 2012. Penetration enhancers. *Advanced Drug Delivery Reviews* 64: 128–137.

Yeoh, T., Modi, N. 2020. Topical formulation: from idea/concept to marketed product. Webinar from American Association of Pharmaceutical Sciences (AAPS), Pfizer, USA, April 24, 2020.

9 Thermal Degradation of Cannabinoids and Cannabis Terpenes
A Review

Jiries Meehan-Atrash and Robert M. Strongin

CONTENTS

9.1   INTRODUCTION

Manufactured cannabis concentrates (cannabis extracts, cannabis oil) are the formulations most often used in e-cigarettes marketed as vape pens. Concentrates are highly enriched in THC (Δ^9-THC) or alternatively, in CBD (Figure 9.1). The second-most abundant class of compounds in concentrates are terpenes.

Two examples of extracts are butane hash oil (BHO) and supercritical fluid extract (SFE). THC levels in commercial extracts are often >50–90% (w/w), while the THC content in cannabis plant material is 10–25%. Vacuum distillation of BHO or SFE to afford an even purer cannabinoid product has become common industry practice. The distilled cannabinoids are then recombined with terpenes (and potentially other additives), affording the popular concentrate products termed distillates, marketed as having the relatively highest levels of THC enrichment.

A related method of vaping concentrates is termed dabbing. Dabbing entails flash vaporizing concentrates on a hot surface at typically ~300–400°C or higher. An analysis of >2.2 million posts on a cannabis-focused Reddit forum found that, from 2010–2016, "dabbing" and "BHO" showed the greatest relative increases in mentions

DOI: 10.1201/9780429274893-9

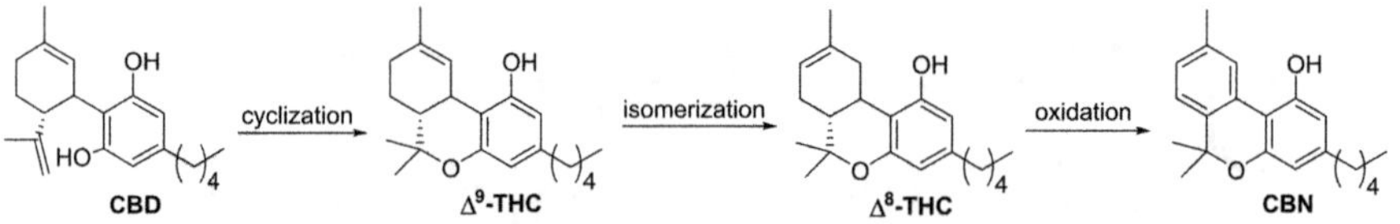

FIGURE 9.1 The structures and selected reactions of the four major cannabis-derived cannabinoids: cannabidiol (CBD), Δ^9-tetrahydrocannabinol (Δ^9-THC), Δ^8-tetrahydrocannabinol (Δ^8-THC), and cannabinol (CBN). CBD is not psychoactive. The CBD drug Epidiolex is approved by the FDA to treat two epilepsy disorders. CBD can cyclize to the main psychoactive constituent of cannabis, Δ^9-THC, under acidic conditions. Δ^9-THC can isomerize to Δ^8-THC. The main degradation product of Δ^9-THC (as well as Δ^8-THC) is CBN. Δ^8-THC has a lower psychotropic potency compared with Δ^9-THC. CBN is non-psychoactive. There are many possible degradation products; however, the determination of the components of aerosols derived from vaping cannabis concentrates has received relatively little attention to date.

about usage patterns (Meacham et al. 2018). A national web survey of cannabis consumers found that nearly 60% of respondents had dabbed at least once and that 38% endorsed its regular use (Daniulaityte et al. 2018).

In addition to THC-containing concentrate products being associated with the 2019–2020 lung injury (EVALI) outbreak, there are ongoing concerns of health officials about these new products and routes of administration. High THC concentrations increase the risks of overdose and psychosis (Di Forti et al. 2019). The long-term health effects of using cannabis concentrates may not be known for several decades after the completion of epidemiological studies.

A common belief among proponents is that aerosols produced by concentrates are less harmful compared with marijuana smoke produced by a cannabis flower cigarette. The rationale includes the lack of combustion during vaping along with the relatively fewer toxic plant constituents present in concentrates (Gieringer 2001).

The lack of evidence-based data about vaping concentrate aerosols must be urgently addressed to better understand the potential risks and harm reduction benefits associated with these prevalent products and routes of administration. Such studies are especially needed for more vulnerable cohorts, such as teens and pre-teens, and chronically ill medical patients with compromised immune systems.

Understanding the relative risks and benefits of concentrate vaping can be initiated by investigations of fundamental chemical and physical attributes, such as aerosol doses of cannabinoids and terpenes, and any potential toxic products that can form during vaping and dabbing. Herein, we describe our recent investigations concerning the chemistry of vaping and dabbing terpenes, THC, and cannabis concentrate materials. The focus is on aerosol emissions, rather than on the concentrates prior to vaping, because of the greater relevance to user exposure. In the following sections (9.2–9.4) (Meehan-Atrash 2021), we describe examples of the earlier research on cannabinoid reactivity, myrcene chemistry, and cannabis vaping. These studies have informed and inspired our recent investigations.

9.2 THERMAL REACTIVITY OF THE CANNABINOIDS

There are several relatively recent reports describing the stability of cannabinoids to storage and processing conditions (Turner and Elsohly 1979; Carbone et al. 2010; Perrotin-Brunel et al. 2011; Repka et al. 2006). However, publications focusing on higher temperature thermal degradation reactions of cannabinoids stopped appearing in the literature nearly 30 years ago.

In 1971, Mikeš and Waser reported one of the earliest cannabinoid chemical reactions occurring during smoking. This work was motivated by findings showing that hashish was more potent when smoked compared with being ingested (Mikes and Waser 1971). Interestingly, it is now known that both oral ingestion and smoking of cannabis produce similar subjective effects despite having very different pharmacokinetic profiles (Wachtel et al. 2002).

Mikeš and Waser proposed that CBD, often present in a one-to-one ratio with THC in hashish, isomerized to THC during smoking. In 1941, Adams had previously reported the acid-catalyzed cyclization of CBD to what was then known as "tetrahydrocannabinols" (Adams et al. 1941), as the precise molecular structure of THC would not be elucidated until over 20 years later. Adams' finding served as the basis of Mikeš and Waser's hypothesis (Figure 9.2). They added THC, CBD, or hashish to a tobacco cigarette, and analyzed the resultant smoke constituents via GC-MS (gas chromatography-mass spectrometry) to monitor THC conversion. In 1973, Quarles clarified that the isomerization reaction required the presence of tobacco, which had a measured pH of 5.72, and that it would not proceed when combusting cannabis alone (pH = 8.14). This was consistent with Adams' 1941 report about the role of acid catalysis (Quarles et al. 1973).

Following the CBD-to-THC conversion studies, a series of cannabinoid pyrolysis experiments were investigated by a pair of research groups with synergistic expertise in organic and analytical chemistry at the University of Utrecht from 1973–1978 (Küppers et al. 1973; Spronck et al. 1978). Their goal was to identify the production of molecules of toxicological concern. After initially studying cannabis smoke, they decided to simplify the research by focusing on a single cannabinoid, CBD (Tjeerdema 1987). CBD was chosen in part due to it being a crystalline solid (mp = 67.5 ± 0.3123) that is easier to handle than THC, which is an extremely sticky, sappy oil at room temperature. In addition, CBD was the most abundant cannabinoid in most preparations at that time (Tjeerdema 1987).

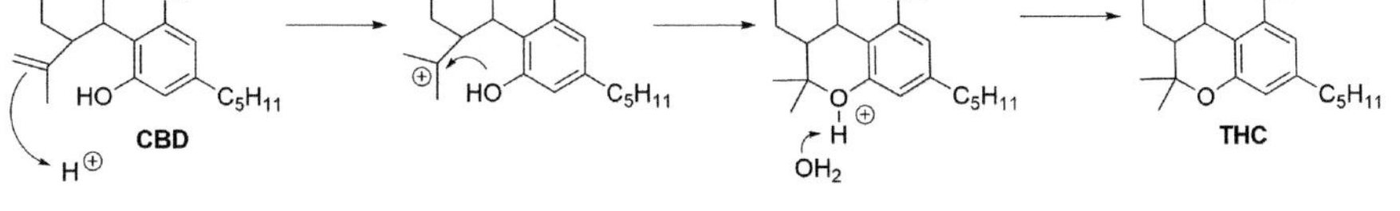

FIGURE 9.2 The acid-catalyzed cyclization of CBD to THC.

The Utrecht researchers performed aerobic and anaerobic pyrolysis experiments by passing air or N_2 through a heated quartz tube containing CBD at temperatures up to 700°C. They collected the pyrolysates in a −80°C cold trap (Küppers et al. 1975b; Küppers et al. 1973; Küppers et al. 1975a; Luteyn et al. 1978; Pronck and Lousberg 1977; Spronck and Salemink 1978). Degradation products were isolated by preparative GC and TLC (thin layer chromatography), and structural assignments were performed using mass spectrometry, ^{1}H NMR (proton nuclear magnetic resonance), and optical rotation (Küppers et al. 1975b; Küppers et al. 1973; Küppers et al. 1975a; Luteyn et al. 1978; Pronck and Lousberg 1977; Spronck and Salemink 1978). They identified many CBD degradation products and divided them into two groups based on their relative elution order with respect to CBD in the GC-MS: early eluting products (also referred to as "cracking products") and later eluting products (Tjeerdema 1987).

Examples of cracking products identified in Kuppers et al. (1975a) are shown in Figure 9.3. The pair of compounds shown in Figure 9.3 contains an intact pentylresorcinol moiety, as do all of the other related cracking products characterized. This suggested that the thermal reactivity of CBD is initiated at the cyclopentenyl terpenoid moiety. Relatively more volatile products, such as the well-known volatile organic compounds (VOCs) isoprene, butadiene, benzene, and so on, were not reported. These likely were either not resolved due to overlap with the large GC-MS solvent peak (pentane; Küppers et al. 1973) or may have evaporated during collection or processing.

Figure 9.4 shows examples of later eluting CBD pyrolysis products. In their initial paper, the researchers had identified cannabielsoin as the major product formed upon

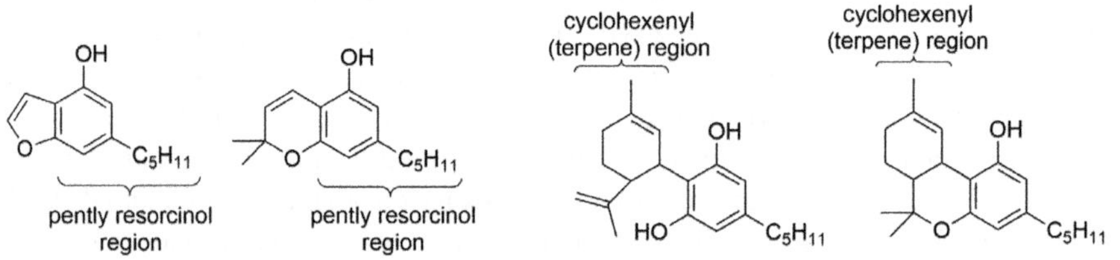

cracking products from CBD pyrolysis **CBD** **THC**

FIGURE 9.3 (Left) Representative cracking products reported by Kuppers (1975) showing loss of the cannabinoid cyclohexenyl region.

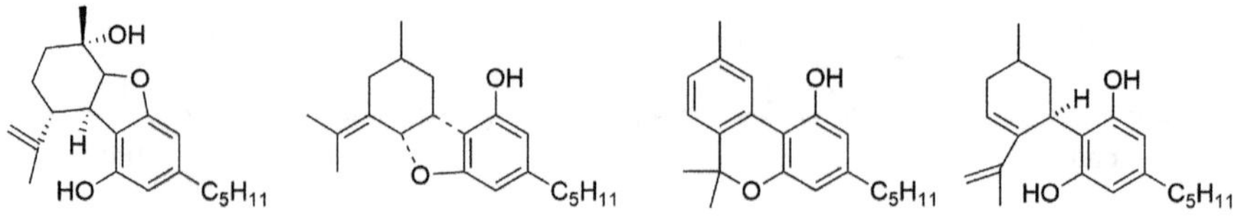

cannabielsoin **314/271** **CBN** **Δ^4-CBD**

FIGURE 9.4 Examples of "later eluting" products of CBD pyrolysis.

aerobic pyrolysis of CBD (Küppers et al. 1973). Several years later, they identified a product that they called 314/271 as the major product of aerobic pyrolysis (Spronck et al. 1978).

The researchers found many other products that were more readily identifiable in O_2-free experiments (Tjeerdema 1987). Given the discrepancy between these two experimental conditions, the group monitored the mainstream smoke of a tobacco cigarette using a polarographic O_2 sensor and determined that anaerobic conditions were a better representation of actual smoking (Spronck et al. 1978).

9.3   THE REACTIVITY OF MYRCENE, A PREVALENT CANNABIS TERPENE

Myrcene is a C_{10} monoterpene terpene first isolated in 1895 from *Myrcia acris* (bay oil) (Behr and Johnen 2009). Myrcene exists as two isomers depending on the position of the double bond on the isopropylidene/isopropenyl moiety: α-myrcene and β-myrcene (Figure 9.5a). The position of the double bond in β-myrcene was first reported in 1924 (Ruzicka and Stoll 1924). Their assignment was later confirmed by IR (infrared) and NMR spectroscopy (Behr and Johnen 2009).

Many reports describing the composition of cannabis essential oil note β-myrcene as one of the most abundant terpenes present in both drug type cannabis (*Cannabis sativa subsp. indica var. indica*) (Al Bakain et al. 2020; Leyva-Gutierrez et al. 2020; Milay et al. 2020; Bueno et al. 2020; Krill, Rochfort, and Spangenberg 2020) and hemp (*C. sativa subsp. sativa var. sativa*) (Mazian et al. 2019; Kwaśnica et al. 2020). One study reported β-myrcene levels accounting for 33% m/m of a distilled essential oil, nearly double the next most abundant terpene, D-limonene (Ross and ElSohly 1996).

The earliest study of the thermal degradation of β-myrcene appears in the 1913 doctoral thesis of Ioan Prodrom at the Swiss Federal Institute of Technology (Prodrom 1913). Among the reactions of terpenes and other hydrocarbons that

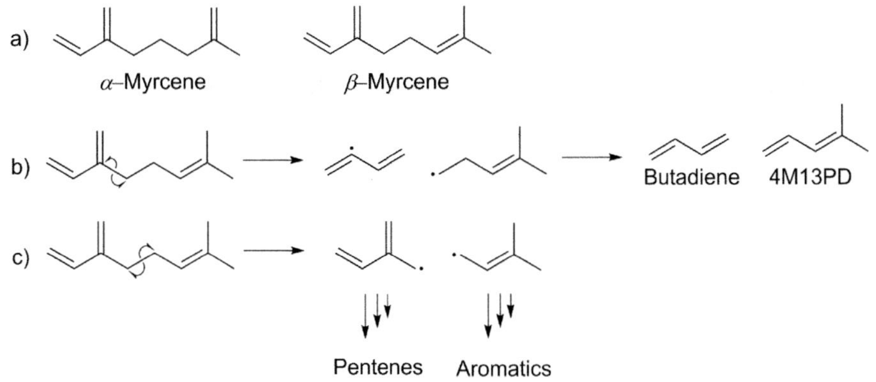

FIGURE 9.5   (a) Structures of α- and β-myrcene. (b) The initially proposed mechanism of β-myrcene decomposition by Kolichescki. (c) Ondruschka's proposed mechanism.

Prodrom explored, he found that β-myrcene produced good yields of isoprene (39%) when pyrolyzed by passing a current through a platinum wire submerged in the myrcene. However, the isoprene was of lower quality than that derived from limonene, and it was suggested this may have been due to impurities in the starting material. In 1946, Davis et al. performed similar pyrolysis experiments to determine which of seven terpenes would be the most practical source of isoprene for the manufacture of synthetic rubber (Davis et al. 1946). Davis et al. also pyrolyzed the terpenes using a resistively heated wire (nickel-chromium). β-Myrcene produced the third-highest yield of isoprene (21%), after β-pinene (23%) and D-limonene (54%).

The most common current production method for β-myrcene is the pyrolysis of β-pinene (Behr and Johnen 2009). Analysis of the degradation products formed during the transformation by GC-MS revealed that the degradation of β-myrcene via alkyl radicals accounted for decreased yields (Kolicheski et al. 2007). The proposed degradation pathway for β-myrcene is shown in Figure 9.5, and would primarily yield butadiene and 4-methyl-1,3-pentadiene, though the researchers did not detect these products. Kolicheski et al. instead detected several known products of butadiene chemistry (benzene, xylenes, ethylbenzene, etc.) along with 4-methyl-1,3-pentadiene constitutional isomers (Kolicheski et al. 2007). Approximately six months after this publication, the journal published a critical commentary stating that the bond homolysis shown in Figure 9.5b proposed by Kolicheski et al. is unlikely given the relative instability of primary and vinyl radicals (Stolle and Ondruschka 2008). Stolle and Ondruschka instead proposed a mechanism which affords two relatively more stable allylic radicals, and suggested these radicals are precursors for isopentene, pentene, and aromatic hydrocarbons.

A further theoretical and experimental study of the synthesis of β-myrcene from β-pinene was published in 2017 (Zheng et al. 2017). Pyrolysis products of not only β-pinene but also D-limonene and β-myrcene were investigated. Zheng et al. characterized and quantified reaction products by GC-MS, proposed reaction mechanisms, and developed a kinetic model that showed good agreement with experimental data. Products of β-myrcene pyrolysis they reported included many that formed via intramolecular ene reactions, as well as C_4, C_5, and C_6 degradation products.

9.4 CANNABIS VAPING CHEMISTRY: BACKGROUND

The use of vaporization to consume cannabis flower (not cannabis concentrates) was reported in 2001 (Gieringer 2001; Hazekamp et al. 2006), predating the invention of the nicotine e-cigarette. Cannabis flower vaping generally consists of a handheld or tabletop device that generates hot air that is blown over milled cannabis flower to create an aerosol that is inhaled by the user (Gieringer et al. 2004; Hazekamp et al. 2006). The work by Gieringer et al. led to the first characterization of the aerosol components emitted by a cannabis flower vaporizer (Gieringer et al. 2004). Aerosol was generated from a Volcano→ tabletop vaporizer and transferred directly to a 250 mL volatile gas trap, from which a headspace syringe was used to inject 2 mL of gas directly into the GC-MS injection port for analysis without preconcentration. The inner surface of the volatile gas trap was rinsed with methanol for collection of the aerosol particulate matter and also analyzed. The authors reported that both particulate and gas samples only contained cannabinoids and terpenes, which led them to conclude that vaporizing with a Volcano→ suppressed the formation of harmful degradation products. Interest in cannabis flower vaporization as a route of pulmonary medical cannabis administration led to a brief flurry of papers characterizing aerosolization parameters of the Volcano→ (Pomahacova et al. 2009) *in vitro* studies (Lanz et al. 2016), and even some small pre-clinical trials with human volunteers (Abrams et al. 2007; Earleywine and Barnwell 2007; Wilsey et al. 2013).

In general, two types of cannabis e-cigarettes exist (additionally, see also Chapter 7 in this volume), top-loading vaporizers (TLVs) and cartridge vaporizers (CVs) (Meehan-Atrash et al. 2019). TLVs consist of an exposed atomizer containing a resistively heated coil upon which a user manually places any cannabis extract, and an attached mouthpiece allowing direct inhalation of the aerosol. CVs also use a resistively heated element to vaporize cannabis concentrate, but the atomizer is embedded within a cartridge that contains the concentrate.

Though the earliest report mentioning the use of an e-cigarette to consume cannabis was in 2011 (Etter and Bullen 2011), the first studies to focus on this topic appeared in 2015 (Etter 2015; Giroud et al. 2015), an internet survey and literature review, respectively. These reports indicated that TLV and CV usage was in an early stage with a considerable "do it yourself" aspect, with mentions of mixing cannabis extracts with glycerol and/or propylene glycol (two solvents used in nicotine e-cigarettes; Jensen et al. 2017) and even self-manufacture of the cannabis extract (Etter 2015; Giroud et al. 2015).

The first investigation into the release of harmful degradation products from cannabis extract vaping was published in 2016 (Varlet et al. 2016). In this study, the authors made BHO, mixed it with propylene glycol, and vaped it in a nicotine e-cigarette. The authors measured VOCs released from the aerosol by passing the aerosol through an activated charcoal filter, which was later eluted with carbon disulfide for analysis by GC-MS. They also measured carbonyls by passing the aerosol through cartridges coated in 2,4-dinitrophenylhydrazine (2,4-DNPH, an aldehyde-derivatizing agent used for quantifying carbonyls in tobacco cigarette and e-cigarette aerosols) eluting any formed aldehyde-2,4-DNPH hydrazones with acetonitrile for analysis by high-performance liquid chromatography with ultraviolet-visible spectroscopy (HPLC-UV). The authors were not able to detect any VOCs apart from two carbonyls, formaldehyde and acetaldehyde (Varlet et al. 2016). They also reported difficulties when dissolving BHO in propylene glycol and were only able to make stable solutions of BHO in propylene glycol of levels of up to 10%. The authors thus questioned the usefulness of vaping cannabis with an e-cigarette, apart from microdosing.

Currently, vaporizing cannabis is one of the most common non-smoking cannabis inhalation methods, with one study reporting that 21.8% of past-30-day cannabis-consuming Colorado high school students reported past-30-day cannabis vaporizing as a use mode in 2015 (Tormohlen et al. 2019), and another reported that 19.5% of surveyed cannabis users from 12 US states from 2016 reported past-month vaping (Schauer et al. 2020). These studies differentiated vaping from dabbing but did not differentiate cannabis flower and concentrate vaping.

Dabbing can be considered another form of cannabis vaping. However, differences between the e-cigarette and dabbing platforms warrant the separation of this method into a class of its own. In its simplest form, dabbing is the flash vaporization of a small amount of cannabis concentrate, a *dab*, when contacted with a heated surface (Meehan-Atrash et al. 2019; Meehan-Atrash et al. 2017). The heated surface may be a small piece of titanium, ceramic, quartz, or glass often called a *nail*, which is attached to a water pipe, pipe, or straw through which the user inhales. Many commercially available nails are made to be heated with a blowtorch, but electrically heated nails, e-nails, are also commonplace and allow for greater temperature control.

Exactly when dabbing emerged as a route of administration for cannabis is unknown, but its first mention in the literature was in a 2014 internet survey that assessed user perceptions of the method and concluded that dabbing appeared to lead to increased drug tolerance to THC, and that the method is more dangerous than other usage modes (Loflin and Earleywine 2014).

Despite the lack of research on dabbing, two studies reported cannabinoid transfer and THCA decarboxylation efficiency during dabbing. A 2015 study partly performed by members of a cannabis industry-associated testing laboratory assessed the transfer efficiency of cannabinoids during dabbing (Elzinga et al. 2015). A "mechanical lung system" was used to pull aerosol generated from 40 mg dabs applied to a nail heated to an estimated 300°C through two chilled methanol traps that were subsequently analyzed by HPLC-UV for cannabinoid detection. The authors reported that ~50% of the available THC was transferred depending on the type of cannabis extract used and that the decarboxylation of THCA proceeded with >90% conversion.

A 2019 study by Swiss and German forensic chemists involved similar dabbing experiments that consisted of placing 160–230 mg portions of cannabis extract onto a nail heated to an unknown temperature, and the resulting aerosol passed through two in-series liquid N_2-cooled aerosol traps filled with glass boiling chip granules (Hädener et al. 2019). After this, the aerosol traps were rinsed with methanol, the solvent evaporated *in vacuo*, the residue reconstituted in a known volume of methanol, and the solution analyzed by HPLC-UV. Though liquid impingers, such as those reported in Elzinga et al., for the analysis of cannabis and tobacco smoke aerosols have been reported many times in the literature (Hädener et al. 2019), and the use of chilled glass boiling chip granules for aerosol capture represented a novel method. Hädener et al. reported a decarboxylation efficiency of >99%, and a THC transfer of 75.5%, slightly higher than that reported by Elzinga et al. Both research groups conclude that the unrecovered THC is likely lost to sidestream smoke, adsorption on the experimental setup, or thermal degradation.

Though the first user survey indicated user hesitation about dabbing (Loflin and Earleywine 2014), dabbing has emerged as an incredibly popular cannabis concentrate consumption technique. In 2015, 4.3% of past-30-day cannabis-consuming Colorado high school students reported past-30-day dabbing (Tormohlen et al. 2019), and in 2016, 14.6% of surveyed cannabis users in 12 US states reported past-month dabbing (Schauer et al. 2020).

Despite the popularity of cannabis concentrate consumption by vaping and dabbing, prior efforts to examine the chemical processes and emission exposures that occur during consumption by these methods have been scarce. The remaining sections of this chapter describe our recent efforts toward addressing this knowledge gap by focusing on the chemical origins, identities, and levels of aerosol emissions resulting from cannabis concentrate vaping and dabbing. Our goal is to identify and understand the chemical changes that occur to concentrate formulations upon heating and aerosolization. The vision is that these studies will help understand the factors that promote the formation of aerosol harmful and potentially harmful constituents (HPHCs). The studies are additionally relevant to understanding the relationship between starting concentrate levels, aerosolization efficiency, and emission of cannabinoids and terpenes.

9.5   THE CHEMISTRY OF TERPENE DABBING

Terpenes and terpenoids are ubiquitous natural products. Apart from their well-known role in cannabis aroma, they are also one of the most prevalent classes of flavor additives used in tobacco e-cigarettes. The chemistry of terpenes has been a long-term focus of atmospheric and environmental chemists (Atkinson and Arey 2003). Although the reactions of terpenes and terpenoids with ozone and nitrogen oxides in the atmosphere are not of direct relevance to tobacco e-cigarettes or cannabis vaping, they serve as a foundation for understanding the chemistry of terpenes under the oxidative thermal conditions of vaping. For example, it is well-known that highly oxidizing hydroxyl radicals are produced during vaping and that oxidation and dehydration reactions are two of the dominant chemical processes that occur (Strongin 2019).

In our initial study of terpene dabbing in 2017 (Meehan-Atrash et al. 2017), we used levels of terpenes that corresponded to those that would be present in a typical concentrate for dabbing. The experimental setup included a nail that was heated with a blowtorch. The nail temperature was monitored for consistency between runs with an infrared camera. The aerosol produced was pulled via a commercial smoking machine through tubing leading from the DMSO-d_6 (for NMR analysis) or a Cambridge filter pad and an ATD cartridge (adsorption/thermal desorption for GC-MS analysis), followed by the smoking machine. We used a ten-second puff duration and a puff volume of 339 mL to ensure complete aerosol collection, better reflecting dabbing topography as opposed to vaping. During the ten-second draw, the nail temperature would drop and a range of initial and final temperatures was recorded for each puff.

Overall, dabbing was more technically challenging to study than e-cigarette vaping. This was due to issues such as overwhelming the smoking machine and the ATD cartridges with the relatively large puff volumes, duration, and related factors. We also encountered some sidestream loss of material that may have led to underestimating aerosol product levels. In subsequent dabbing studies, as described in the next section, we modified the setup used in this initial work to better address these issues, but the overall concept was the same, wherein we connected a nail, a cartridge, or impinger, and a vacuum source in series.

Determining the levels of aerosol products arising from dabbing myrcene as a function of temperature was the main focus since it is the most abundant cannabis terpene (Martin 2007). As expected, the levels of HPHC and related degradation products were proportional to temperature. Interestingly, the products produced upon dabbing all of the terpenes studied were consistent with their major known products formed during atmospheric degradation (Atkinson and Arey 2003). All of the terpenes produced isoprene, which is known to undergo atmospheric oxidation (via O_2 or OH radical) to methacrolein, methyl vinyl ketone, and formaldehyde. Products identified by GC-MS included methacrolein, methyl vinyl ketone, and 3-methylfuran, as well as 1,3-butadiene and several cyclic and acyclic dienes, polyenes, and aromatics (Figure 9.6).

The NMR spectra of the aerosols revealed highly resolved peaks with relatively high integral areas corresponding to benzene and methacrolein. Benzene, alkylbenzenes, and polycyclic aromatic hydrocarbons are known to form during terpene thermolysis (Britt et al. 2001) (Kolicheski et al. 2007; Moir et al. 2008). Benzene exposure is always of concern. It is present in the air and is reported to embody the greatest cancer risk of any compound in air (George et al. 2011). The levels determined in the aerosols were greater than those in ambient air controls; however, they are relatively very low compared with other sources of exposure such as cigarettes. In addition, benzene was only detectable at the highest temperature range used when dabbing myrcene and limonene, and it was not detected at all in the linalool-derived aerosol.

In summary, this initial report focusing on the reactions of terpene upon dabbing revealed that the products observed were consistent with those produced by

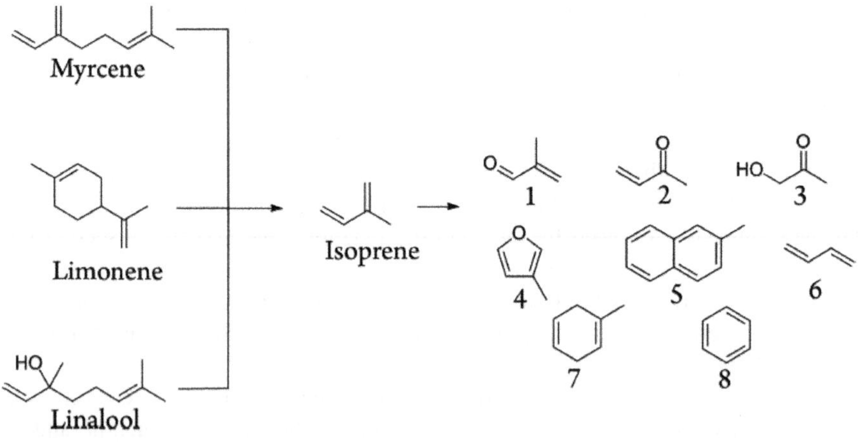

FIGURE 9.6 Terpene degradation products produced by dabbing, identified by GC-MS. 1, methacrolein; 2, methyl vinyl ketone; 3, hydroxyacetone; 4, 3-methylfuran; 5, 2-methylnapthalene; 6, 1,3-butadiene; 7, 1-methylcyclohexa-1,4- diene; 8, benzene. These and additional products were produced from pure samples of each of limonene, linalool, and myrcene. Reproduced from Meehan-Atrash et al. (2017) and used with permission from the American Chemical Society.

terpenes upon atmospheric oxidation. In addition, the levels of aerosol benzene differed depending on the specific terpene used, which indicates that specific terpenes have characteristic risk profiles. Although benzene and other chemicals of concern, such as methacrolein, isoprene, methyl vinyl ketone, and others were found, their emission levels were moderated at lower dab temperatures.

9.6 THC AND TERPENE VAPING CHEMISTRY

In a study published in 2019 (Meehan-Atrash et al. 2019), we investigated both the dabbing and vaping chemistry of concentrates. Samples were prepared to model high potency distillates (synthetic distillates, SNDs) with 9:1 THC:terpene formulations. The goal was to discover the gaseous products arising from THC as well as THC and terpene mixtures. The gas-phase emission fraction contains HPHCs. These are the compounds contained in tobacco smoke or aerosols where the emissions have been determined to carry the greatest human health risks by the Food and Drug Administration (FDA). For more information and a listing of the current (nearly 100) HPHCs, see Chapter 7. In addition, the researchers at the University of Utrecht (Section 9.2) did not report the gas-phase pyrolysis products of CBD. Although the HPHCs found in cannabis smoke are known and are similar to those found in tobacco cigarettes, it is not clear which derive from the plant material and which derive from cannabinoids or terpenes (Meehan-Atrash et al. 2019). By focusing on vaping and dabbing THC and terpenes one can thus determine the identities and levels of HPHCs deriving from them without the confounding presence of additional plant material. Moreover, dabbing is a platform where one can study the aerosolization of either pure THC or pure terpenes without concern for viscosity, and thus compare their unique chemistry.

We replaced the smoking machine with a flow control valve, mass flow meter, and a vacuum source, and added a by-pass line for additional control of the flow. In addition, the nail was replaced with an e-nail, affording more facile temperature control. For the vape pen investigations, we used a CCell device and vaped with a setup that is essentially the same used for standard tobacco e-cigarette studies.

The data in Table 9.1 was obtained from the equivalent of one 40 mg dab or one puff of a vape pen. That similar gas-phase products are derived from both terpenes and THC is reasonable, given that cannabinoids are terpenophenols. Benzene, methacrolein, and isoprene are present in the smoke from combusted plant cannabis cigarettes, but their origin from THC had not been previously known.

Although the levels of the HPHCs are generally lower than those found in smoke from cannabis plant material, they are still of concern. For example, unlike cancer, exposure to relatively lower levels of toxicants over time does not necessarily translate to lower cardiovascular health risk (Bhatnagar 2016). In addition, many more gas-phase compounds were observed by GC-MS but were not identifiable.

As expected, dabbing resulted in relatively higher levels of HPHCs, as did increasing the power levels of the vape pen. The dabbing experiments showed that terpenes contribute greater levels of HPHCs to the aerosol compared with THC, even when there is a 9-fold excess of THC present. Although, as mentioned, many of the

TABLE 9.1

Levels of Gas-Phase HPHCs Found in Aerosols

Compound, unit	THC dab	SND dab	Vape 3.2 V	Vape 4.0 V	Vape 4.8 V
Methacrolein, μg	2.7 ± 0.8	12 ± 0.82	5.6 E−3	3.2 E−2	1.9 E−1
Benzene, ng	33 ± 14	360 ± 120	9.9 E−1	2.7 E+0	3.6 E+1
Xylenes, μg	0.33 ± 0.20	0.85 ± 0.30	1.0 E−3	1.5 E−2	1.8 E−1
Toluene, μg	0.44 ± 0.22	1.4 ± 0.42	7.0 E−4	1.0 E−2	1.6 E−1
Styrene, ng	0.88 ± 0.72	27 ± 14	9.3 E−2	2.7 E−1	ND*
Ethylbenzene, ng	1.5 ± 0.99	55 ± 30	3.7 E−2	2.5 E−1	2.7 E+0
Isoprene, μg	9.6 ± 1.7	44 ± 3.5	3.0 E−2	8.3 E−1	6.0 E+0
Other HCs,[†] μg	5.3 ± 0.7	21 ± 11	4.2 E−2	7.2 E−1	7.9 E+0
Total VOCs,[‡] μg	2.0 E+01	7.7 E+01	9.4 E−2	1.5 E+0	1.2 E+1

For dabbing experiments, HPHCs were quantified with internal standard, and represent normalized levels from a (realistic) 40 mg dab ± SEM (duplicate runs). Isoprene in dabbing was estimated by internal standard response factor analysis (IS-RF). Gas-phase components found by vaping at three voltages are from single puff measurements, estimated via IS-RF. *Styrene was not detected in CV vaping at 4.8 V due to the overlap of alkene terpene degradation products in the chromatogram. [†]Non-targeted HCs not specified in this table. [‡]Total of all VOCs quantified. 9:1 THC:terpenes.

gas-phase aerosol components could not be identified, and studying the particulate phase compounds was beyond the scope of the study, we performed quantitative risk assessments for each of the conditions shown in Table 9.1.

Keeping in mind the limitations, we were able to do these estimations because, unlike many other aerosol components identified in e-cigarette and aerosols produced by vaping, the HPHCs shown in Table 9.1 have been relatively well-characterized by toxicologists. Both a hazard index (HI, non-cancer risk) and excess lifetime cancer risk (ELCR), estimates of long-term health risks, were calculated based on the data corresponding to each of the experimental conditions shown in Table 9.1 and also compared with smoking (based on data compiled via an extensive literature search). As expected, ELCR and HI values increased for dabbing versus smoking, and with higher power levels when using the vape pen. Cannabis flower smoking had the highest chronic risk estimate compared with all other routes of exposure. This latter finding is in keeping with the general assumption that vaping is less harmful than smoking; however, more work needs to be done to confirm this, especially given the limitations noted.

9.7   THC AND MYRCENE REACTION SYNERGY AND MECHANISMS

Our third paper on concentrate vaping is focused on the mechanism of VOC formation from myrcene and THC, as well as the influence of myrcene on THC reactivity and dosing (i.e., transfer to the aerosol) (Meehan-Atrash et al. 2021). The investigation began with a rigorous study of the products formed upon dabbing a pure myrcene-d_6 sample. Of the numerous product peaks displayed in the GC-MS data, and based on isotopic labeling, we proposed a reaction mechanism to account for ~30% of the total aerosol VOCs (Figure 9.7).

For comparison, pure THC was dabbed and vaped using a CCELL TH2 vaporizer. Non-targeted chromatographic analysis of the aerosol components revealed elevated levels of isoprene, substituted C_6–C_{10} dienes, and aromatics including toluene and xylenes. As a control, CBN (Figure 9.4) was also vaped under the same conditions as THC. This was done to investigate the role of THC's cyclohexenyl ring (Figure 9.3) as an originating site of gas-phase degradation products since the same ring in CBN is aromatic.

CBN vaping afforded a 10-fold lower level of total VOCs compared with THC. Moreover, the gas-phase products consisted nearly entirely of 1-butene, 1-propene, 1-pentene, butanal, propanal, and pentanal. The absence of isoprene and related terpene products, as well as and the production of overall fewer degradation products, embodies evidence that the substituted cyclohexenyl of THC is the most labile part of the molecule, and accounts for the majority of the gas-phase aerosol products derived from THC.

Based on the product distributions of the THC and CBN experiments, a mechanism accounting for ~22% of the formation of THC degradation products can be proposed, as shown in Figure 9.8. It is noteworthy that the same four products, 3-methylcrotonaldehyde, 2-methyl-2-butene, isoprene, and 3-methyl-1-butene, account for approximately 30% and 22% of the total gas-phase products resulting from vaping myrcene and THC, respectively. This is also consistent with the results of the CBN vaping experiment, which supports the fact that the substituted cyclohexenyl moiety of THC

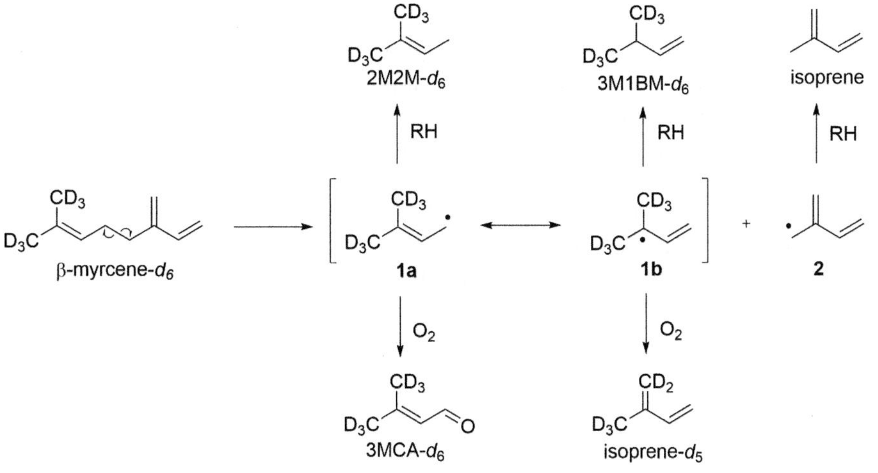

FIGURE 9.7 Proposed mechanism for the thermal degradation of β-myrcene-d_6. 3MCA = 3-methylcrotonaldehyde; 2M2B = 2-methyl-2-butene; 3M1B = 3-methyl-1-butene. Reproduced from Meehan-Atrash et al. (2021) and used with permission from the Royal Society of Chemistry.

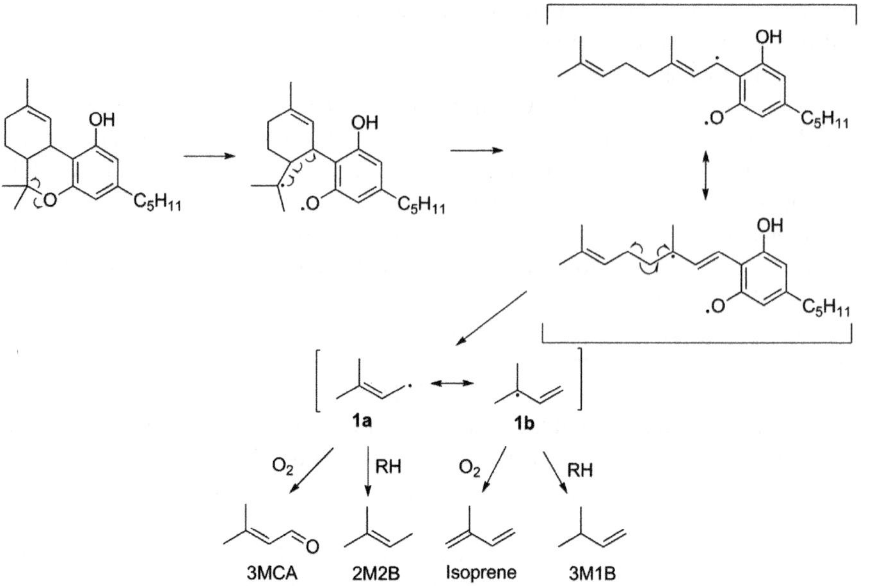

FIGURE 9.8 Proposed thermal degradation mechanism of THC under vaping and dabbing conditions via the cyclohexenyl moiety. 3MCA = 3-methylcrotonaldehyde; 2M2B = 2-methyl-2-butene; 3M1B = 3-methyl-1-butene. Reproduced from Meehan-Atrash et al. (2021) and used with permission from the Royal Society of Chemistry.

produces the terpene-related aerosol products, and accounts for a majority of the THC chemistry occurring during vaping or dabbing.

During the course of this study, dabbing a mixture of 5% deuterium-labeled myrcene and 95% THC enabled us to show that myrcene produces 5-fold higher levels of aerosol isoprene compared with THC, despite the excess THC. When the amount of myrcene was increased to 9%, a >6-fold higher level of aerosol isoprene derived from myrcene was found. The higher yields of isoprene during vaping compared with THC are consistent with the studies described in Section 9.6. Several reasons for this are plausible, one of which includes (i) the greater lability of terpenes compared with THC and (ii) that myrcene partitions into the gas phase and is thus more amenable to reactions known to occur in the gaseous state (Atkinson and Arey 2003). In contrast, THC only has appreciable access to the gas phase at the elevated temperatures directly surrounding the nail before its rapid partitions into the particulate phase.

Interestingly, we found that, in analogous experiments conducted using the CCell vaporizer instead of the dab platform, successively increasing the levels of myrcene (0%, 7%, and 14%) in the model concentrate samples resulted in *higher* transfer efficiency of THC and myrcene into the aerosol, while affording *lower* overall yields of isoprene and other VOC degradation products.

This trend is not consistent with our earlier dabbing experiments, in which myrcene (and other terpenes) clearly promoted the formation of isoprene and related degradation products (Meehan-Atrash et al. 2019). We attribute this to the physical properties of terpenes and cannabinoids and the differences in dabbing and vaping. For example, the lower boiling point of β-myrcene (167°C; Luo and Cheng 2015) compared with THC (417°C; Lovestead and Bruno 2017) may translate to a reduced boiling point of the mixture, lowering the aerosolization temperature. In addition, terpenes moderate THC viscosity, which facilitates wicking and thus improves heat transfer efficiency in vape pens, a well-known major factor that influences e-cigarette HPHC aerosol yields (Strongin 2019).

As expected, keeping myrcene levels fixed while increasing vaporizer power levels enhanced VOC production and reduced the aerosol transfer efficiency of myrcene and THC. Analysis of the effects of varying power levels on the formation of specific products revealed that increasing power levels lowers the ratio of **1a**-derived products to **1b**-derived products (Figure 9.8) in a process mainly governed by a relative decrease in the formation of 3-methylcrotonaldehyde relative to isoprene; 3-methylcrotonaldehyde is envisioned to form via addition of oxygen to **1a** followed by β-scission and the release of a hydroxyl radical. Isoprene forms from **1b** via addition of oxygen followed by the release of a hydroperoxyl radical. At higher temperatures, the barrier for O_2 addition to any carbon becomes nearly nonexistent (Taatjes 2006). This favors oxidation via the more significant resonance contributor (**1b**) pathway at higher temperatures. In addition, lower temperatures cannot overcome the relatively larger energy barrier for the back reaction of 3-methylcrotonaldehyde to **1a**. The experimental results thus show that the aerosol ratios of 3-methylcrotonaldehyde to isoprene formation can be controlled in a predictable manner by varying the temperature. Moreover, increasing concentrate myrcene mass percentages increased the formation of 3-methylcrotonaldehyde compared with isoprene, which is in keeping with myrcene lowering aerosolization temperatures as a viscosity modifier or by depressing the boiling point of myrcene-THC mixtures.

9.8 CONCLUSION

A greater understanding of the risks of exposure to emissions from vaping or dabbing cannabis concentrates is needed. The HPHCs in the smoke from marijuana cigarettes have been known for decades. However, the evaluation of the origins and identities of chemicals of concern present in aerosols derived from cannabis concentrate vaping and dabbing is in the early stages. Building upon pioneering studies of terpene and cannabinoid chemistry mainly from the pre-vaping era, we set out to address this important knowledge gap.

Initial findings from investigating terpene dabbing revealed aerosol HPHC product profiles consistent with prior investigations of terpene atmospheric chemistry. This is also in keeping with relatively recent tobacco e-cigarette studies showing that oxidation and free radical chemistry are common reaction pathways promoted during heating and aerosolization.

Subsequent investigations involving dabbing and vaping model concentrate formulations (9:1 THC:terpenes, SNDs) showed that THC and terpenes afford similar gas HPHC product profiles.

The results also showed that smoking cannabis versus vaping or dabbing concentrates afforded significantly different aerosol emission profiles. Lower levels of select HPHCs compared with traditional smoking were found regardless of the vaping or dabbing conditions studied. However, much more work is needed to understand the relative health risks and harm reduction properties of these products. Although the findings are promising, only a limited percentage of the total HPHCs and VOCs were identified and quantified, and particle phase aerosol components remain to be determined. The particle phase, where the cannabinoids and relatively larger and less polar non-gaseous molecules are partitioned, can have a significant impact on health-related properties.

In order to gain a more complete understanding of the mechanistic origins of HPHCs formed during cannabis vaping, product distributions deriving from isotopically labeled myrcene, THC, and CBN were investigated. This enabled us to elucidate which specific atoms from myrcene and THC are incorporated into HPHC structures, enabling a deeper understanding of how concentrate ingredients react and interact.

Dabbing afforded higher levels of HPHCs derived from myrcene compared with THC. However, the opposite was true in the case of vaping. Increasing myrcene concentrate levels led to more efficient aerosol delivery of both THC and myrcene, as well as lower HPHC levels. The relative aerosol levels of the products isoprene and 3-methylcrotonaldehyde were found to be temperature dependent, with isoprene formation favored at relatively higher power levels. Increasing myrcene levels resulted in enhanced levels of 3-methylcrotonaldehyde, in keeping with the finding that myrcene lowers the aerosolization temperature during vaping as opposed to dabbing. As research continues, additional insights into the chemical and physical factors that impact HPHC aerosol profiles and other health-relevant properties of concentrate aerosols will help guide the development of products that can optimize harm reduction and mitigate risks.

REFERENCES

Abrams, Donald I, Hector P Vizoso, Starley B Shade, Cheryl Jay, Mary Ellen Kelly, and Neal L Benowitz. 2007. 'Vaporization as a smokeless cannabis delivery system: a pilot study', *Clinical Pharmacology & Therapeutics*, 82: 572–8.

Adams, Roger, CK Cain, WD McPhee, and RB Wearn. 1941. 'Structure of Cannabidiol. XII. Isomerization to tetrahydrocannabinols', *Journal of the American Chemical Society*, 63: 2209–13.

Al Bakain, Ramia Z, Yahya S Al-Degs, James V Cizdziel, and Mahmoud A Elsohly. 2020. 'Comprehensive chromatographic profiling of cannabis from 23 USA States marketed for medical purposes', *Acta Chromatographica*, 33: 78–90.

Atkinson, Roger, and Janet Arey. 2003. 'Atmospheric degradation of volatile organic compounds', *Chemical Reviews*, 103: 4605–38.

Behr, Arno, and Leif Johnen. 2009. 'Myrcene as a natural base chemical in sustainable chemistry: a critical review', *ChemSusChem: Chemistry & Sustainability Energy & Materials*, 2: 1072–95.

Bhatnagar, Aruni. 2016. 'E-cigarettes and cardiovascular disease risk: evaluation of evidence, policy implications, and recommendations', *Current Cardiovascular Risk Reports*, 10: 1–10.

Britt, PF, AC Buchanan III, MM Kidder, C Owens, JR Ammann, JT Skeen, and L Luo. 2001. 'Mechanistic investigation into the formation of polycyclic aromatic hydrocarbons from the pyrolysis of plant steroids', *Fuel*, 80: 1727–46.

Bueno, Justin, Emily Leuer, Michael Kearney, Edward H Green, and Eric A Greenbaum. 2020. 'The preservation and augmentation of volatile terpenes in cannabis inflorescence', *Journal of Cannabis Research*, 2: 1–11.

Carbone, Marianna, Francesco Castelluccio, Antonella Daniele, Alan Sutton, Alessia Ligresti, Vincenzo Di Marzo, and Margherita Gavagnin. 2010. 'Chemical characterisation of oxidative degradation products of Δ^9-THC', *Tetrahedron*, 66: 9497–501.

Daniulaityte, Raminta, Mussa Y Zatreh, Francois R Lamy, Ramzi W Nahhas, Silvia S Martins, Amit Sheth, and Robert G Carlson. 2018. 'A Twitter-based survey on marijuana concentrate use', *Drug and Alcohol Dependence*, 187: 155–9.

Davis, BL, LA Goldblatt, and S Palkin. 1946. 'Production of isoprene from turpentine derivatives', *Industrial & Engineering Chemistry*, 38: 53–7.

Di Forti, Marta, Diego Quattrone, Tom P Freeman, Giada Tripoli, Charlotte Gayer-Anderson, Harriet Quigley, Victoria Rodriguez, Hannah E Jongsma, Laura Ferraro, and Caterina La Cascia. 2019. 'The contribution of cannabis use to variation in the incidence of psychotic disorder across Europe (EU-GEI): a multicentre case-control study', *The Lancet Psychiatry*, 6: 427–36.

Earleywine, Mitch, and Sara Smucker Barnwell. 2007. 'Decreased respiratory symptoms in cannabis users who vaporize', *Harm Reduction Journal*, 4: 1–4.

Elzinga, Sytze, Oscar Ortiz, and Jeffrey C Raber. 2015. 'The conversion and transfer of cannabinoids from cannabis to smoke stream in cigarettes', *Natural Products Chemistry & Research*, 3: 163.

Etter, Jean-Francois. 2015. 'Electronic cigarettes and cannabis: an exploratory study', *European Addiction Research*, 21: 124–30.

Etter, Jean-François, and Chris Bullen. 2011. 'Electronic cigarette: users profile, utilization, satisfaction and perceived efficacy', *Addiction*, 106: 2017–28.

George, Barbara Jane, Bradley D Schultz, Ted Palma, Alan F Vette, Donald A Whitaker, and Ronald W Williams. 2011. 'An evaluation of EPA's National-Scale Air Toxics Assessment (NATA): comparison with benzene measurements in Detroit, Michigan', *Atmospheric Environment*, 45: 3301–8.

Gieringer, Dale H. 2001. 'Cannabis "Vaporization" a promising strategy for smoke harm reduction', *Journal of Cannabis Therapeutics*, 1: 153–70.

Gieringer, Dale, Joseph St. Laurent, and Scott Goodrich. 2004. 'Cannabis vaporizer combines efficient delivery of THC with effective suppression of pyrolytic compounds', *Journal of Cannabis Therapeutics*, 4: 7–27.

Giroud, Christian, Mariangela De Cesare, Aurélie Berthet, Vincent Varlet, Nicolas Concha-Lozano, and Bernard Favrat. 2015. 'E-cigarettes: a review of new trends in cannabis use', *International Journal of Environmental Research and Public Health*, 12: 9988–10008.

Hädener, Marianne, Sina Vieten, Wolfgang Weinmann, and Hellmut Mahler. 2019. 'A preliminary investigation of lung availability of cannabinoids by smoking marijuana or dabbing BHO and decarboxylation rate of THC-and CBD-acids', *Forensic Science International*, 295: 207–12.

Hazekamp, Arno, Renee Ruhaak, Lineke Zuurman, Joop van Gerven, and Rob Verpoorte. 2006. 'Evaluation of a vaporizing device (Volcano®) for the pulmonary administration of tetrahydrocannabinol', *Journal of Pharmaceutical Sciences*, 95: 1308–17.

Jensen, R Paul, Robert M Strongin, and David H Peyton. 2017. 'Solvent chemistry in the electronic cigarette reaction vessel', *Scientific Reports*, 7: 1–11.

Kolicheski, MB, LC Cocco, DA Mitchell, and M Kaminski. 2007. 'Synthesis of myrcene by pyrolysis of β-pinene: analysis of decomposition reactions', *Journal of Analytical and Applied Pyrolysis*, 80: 92–100.

Krill, Christian, Simone Rochfort, and German Spangenberg. 2020. 'A high-throughput method for the comprehensive analysis of terpenes and terpenoids in medicinal cannabis biomass', *Metabolites*, 10: 276.

Küppers, FJEM, CAL Bercht, CA Salemink, and RJJ Lousberg. 1975a. 'Cannabis. XIV. Pyrolysis of cannabidiol—analysis of the volatile constituents', *Journal of Chromatography A*, 108: 375–9.

Küppers, FJEM, CAL Bercht, CA Salemink, RJJ Ch Lousberg, JK Terlouw, and W Heerma. 1975b. 'Cannabis—XV: pyrolysis of cannabidiol. Structure elucidation of four pyrolytic products', *Tetrahedron*, 31: 1513–16.

Küppers, FJEM, RJJ Ch Lousberg, CAL Bercht, CA Salemink, JK Terlouw, W Heerma, and A Laven. 1973. 'Cannabis—VIII: pyrolysis of Cannabidiol. Structure elucidation of the main pyrolytic product', *Tetrahedron*, 29: 2797–802.

Kwaśnica, Andrzej, Natalia Pachura, Klaudia Masztalerz, Adam Figiel, Aleksandra Zimmer, Robert Kupczyński, Katarzyna Wujcikowska, Angel A Carbonell-Barrachina, Antoni Szumny, and Henryk Różański. 2020. 'Volatile composition and sensory properties as quality attributes of fresh and dried hemp flowers (Cannabis sativa L.)', *Foods*, 9: 1118.

Lanz, Christian, Johan Mattsson, Umut Soydaner, and Rudolf Brenneisen. 2016. 'Medicinal cannabis: in vitro validation of vaporizers for the smoke-free inhalation of cannabis', *PLoS One*, 11: e0147286.

Leyva-Gutierrez, Francisco MA, John P Munafo Jr, and Tong Wang. 2020. 'Characterization of by-products from commercial cannabidiol production', *Journal of Agricultural and Food Chemistry*, 68: 7648–59.

Loflin, Mallory, and Mitch Earleywine. 2014. 'A new method of cannabis ingestion: the dangers of dabs?', *Addictive Behaviors*, 39: 1430–3.

Lovestead, Tara M, and Thomas J Bruno. 2017. 'Determination of cannabinoid vapor pressures to aid in vapor phase detection of intoxication', *Forensic Chemistry*, 5: 79–85.

Luo, YR, and JP Cheng. 2015. 'Physical constants of organic compounds'. In: WM Haynes (ed), *CRC Handbook of Chemistry and Physics*. Boca Raton, FL: Taylor & Francis, CRC Press.

Luteyn, JM, HJW Spronck, and CA Salemink. 1978. 'Cannabis XVIII: isolation and synthesis of olivetol derivatives formed in the pyrolysis of cannabidiol', *Recueil des Travaux Chimiques des Pays-Bas*, 97: 187–90.

Martin, Billy R. 2007. 'The endocannabinoid system and the therapeutic potential of cannabinoids'. In: Mahmoud A ElSohly (ed), *Marijuana and the Cannabinoids*. Totowa, NJ: Humana Press.

Mazian, Brahim, Stéphane Cariou, Mathilde Chaignaud, Jean-Louis Fanlo, Marie-Laure Fauconnier, Anne Bergeret, and Luc Malhautier. 2019. 'Evolution of temporal dynamic of volatile organic compounds (VOCs) and odors of hemp stem during field retting', *Planta*, 250: 1983–96.

Meacham, Meredith C, Michael J Paul, and Danielle E Ramo. 2018. 'Understanding emerging forms of cannabis use through an online cannabis community: an analysis of relative post volume and subjective highness ratings', *Drug and Alcohol Dependence*, 188: 364–9.

Meehan-Atrash, Jiries, Wentai Luo, Kevin J McWhirter, David G Dennis, David Sarlah, Robert P Jensen, Isaac Afreh, Jia Jiang, Kelley C Barsanti, and Alisha Ortiz. 2021. 'The influence of terpenes on the release of volatile organic compounds and active ingredients to cannabis vaping aerosols', *RSC Advances*, 11: 11714–23.

Meehan-Atrash, Jiries, Wentai Luo, Kevin J McWhirter, and Robert M Strongin. 2019. 'Aerosol gas-phase components from cannabis e-cigarettes and dabbing: mechanistic insight and quantitative risk analysis', *ACS Omega*, 4: 16111–20.

Meehan-Atrash, Jiries, Wentai Luo, and Robert M Strongin. 2017. 'Toxicant formation in dabbing: the terpene story', *ACS Omega*, 2: 6112–17.

Mikes, Frantisek, and Peter G Waser. 1971. 'Marihuana components: effects of smoking on delta-9-tetrahydrocannabinol and cannabidiol', *Science (New York, NY)*, 172: 1158–9.

Milay, Looz, Paula Berman, Anna Shapira, Ohad Guberman, and David Meiri. 2020. 'Metabolic profiling of cannabis secondary metabolites for evaluation of optimal post-harvest storage conditions', *Frontiers in Plant Science*, 11: 1556.

Moir, David, William S Rickert, Genevieve Levasseur, Yolande Larose, Rebecca Maertens, Paul White, and Suzanne Desjardins. 2008. 'A comparison of mainstream and side-stream marijuana and tobacco cigarette smoke produced under two machine smoking conditions', *Chemical Research in Toxicology*, 21: 494–502.

Perrotin-Brunel, Helene, Wim Buijs, Jaap Van Spronsen, Maaike JE Van Roosmalen, Cor J Peters, Rob Verpoorte, and Geert-Jan Witkamp. 2011. 'Decarboxylation of Δ^9-tetrahydrocannabinol: kinetics and molecular modeling', *Journal of Molecular Structure*, 987: 67–73.

Pomahacova, Barbora, F Van der Kooy, and Robert Verpoorte. 2009. 'Cannabis smoke condensate III: the cannabinoid content of vaporised Cannabis sativa', *Inhalation Toxicology*, 21: 1108–12.

Prodrom, Ioan. 1913. *Untersuchungen über Autoxydation und über Umwandlung verschiedener Terpene in Isopren*. Zurich: ETH Zurich.

Pronck, HJW, and RJJ Ch Lousberg. 1977. 'Pyrolysis of cannabidiol. Structure elucidation of a major pyrolytic conversion product', *Experientia*, 33: 705–6.

Quarles, William, George Ellman, and Reese Jones. 1973. 'Toxicology of marijuana: conditions for conversion of cannabidiol to THC upon smoking', *Clinical Toxicology*, 6: 211–16.

Repka, Michael A, Manish Munjal, Mahmoud A ElSohly, and Samir A Ross. 2006. 'Temperature stability and bioadhesive properties of Δ^9-tetrahydrocannabinol incorporated hydroxypropylcellulose polymer matrix systems', *Drug Development and Industrial Pharmacy*, 32: 21–32.

Ross, Samir A, and Mahmoud A ElSohly. 1996. 'The volatile oil composition of fresh and air-dried buds of Cannabis sativa', *Journal of Natural Products*, 59: 49–51.

Ruzicka, L, and M Stoll. 1924. 'Höhere Terpenverbindungen XVIII. Über die Konstitution des Cadinens', *Helvetica Chimica Acta*, 7: 84–94.

Schauer, Gillian L, Rashid Njai, and Althea M Grant-Lenzy. 2020. 'Modes of marijuana use–smoking, vaping, eating, and dabbing: results from the 2016 BRFSS in 12 States', *Drug and Alcohol Dependence*, 209: 107900.

Spronck, HJ, CA Salemink, F Alikaridis, and D Papadakis. 1978. 'Pyrolysis of cannabinoids: a model experiment in the study of cannabis smoking', *Bulletin on Narcotics*, 30: 55–9.

Spronck, HJW, and CA Salemink. 1978. 'Cannabis XVII: pyrolysis of cannabidiol. Structure elucidation of two pyrolytic conversion products', *Recueil des Travaux Chimiques des Pays-Bas*, 97: 185–6.

Stolle, A, and B Ondruschka. 2008. 'Comment to the paper "Synthesis of myrcene by pyrolysis of β-pinene: analysis of decomposition reactions" by MB Kolicheski et al. [J. Anal. Appl. Pyrol. 80 (2007) 92–100]', *Journal of Analytical and Applied Pyrolysis*, 81: 136–8.

Strongin, Robert M. 2019. 'E-cigarette chemistry and analytical detection', *Annual Review of Analytical Chemistry*, 12: 23–39.

Taatjes, Craig A. 2006. 'Uncovering the fundamental chemistry of alkyl+ O2 reactions via measurements of product formation', *The Journal of Physical Chemistry A*, 110: 4299–312.

Tjeerdema, RS. 1987. 'The pyrolysis of cannabinoids'. In: GW Ware (ed), *Reviews of Environmental Contamination and Toxicology: Continuation of Residue Reviews*. New York: Springer, pp. 61–81.

Tormohlen, Kayla N, Ashley Brooks-Russell, Ming Ma, Kristin E Schneider, Arnold H Levinson, and Renee M Johnson. 2019. 'Modes of marijuana consumption among Colorado high school students before and after the initiation of retail marijuana sales for adults', *Journal of Studies on Alcohol and Drugs*, 80: 46–55.

Turner, Carlton E, and Mohmoud A Elsohly. 1979. 'Constituents of cannabis sativa L. XVI. A possible decomposition pathway of Δ^9-tetrahydrocannabinol to cannabinol', *Journal of Heterocyclic Chemistry*, 16: 1667–8.

Varlet, Vincent, Nicolas Concha-Lozano, Aurélie Berthet, Grégory Plateel, Bernard Favrat, Mariangela De Cesare, Estelle Lauer, Marc Augsburger, Aurélien Thomas, and Christian Giroud. 2016. 'Drug vaping applied to cannabis: is "Cannavaping" a therapeutic alternative to marijuana?', *Scientific Reports*, 6: 1–13.

Wachtel, S, M ElSohly, S Ross, J Ambre, and H De Wit. 2002. 'Comparison of the subjective effects of Δ^9-tetrahydrocannabinol and marijuana in humans', *Psychopharmacology*, 161: 331–9.

Wilsey, Barth, Thomas Marcotte, Reena Deutsch, Ben Gouaux, Staci Sakai, and Haylee Donaghe. 2013. 'Low-dose vaporized cannabis significantly improves neuropathic pain', *The Journal of Pain*, 14: 136–48.

Zheng, Huidong, Jinliang Chen, Chao Li, Jingjing Chen, Yingshu Wang, Suying Zhao, and Yanru Zeng. 2017. 'Mechanism and kinetics of the pyrolysis of β-pinene to myrcene', *Journal of Analytical and Applied Pyrolysis*, 123: 99–106.

10 Cannabis Pharmacokinetics and Pharmacodynamics

Ted W. Simon

CONTENTS

10.1 INTRODUCTION

Cannabinoids are the biologically active molecules in *Cannabis sativa* plants. Synthetic cannabinoids have also been produced. Both types of exogenous cannabinoids mimic the signaling of endogenous ligands, the endocannabinoids produced by the metabolism of arachidonic acid. Endocannabinoids and genes involved in

DOI: 10.1201/9780429274893-10

endocannabinoid signaling have been found in diverse species including mammals, fish, arthropods, mollusks, annelids, Cnidaria, Protista, and bacteria (McPartland et al. 2006).

Cannabinoid receptors are located throughout the body and produce a variety of effects in addition to the euphoric state associated with the psychotropic effects of Δ^9-tetrahydrocannabinol (THC) and the calming effects of cannabidiol (CBD). The most widely characterized endocannabinoids are 2-arachidonoylglycerol (2-AG) and anandamide (AEA). The cannabinoid receptors, the endocannabinoid ligands (ECs), and the enzymes that produce and metabolize the ECs are collectively known as the endocannabinoidome (Cristino et al. 2020). The endocannabinoids modulate synaptic transmission throughout the brain via inhibitory GABAergic or excitatory glutamatergic synapses in the hippocampus, nucleus accumbens, and other brain regions (Devinsky et al. 2014; Hwang and Lupica 2020; Lupica et al. 2017).

The potential medicinal uses of cannabinoids have been explored by humans for over 10,000 years (Schurman et al. 2020). Cannabinoids can be classified into three groups:

1. Phytocannabinoids derived from plants
2. Synthetic cannabinoids produced by laboratory synthesis
3. Endocannabinoids that are produced within the body (Schurman et al. 2020; Wiley et al. 2014)

Phytocannabinoids include THC, CBD, cannabigerol (CBG), cannabichromene (CBC), and tetrahydrocannabivarin (THCV). In living plants, these exist as acids, such as tetrahydrocannabinolic acid (THCA). Once the plant is harvested, the acids are decarboxylated during drying and/or application of heat (Elzinga et al. 2015; Citti et al. 2018). Figure 10.1 shows the most common endocannabinoids and phytocannabinoids.

In this chapter, both the pharmacokinetics and pharmacodynamics of THC and CBD cannabinoids will be considered with a focus on consumer use and forensic considerations and less on the use in the pharmacopeia. The two takeaways for the reader will be a basic understanding of how cannabinoids affect physiology and behavior at a range of organization levels; knowledge of the links between this basic biology and effects on health and wellbeing will also be considered.

10.2 PHARMACOKINETICS OF CANNABINOIDS

To exert biological effects, exogenous substances must distribute from the site of application to the site of action in the target tissue. Pharmacokinetics or ADME is the study of Absorption, Distribution, Metabolism, and Elimination of substances from the body. The ubiquity of the endocannabinoidome throughout the body and in proximity to the site of action means that pharmacokinetic considerations are much less applicable to endocannabinoids than to exogenous cannabinoids such as THC or CBD.

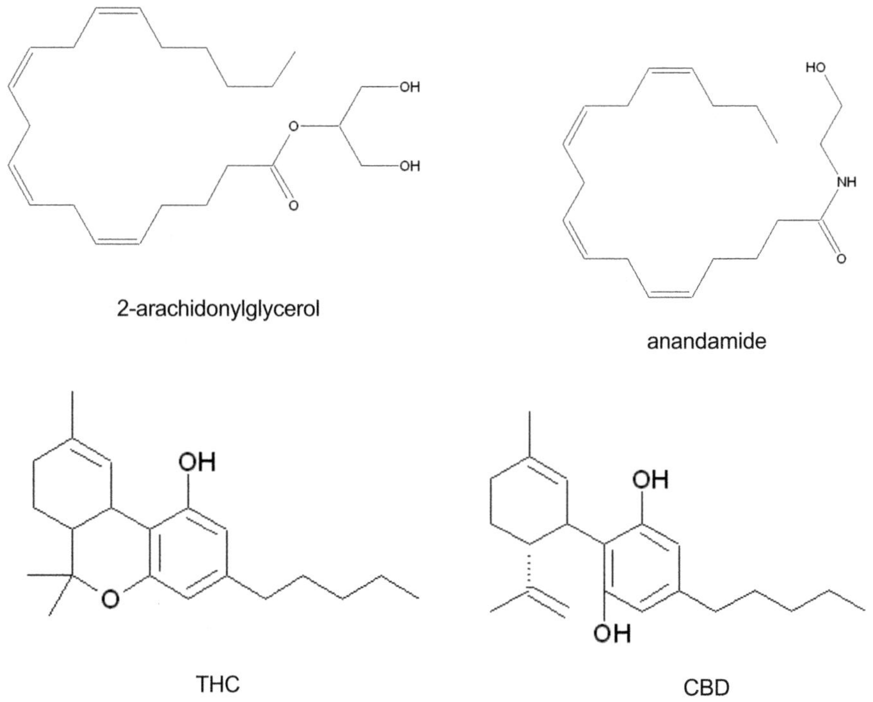

2-arachidonylglycerol

anandamide

THC

CBD

FIGURE 10.1 Chemical structures of the common endocannabinoids and cannabinoids from *cannabis*.

10.2.1 ABSORPTION OF CANNABINOIDS

THC was originally taken through combustible smoking and has evolved into other dosage forms and routes of administration. Smoking THC is still common with an increase in CBD strains for smoking on the rise. Both CBD and THC are commonly inhaled by vaping or taken orally in capsules, food products, or liquids via oral or sublingual administration. While some amounts of these substances occur in plant material, the acidic forms, tetrahydrocannabinolic acid and cannabidiolic acid, are also present and are decarboxylated by heat to form THC and CBD (Citti et al. 2018; Dussy et al. 2005). Both THC and CBD are uncharged at physiological pH and are lipophilic with logP values around six, which results in their high lipophilicity. When absorption occurs through the gastrointestinal tract following oral administration, phase I and phase II metabolic enzymes present in the enterocytes and in the liver account for a first-pass effect that limits the amount of either THC or CBD that reaches the central circulation.

10.2.2 DISTRIBUTION OF CANNABINOIDS

Distribution of either THC or CBD occurs rapidly into richly perfused organs such as the brain, heart, and liver. A second less-rapid phase also occurs to less vascularized tissues that serve as reservoirs (Lucas et al. 2018). This rapid distribution is the reason that psychoactive effects and driving impairment by THC cannot be readily predicted from blood concentrations (Compton 2017).

Cannabinoids and their metabolites bind strongly to plasma proteins, including albumin, and this binding represents yet another reservoir (Widman et al. 1974; Widman et al. 1973; Klausner et al. 1975; Skopp et al. 2002; Fanali et al. 2011; Wolowich et al. 2019). Both high lipid solubility and strong binding to plasma proteins greatly hinder the development of pharmacokinetic models for cannabinoids (Schwilke et al. 2009; Poulin and Haddad 2015; Ye et al. 2016; Poulin et al. 2016; Korzekwa and Nagar 2017; Chan et al. 2018). As a result, the majority of the models are empirical—based solely on the observed time courses of these substances in blood or plasma. Physiologically based pharmacokinetic (PBPK) models that track the amounts or concentrations of substances in specific organs such as the brain, liver, or kidney present a much greater challenge than empirical models.

10.2.3 METABOLISM OF CANNABINOIDS

The first phase of the metabolism of cannabis occurs through the action of enzymes known as cytochrome p450 mixed-function oxidases or CYPs. THC is metabolized to the psychoactive metabolite 11-hydroxy-Δ^9-tetrahydrocannabinol (THCOH) by CYP2C9, CYP2C19, and CYP3A4 (Bland et al. 2005), These same enzymes metabolize THC-OH to inactive 11-nor-9-carboxy-Δ^9-tetrahydrocannabinol (THCCOOH). Figure 10.2 shows the metabolism of THC including glucuronide conjugation of metabolites.

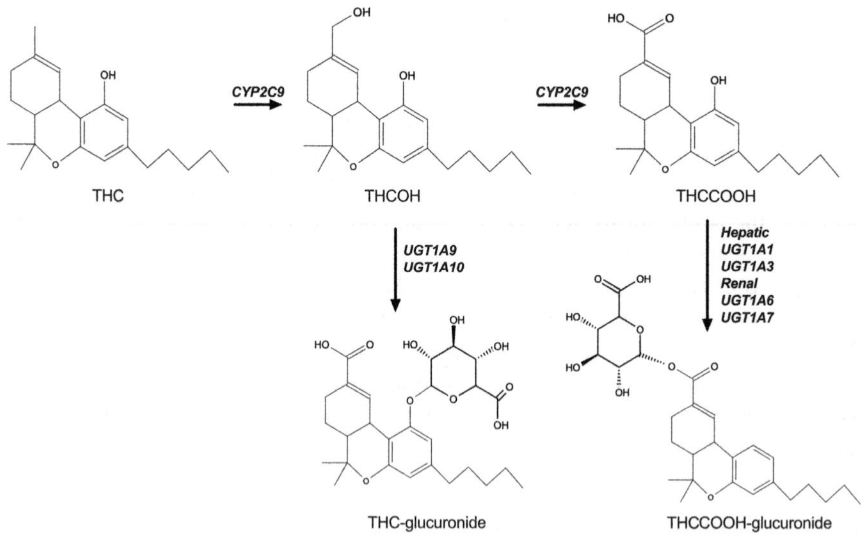

FIGURE 10.2 Metabolism of delta-9-tetrahydrocannabinol. The arrows show the metabolic transformations with the enzymes involved shown in bold.

Seven different phase I enzymes metabolize CBD to various extents, including CYP1A1, CYP1A2, CYP2C9, CYP2C19, CYP3A4, and CYP3A5 (Jiang et al. 2011). A large number of metabolites formed from phase I oxidation of CBD with the most common being carboxylic acids (Ujváry and Hanuš 2016; Harvey and Mechoulam 1990). Figure 10.3 shows the phase I metabolism of CBD.

Considerable genetic variation exists between individuals in the activity of the enzymes that metabolize both THC and CBD (Bland et al. 2005; Ujváry and Hanuš 2016; Bornheim et al. 1992; Sachse-Seeboth et al. 2009). In addition, the activity of these enzymes may be modulated within a single individual by diet, use of pharmaceuticals, and possibly other factors, and these variations result in drug-drug interactions between cannabinoids and prescribed pharmaceuticals (Bland et al. 2005; Alsherbiny and Li 2019; Anderson and Chan 2016; Brown and Winterstein 2019; MacCallum and Russo 2018).

Phase II metabolism involves the conjugation of a polar moiety to enhance excretion via both bile and urine. The most common conjugates are glucuronic acid and sulfate. Cannabinoids are glucuronidated via the action of specific uridine diphosphate-glucuronyl transferase enzymes (UGTs) present in the liver, kidney, and intestine. The human genome codes for 22 different UGTs, and alternative splicing and heterotypic oligomerization provide large variability in substrate specificities (Kasteel et al. 2020; Meech et al. 2019; Hu et al. 2019).

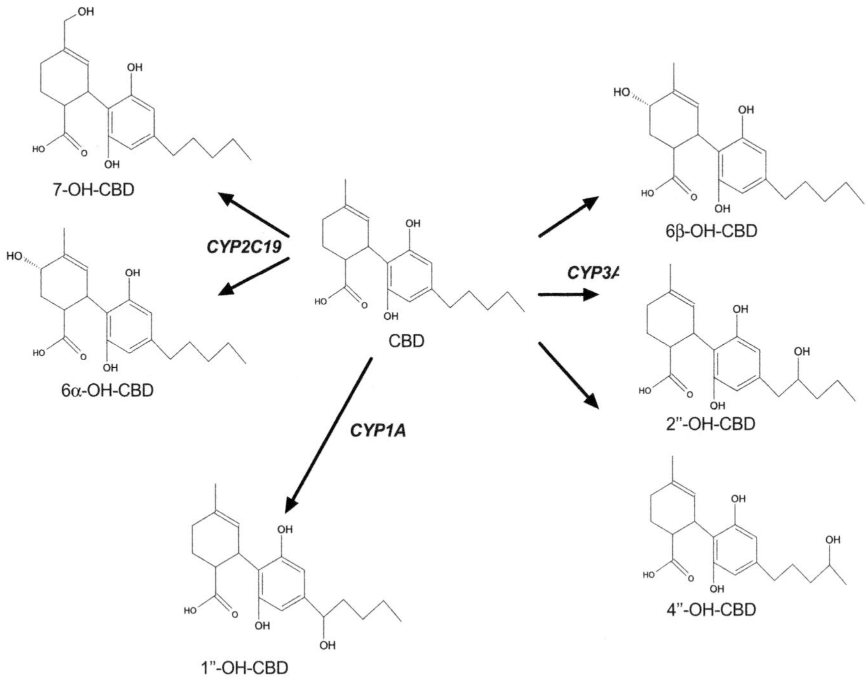

FIGURE 10.3 Metabolism of cannabidiol. The arrows show the metabolic transformations with the enzymes involved shown in bold.

The active metabolite of THC is glucuronidated to a small extent by UGT1A9 and 1A10 to produce THC-glucuronide. THCCOOH is extensively glucuronidated by UGT1A1 and 1A3. Additional glucuronidation occurs via UGT1A7 and 1A6. CBD is glucuronidated by UGT1A9, 2B7, 2B15, and 2B17 (Mazur et al. 2009). The extensive hepatic glucuronidation of THCCOOH is the reason that the majority of this metabolite is excreted in bile and feces. CBD itself is glucuronidated. Information is not yet available about which CBD metabolites are subject to glucuronidation (Ujváry & Hanuš 2016).

10.2.4 ELIMINATION OF CANNABINOIDS

THC is eliminated from plasma with observed half-lives of 2–60 hours (Grotenhermen 2003). The high variability is due to the multi-phasic redistribution into the plasma from reservoir tissues and slow dissociation from plasma proteins. The elimination half-life of THCOH is also relatively short and highly variable for the same reasons. THCCOOH is eliminated from plasma with a half-life of around five to seven days (Kelly and Jones 1992).

The majority of THCCOOH is excreted in bile and feces with about 90% as the glucuronide (Grotenhermen 2003; Fabritius et al. 2013; Gronewold and Skopp 2011). Enterohepatic recirculation contributes to the longevity of THCCOOH in plasma. In consequence, urinary excretion of THCCOOH may last for many days, especially in chronic users who have accumulated THC in their fat stores (Bergamaschi et al. 2013; Lowe et al. 2009; Odell et al. 2015). As a molar ratio, about 65% of total THCCOOH in plasma occurs as the glucuronide conjugate, whereas this fraction in urine is about 95% (Kelly and Jones 1992; Desrosiers et al. 2014a; Schwope et al. 2011). The renal half-lives and excretion rates in urine are similar in value for the free form and the conjugate (Dietz et al. 2007); observation suggests that glucuronidation may occur in the kidney during the renal clearance of free THCCOOH, similar to propofol (Bleeker et al. 2008; Gill et al. 2012; Knights et al. 2016; Margaillan et al. 2015). A smaller fraction of CBD and its metabolites are excreted in feces. Urinary excretion of unchanged CBD and glucuronide are also observed (Ujváry and Hanuš 2016).

10.3 PHARMACOKINETIC MODELS OF CANNABINOIDS

Unfortunately, the rapid distribution, multi-phasic redistribution to plasma, binding to plasma proteins, and enterohepatic recirculation of THC metabolites render the development of a comprehensive PBPK model for cannabinoids and their metabolites a Sisyphean nightmare. A single PBPK model of THC has been published based on allometric scaling from a mouse model (Methaneethorn et al. 2020b; Methaneethorn et al. 2020a). A practical example illustrating this difficulty is the observation of increasing urinary concentrations of THCCOOH accompanying weight loss in abstinent former chronic marijuana users: THC stored in adipose tissue is mobilized to plasma, metabolized, and excreted. Sadly, many of those with the power to change lives, such as medical review officers or personnel in child protective services, are blithely unaware of such nuances.

Nonetheless, pharmacokinetic modeling of THC has advanced in the 21st century with the use of NONMEM and similar phenomenological Bayesian population models (Zhang et al. 2003; Mandema et al. 1992). As of this writing, two pharmacokinetic models of CBD have been developed (Lim et al. 2020; Liu et al. 2020).

10.3.1 PHARMACOKINETIC MODELING OF THC AND METABOLITES

Strougo et al. (2008) developed a pharmacokinetic-pharmacodynamic (PK-PD) model for THC and its active metabolite, THCOH. The kinetic portion for each substance was a two-compartment model and the pharmacodynamic model could predict changes in heart rate, body sway, and several visual analog scale (VAS) measures, including "feeling high" using an effect compartment E_{max} model. Unfortunately, the model description provided in the paper was so sparse that reproducing the model was impossible.

Heuberger et al. (2015) published a three-compartment model for THC based on prior studies of oral, intravenous, and inhalation dosing (68Ohlsson et al. 1981, 1982; Wall et al. 1983). Elimination was modeled as a first-order rate constant rather than as clearance (Heuberger et al. 2015).

Awasthi et al. (2017) developed a three-compartment sub-model for THC linked to a two-compartment sub-model for THCOH, which was also with transfer rate constants for metabolism based on previous intravenous dosing studies of THC (Hollister et al. 1981; Naef et al. 2004). Both of these sub-models were linked to an effect compartment E_{max} model. The overall model was able to reproduce the reported feeling of being "high" (Awasthi et al. 2018).

Marsot et al. (2017) developed a three-compartment model for THC, also with first-order elimination. The model was based on these same authors' study of ad libitum cannabis smoking in 12 volunteers. The first-order elimination rate was calculated as proportional to the clinical measure alanine aminotransferase (ALT), but these ALT results were not reported in the smoking study. In addition, the plasma concentrations and urinary results were presented as useless plots with grayscale differences between the individuals, thus rendering impossible any understanding of the individual variation from viewing these plots.

Wolowich et al. (2019) used data from a large (n=306) but yet unpublished IV study and a smaller oral study to develop linked three-compartment models for THC, THCOH, and THCCOOH as well as a minimal PBPK model with compartments consisting of liver, lumped brain, heart and kidneys, lumped muscle and skin, subcutaneous adipose tissue, other adipose tissue, and the rest of the body (Vandrey et al. 2017). In addition, the influence of genetic variation in CYP2C9 was included.

Sempio et al. (2019) developed linked three-compartment sub-models for THC and THCOH and a one-compartment model for THCCOOH. Elimination of all three substances was modeled as clearance. The model was based on data collected from six male cannabis smokers (Huestis et al. 1992a, 1992b).

Methaneethorn et al. (2020) developed a PBPK model for THC by interspecies extrapolation to humans of a rodent PBPK model developed by the same authors (Methaneethorn et al. 2020a, 2020b). The model was able to reproduce plasma concentrations from several studies of intravenous, oral, and inhalation dosing (Naef et al. 2004; Huestis et al. 1992a; Hunault et al. 2008; Newmeyer et al. 2016; Wall and Perez-Reyes 1981). The model was comprised of seven compartments including brain, liver, kidneys, lungs, fat, and slowly perfused and rapidly perfused tissues. THC was the only substance included in the model. One interesting aspect of the model is the clearance of THC from the brain via P-glycoprotein excretion (Zhu et al. 2006). Because this model includes only THC and not the psychoactive metabolite THCOH, any attempt to use it alone for pharmacodynamic predictions will be incomplete.

Glaz-Sandberg and colleagues conducted observations of ten individuals after intravenous dosing with THCCOOH and developed a three-compartment model for this inactive metabolite (Glaz-Sandberg et al. 2007). Elimination of THCOOH from plasma occurs by at least three processes—urinary clearance, hepatic glucuronidation, and renal glucuronidation. In the model, these three processes were lumped together in a single first-order rate constant. From the same study participants, Dietz et al. (2007) analyzed the urinary excretion kinetics of both THCCOOH and its glucuronide conjugate. The mean urinary half-life of the unconjugated form was 16.0 hours with a range of 10.7 to 27.6 hours. The mean urinary half-life of the conjugate was 17.3 hours with a range of 9.0 to 27.4 hours. Another publication from the same observational study reported the effects of reducing enterohepatic recirculation by oral pre-dosing with activated charcoal. In the intestine, the charcoal absorbs a portion of any material present thus either reducing the amount of glucuronide available to the gut bacteria and reducing de-conjugation or reducing the amount of free THCCOOH available for reabsorption. The authors did observe an increase in plasma concentrations of free THCCOOH in the presence of activated charcoal (Böhnke et al. 2013).

10.3.2 Pharmacokinetic Modeling of CBD and Metabolites

A three-compartment model for CBD was developed from data extracted from 15 studies of CBD with oral dosing that included oral solutions, capsules, and oral mucosal spray (Lim et al. 2020). Absorption from the gastrointestinal tract was modeled using both a zero-order model that assumes a constant rate of absorption and a Weibull model with an increasing rate of absorption over time (Zhou 2003). The physiological aspects represented by the Weibull model are a low rate of gastric absorption and a higher rate of absorption from the intestine with total absorption changing along with gastric emptying.

A model of both CBD and THC was developed from blood sampling from 36 cannabis users administered CBD alone, THC alone, or mixtures of the two by vaporization from an alcoholic solution (Liu et al. 2020). THC pharmacokinetics could be modeled with a three-compartment model and CBD with a two-compartment model. The stated purpose of both these models was to gain a better understanding of cannabinoid dosing for clinical purposes. Neither model considered metabolism or elimination.

10.3.3 SIGNIFICANCE AND DEVELOPMENT OF A UNIFIED THC MODEL

While the models discussed previously represent a considerable effort on the part of the authors, none of them is a comprehensive model that includes concentrations of THC and all three metabolites—THC, THCOH, THCCOOH, and THCCOOH-glucuronide—in plasma as well as THCCOOH and THCCOOH-glucuronide in urine.

What also has not been investigated at all is renal glucuronidation of THCCOOH. As noted, the molar fraction of THCCOOH-glucuronide of total THCCOOH in plasma is about 60% (Kelly and Jones 1992; Desrosiers et al. 2014a; Schwope et al. 2011; Law et al. 1984). In contrast, the molar fraction of glucuronide in urine is about 95% (Kelly and Jones 1992; Andersson et al. 2016; Desrosiers et al. 2014b; Scheidweiler et al. 2012). What this difference suggests is that, similar to the anesthetic propofol, free THCCOOH is glucuronidated in the renal tubular cells and secreted into the tubular urine. While renal glucuronidation of THCCOOH has not yet been measured, the UGT isoforms capable of conjugating THCCOOH are expressed in the kidney (Mazur et al. 2009; Knights et al., 2016; Knights and Miners 2010).

An idea of the relative magnitude of hepatic and renal glucuronidation *in vivo* can be obtained within *in vitro* to *in vivo* extrapolation (IVIVE). Using this method (Box 10.1), hepatic glucuronidation is estimated to be about 7-fold greater than renal glucuronidation (Mazur et al. 2009).

BOX 10.1   IVIVE Extrapolation for Glucuronidation of THCCOOH

Data on the enzyme activities of Mazur et al. (2009) used recombinant uridine diphosphate (UDP) glucuronosyltransferases (UGTs) in a heterologous expression system to measure the enzyme kinetics of individual isoforms that conjugate cannabinoids (Mazur et al. 2009). These data along with data on plasma protein binding of THCCOOH and concentrations on microsomal protein in liver and kidney were used to calculate clearance by glucuronidation (Barter et al. 2007; Gibson et al. 2013; Knights and Miners 2010; Knights et al. 2016; Lipscomb and Kedderis 2002; Lipscomb et al. 2003; Patilea-Vrana et al. 2019).

Michaelis–Menten kinetic parameters for glucuronidation of both THC-OH and THC-COOH can be determined from *in vitro* data. The Michaelis–Menten equation is as follows:

Vmax is the maximum reaction velocity given in pmol/mg protein/min and K_m is the substrate concentration at half the maximum velocity given in umol. For most enzymes, the maximal intrinsic clearance or $CL_{int,max}$ is the ratio of V_{max}/K_m. Estimated unbound intrinsic clearance or $CL_{int,u}$ can be calculated as the product of $CL_{int,max}$, liver weight, microsomal protein concentration, and the relative activity factor between the recombinant enzyme and a microsomal preparation.

Actual clearance is given by the following equation from Gibson et al. (2013):

Micaelis–Menten

$$v = \frac{V_{max} x [S]}{K_m + [S]}$$

And clearance

$$CL = \frac{Q * fu_{plasma} * CL_{int,u}}{Q + fu_{plasma} * CL_{int,u} / BP}$$

where Q is the blood flow to the kidney or liver, fu_{plasma} is the fraction of unbound substrate in plasma, and BP is the blood-to-plasma concentration ratio of substrate.

The median estimate for hepatic clearance via glucuronidation of THCCOOH 1.5 L/hr and that for THCOH is 0.0073 L/hr. The median estimate for renal clearance of THCCOOH via glucuronidation is 0.18 L/hr. The geometric standard deviations for these three clearance values are 2.3, 1.4, and 3.1, respectively, indicating high variability in clearance of these THC metabolites.

The reason all these considerations are important is the reliance by decision-makers on urine drug screening results. The antibodies used in these tests developed against free THCCOOH either cross-react to a significant extent with the glucuronide or hardly at all. Examination of the 510(K)-pre-manufacturing database from the FDA indicates about half the assays in commercial use show this cross-reactivity. This variation in assay performance along with the high variation in phase I and phase II metabolism of THC suggests that the results of these screening assays are inaccurate, a fact that goes unrecognized by decision-makers.

10.3.4 PHARMACOKINETIC MODEL FOR THC AND METABOLITES INCLUDING ELIMINATION

The model shown later includes THC and its major metabolites except for THC-glucuronide; neither is this model comprehensive—pharmacodynamic considerations are not included. Nonetheless, this model can predict the concentrations of THC and its three major metabolites in plasma as well as the concentrations of both the free and conjugated forms of THCCOOH in urine. Figure 10.4 shows the structure of the model. The model parameters are a combination of those in the models discussed previously.

For THC, a three-compartment sub-model was used with a central compartment representing plasma and two peripheral compartments, one a reservoir and the other an exchange. The ratio between the rate constants for inflow and outflow determine

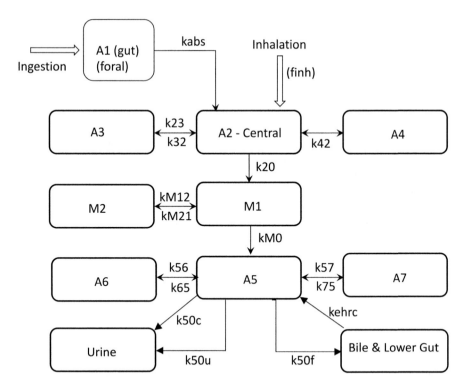

FIGURE 10.4 Graphic scheme of the Pharmacokinetic model used for the simulations shown in Figures 10.5 and 10.6. The compartments are numbers and the first order inter-compartmental transfers are shown as double-headed arrows. Compartments A2, A3, and A4 represent the distribution of THC. THC-OH is produced by transfer k20 and the distribution of THC-OH is represented by compartments M1 and M2. THC-COOH is produced by transfer kM0 and compartments A5, A6, and A7 represent the distribution of THC-COOH. Glucuronide conjugation occurs with A5 and is excreted into urine by a separate process than free THC-COOH. The return of THC-COOH by enterhepatic recirculation is shown as transfer kehrc.

which peripheral compartment is which: the reservoir compartment had the higher ratio. Outflows from the central compartment are expressed as first-order rate constants. Clearance values were converted to rates by dividing by the volume of distribution. All parameters were generally expressed as lognormal distributions to keep all parameter values positive. For additional information and R code for the model shown in Figure 10.4, please contact the author.

The models of Heuberger et al. (2015), Awasthi et al. (2017), Marsot et al. (2017), Wolowich et al. (2019), and Sempio et al. (2019) provided three-compartment models for THC. Based on the ratios of the rate constants between transport from and return to the central compartment, the two peripheral compartments were considered to be a storage compartment and a distribution compartment. The storage compartment is defined as the one with a higher ratio of transport out of the central compartment and returns to the central compartment. All of these PK studies used NONMEM software to develop distributions and provided the central value as an arithmetic mean and the variance as either a coefficient of variation (CV) or an ω^2 value. The CV can be obtained from ω^2 as:

$$CV = \sqrt{exp\left(\omega^2\right) - 1}$$

(Eq. 10.1)

The arithmetic mean and variance were converted to the lognormal parameters (μ) or log-mean and (σ) or log standard deviation; 1000 random deviates from each of the five lognormal distributions were combined and fit to a combination lognormal distribution.

The two-compartment sub-model in Awasthi et al. (2017) was used to model THCOH kinetics. The three-compartment sub-model of Glaz-Sandberg et al. was used to model the kinetics of THCCOOH. The fraction in plasma of conjugated THCCOOH was modeled as a fraction of total THCCOOH and was represented as a beta distribution. All these parameter values are shown in Table 10.1.

10.3.5 MODELING URINE FLOW RATE AND VOID VOLUME USING NHANES DATA

Measured values in urine flow, void interval, and creatinine concentration, as well as details on age, height, weight, ethnicity, drug use, and existing medical conditions, are available from CDC-NHANES (Aylward et al. 2017; Hays et al. 2015; Middleton et al. 2016; Yeh et al. 2015). NHANES data published from 2009 through 2018, providing a dataset of 41,247 individuals. This dataset was used to obtain measurements of age, body weight, height, body mass index, urine flow rate, and void interval. In addition, information on ethnicity and self-reported drug use were also included. This database was used to select populations that either matched the study participants as closely as possible or represented the general population.

The outputs of the PK model were the amounts over time of THC-COOH and the glucuronide conjugate in the urine. Urine concentrations could then be simulated using these model outputs and NHANES data.

CDC-NHANES data were used to obtain representative data on urine flow, void volume, and void interval. These data from 2011 through 2018 provided a set of 41,275 individuals. Subsets of the NHANES data corresponding in age, height, weight, BMI, and other factors to the study population could be easily obtained. Once a subset was selected, correlations between age, height, body mass, BMI, void interval, and urine flow were used to simulate multivariate lognormal distributions of these factors to represent a hypothetical population.

Intra-individual variation in urine flow and void interval were obtained from the 63 men and 103 women in the NHANES data who provided three consecutive urine samples; these were used to calculate the log standard deviation for both urine flow and void interval for each individual. These were used in a bivariate distribution with log SD for urine flow and void interval modeled as a gamma distribution and a

Weibull distribution, respectively. For each simulated individual, void volume was calculated as the product of urine flow and void interval immediately preceding the urination event. To ensure the void volume remained within biologically plausible limits, at each urination event, the volume was adjusted to remain within the limits specified as the mid-point between highest and lowest volumes observed in the subset of the NHANES data after removal of outliers identified with a random forest method.

10.3.6   MODEL EVALUATION

The combined PK and urine flow model can reproduce the plasma and urine concentrations observed in following an inhalation study of 11 occasional cannabis users smoking cannabis containing 6.8% THC (Desrosiers et al. 2014a, 2014b) (Figures 10.5 and 10.6).

10.4   PHARMACODYNAMICS OF CANNABINOIDS

In this section, the biology of the endocannabinoidome will be considered first as a basis for understanding how the phytocannabinoids THC and CBD modulate and/ or disrupt the normal function of the cannabinoidome. Next, the specific cellular and molecular effects of THC and CBD will be discussed. Finally, several specific examples of the effects of THC and CBD at the organ, tissue, and individual level will be presented to understand how these cellular effects modify both physiology and behavior.

10.4.1   ENDOCANNABINOIDOME AND ENDOCANNABINOID SIGNALING

Presently, two cannabinoid receptors have been identified and a third may be added. CB1 and CB2 respond to endogenous ligands including 2-AG, arachidonyletha-nolamine (anandamide or AEA), and other similar fatty acid derivatives including eicosanoids and prostaglandins (Burstein 2019) (Figure 10.1); 2-AG is considered a full agonist and AEA a partial agonist at both receptors. Distinct biosynthetic and degradation pathways exist for the endocannabinoids and may represent a means of modulating the endocannabinoidome (Tsuboi et al. 2018).

CB1 and CB2 are G protein-coupled receptors expressed on cell surfaces. Following agonist ligand binding, the heterotrimeric receptor binds guanosine tri-phosphate (GTP) and releases one or more subunits with the result of reduction of cAMP via protein kinases. The reduction in cAMP serves to regulate synaptic transmission and plasticity (Kano 2014; Lu and Mackie 2016).

CB1R activation also modulates calcium currents, increases potassium currents, and activates mitogen-activated protein kinase (MAPK) (van der Stelt and Di Marzo 2005; Lozovaya et al. 2009). CB1R itself is regulated via phosphorylation by other kinases and leads to internalization and inactivation of the receptors at the cell surface by interactions with scaffolding proteins known as β-arrestins (Schurman et al. 2020). CB1Rs are located in GABAergic and glutamatergic presynaptic terminals

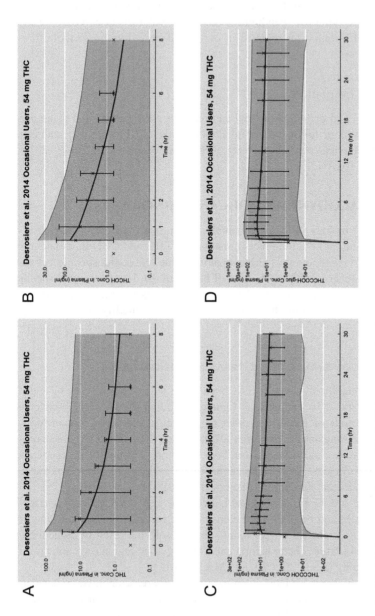

FIGURE 10.5 Modeled concentrations of THC-COOH and THC-COOH glucuronide in plasma and urine compared with those from occasional users in Desrosiers et al. (2014). (A) Timecourse of THC concentrations in plasma. (B) Timecourse of THCOH concentrations in plasma. (C) Timecourse of THCCOOH concentrations in plasma. (D) Timecourse of THCCOOH-glucuronide in plasma. The x-marks and error bars show the measured values in users following smoking a single cannabis cigarette containing 54 mg THC. The blue line and the gray envelope show the median and 95% modeled interval.

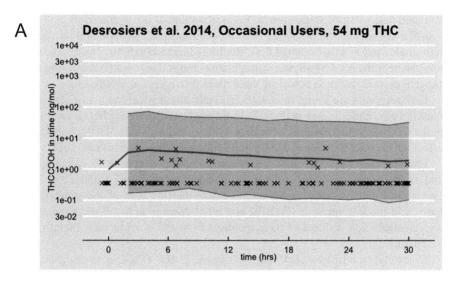

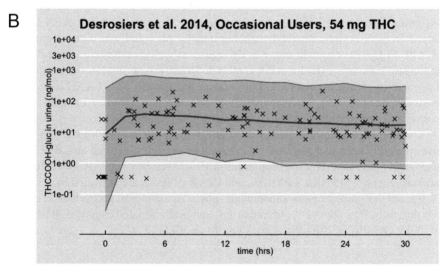

FIGURE 10.6 Modeled concentrations of THCCOOH and THCCOOH-glucuronide in urine compared with those from occasional users in Desrosiers et al. (2014). (A) Timecourse of THCCOOH concentrations in urine. (B) Timecourse of THCCOOH-glucuronide concentrations in urine. The x-marks show individual measurements. The green line shows the modeled median value and the gray envelope shows the 95% modeled interval. The measured values below the limit of detection are shown at this limit (0.5 ng/ml).

and modulate synaptic transmission. Endocannabinoids are synthesized in the post-synaptic cell and act presynaptically to reduce transmitter release and thus act in a retrograde direction to the signal flow. Binding of ligands to both cannabinoid receptors can be influenced by allosteric modulation and active research is ongoing to find exogenous modulators as new drug candidates (Slivicki et al. 2018).

CB2 receptors are found in endothelial cells, the myocardium, vascular smooth muscle cells, and immune cells including lymphocytes, macrophages, and neutrophils. CB2 activation inhibits adenylate cyclase and activates MAPK but does not affect ion channel function (Demuth and Molleman 2006; Sierra et al. 2018).

Endocannabinoids are produced enzymatically in response to calcium influx and from membrane phospholipids by phospholipase-C (del Caño et al. 2014). Endocannabinoids are hydrophobic and act in the tiny area of the synaptic cleft. Fatty acid-binding proteins (FABPs) and other carriers may aid the movement of endocannabinoids within and their reuptake from the synaptic cleft (Schurman et al. 2020).

Diacylglycerol lipases (DAGLs) synthesize 2-AG. DAGL-α is expressed primarily in the nervous system and DAGL-β primarily in immune cells. Hydrolysis of 2-AG occurs mainly via monoacylglycerol lipase (MAGL) and other enzymes including cytochrome p450; cyclooxygenase may also remove 2-AG. AEA is produced from N-acylphosphatidylethanolamines by phospholipase D-type enzymes (NAPE-PLD) that occur in many body organs as well as the brain. Several other redundant pathways exist for AEA synthesis. Deactivation of AEA occurs through fatty acid amide hydrolase (FAAH) to produce arachidonic acid. FAAH is bound in postsynaptic neurons in the cortex, cerebellum, and hippocampus. AEA may also be converted by cytochrome p450 to inflammatory eicosanoids (Schurman et al. 2020).

The transient receptor potential vanilloid type 1 protein (TRPV) is a non-selective cation channel also activated by AEA and has been suggested as CB3R (Joshi and Onaivi 2019). Peroxisome proliferator-activated receptors (PPARs) include three nuclear receptors: PPARα, PPARβ/δ, and PPARγ. PPARs are activated by a variety of ligands that include endocannabinoids, phytocannabinoids, and synthetic cannabinoids, as well as phthalates, fibrate drugs, and perfluorinated chemicals (Oshida et al. 2015; O'Sullivan 2016; Pistis and O'Sullivan 2017).

10.4.2 Localization of Cannabinoid Receptors

CB1R is found in presynaptic terminals in almost all regions of the brain and the mitochondrial outer membrane. In contrast, CB2R is expressed largely in the cells of the immune system. Both receptors are throughout the body (Joshi and Onaivi 2019; Schurman et al. 2020).

10.5 ORGANISM-LEVEL EFFECTS OF CANNABINOIDS

In late 2020, the detailed knowledge of cannabinoid pharmacodynamics is not yet sufficient to detail the pathway links to various effects. Three effects are discussed following: (1) the effect of THC and THCOH in producing driving impairment; (2)

the association of THC and THCOH with heart attacks by their effects on CB1R; and (3) the anxiolytic effect of CBD through activation of CB2R and possibly serotonin-like effects.

10.5.1 EFFECTS OF CANNABIS ON DRIVING SKILLS

The cannabis literature in the 21st century is replete with observational studies of the association of cannabis use, specifically THC, and crash risk in drivers (Ramaekers et al. 2000; Teixeira et al. 2004; Ramaekers et al. 2004; Drummer et al. 2004; Laumon et al. 2005; Asbridge et al. 2005; Khiabani et al. 2006; Jones et al. 2008; Ronen et al. 2008; Sewell et al. 2009; Gadegbeku et al. 2011; Asbridge et al. 2012; Elvik 2013). Several studies attempted to determine a blood level of cannabis that correlated to driving impairment. Some have even attempted to define a threshold blood concentration for driving impairment. Grotenhermen et al. (2007) proposed a range of 7–10 ng/ml in blood for THC based on polynomial regression of the odds ratio for crash risk and whole blood THC concentrations (Drummer et al. 2004; Grotenhermen 2003). Colorado considers a whole blood THC concentration of 5 ng/ml as "reasonable inference of impairment," whereas Idaho, Montana, and Washington consider 5 ng as per se impairment. Ohio and Nevada consider 2 ng/ml as per se impairment.

The 2017 Report to Congress on Marijuana Impaired Driving goes on (ad nauseam at times) on the differences between the effects of alcohol and marijuana on driving skills but also concludes correctly that that blood levels of THC and impairment are not correlated (Compton 2017). The rapid distribution of THC into lipid-rich body reservoirs, such as the brain and adipose tissue, is the reason. What remains evident is that the odds of culpability in a motor vehicle crash are two to three times greater for drivers with detectable blood THC (Drummer et al. 2004; Asbridge et al. 2012; Li et al. 2012; Huestis 2015).

Standard deviation of lateral position (SDLP) is often considered the reference outcome for assessment of impaired driving (Verster and Roth 2011; Verster and Roth 2014). Steering and tracking require integration of sensory information, judgment of the information, and appropriate motor response. Function magnetic resonance imaging (fMRI) can be used to determine activity in specific brain regions as changes in the blood oxygen level dependent (BOLD) response (Beckmann et al. 2005). BOLD measurements have been used to define resting-state connectivity between different brain regions.

A prominent or noticeable stimulus is considered to be salient and cognitive resources including attention are allocated to detecting salience. An unexpected stimulus with attentional salience will interrupt ongoing cognitive processes to focus attention on this salient event. For example, a deer running across the road in front of a vehicle will instantly become salient to the driver who then takes action to avoid hitting the deer. The salience network in the cerebral cortex includes the anterior cingulate cortex and the anterior insula as well as parts of the thalamus and striatum (Peters et al. 2016).

Klumpers et al. (2012) measured resting-state BOLD responses in 12 volunteers following three consecutive inhalation doses of THC in amounts of 2, 6, and 6 mg at

1.5-hour intervals (Klumpers et al. 2012). The act of driving itself produces dynamic changes in the activation of six distinct groups of brain regions that include parts of the salience network (Calhoun et al. 2002). Considerable overlap exists between these groups and those demonstrated to be altered by THC during the resting state.

A single publication attempted to measure differences in brain activity with fMRI in a visuomotor tracking task, an activity specifically related to driving (Battistella et al. 2013). There was a decrease in the BOLD response in several of the primary cognitive networks involved in salience and executive function after smoking cannabis containing 11% THC. A concomitant increase in the BOLD response was observed in the ventromedial prefrontal cortex and anterior cingulate cortex, a part of the salience network. The author concluded that, when influenced by THC, the participants tended to focus on their self-oriented thoughts rather than the external task, resulting in poorer performance—in other words, misplaced salience.

This misplaced salience results in increased reaction time, inability to track, and decrements in decision making. These effects have been observed in a number of studies of the effect of cannabis on attention and tracking, necessary abilities for safe driving (Ronen et al. 2008; Bondallaz et al. 2016; Busardò et al. 2017; Desrosiers et al. 2015; Hartley et al. 2019; Hartman and Huestis 2013; Hartman et al. 2015; Hartman et al. 2016b; Micallef et al. 2018; Ménétrey et al. 2005; Newmeyer et al. 2017; Ramaekers et al. 2006b). Epidemiologic studies of motor vehicle accidents uniformly reveal an association between THC or metabolites in body fluids and crash risk or fatality (Ramaekers et al. 2004; Laumon et al. 2005; Khiabani et al. 2006; Gadegbeku et al. 2011; Asbridge et al. 2012; Elvik 2013; Li et al. 2012; Del Balzo et al. 2018; Gjerde and Mørland 2016; Hasin 2018; Martin et al. 2017; Rogeberg and Elvik 2016; Romano et al. 2017; Scherer et al. 2015).

Measurements of driving capability generally include skills related to attentional salience. These skills include the ability to track/steer and the ability to react quickly as a measure of attention or vigilance. Laboratory testing methods for these skills are the critical tracking test and the stop signal task. The corresponding measures in a driving simulator are SDLP and mean reciprocal reaction time. Dose-related decreases in performance have been observed repeatedly in these laboratory tests (Battistella et al. 2013; Desrosiers et al. 2015; Ramaekers et al. 2006b; Ramaekers et al. 2009; Ramaekers et al. 2006a; Schwope et al. 2012). In one study, these deficits occurred concurrently with changes in event-related potentials and other electrical activity in the brain (Böcker et al. 2010). Observations in driving simulators and actual driving situations demonstrate similar effects of THC on attention and motor control (Bondallaz et al. 2016; Busardò et al. 2017; Hartley et al. 2019; Hartman et al. 2016b; Ménétrey et al. 2005; Micallef et al., 2018; Bosker et al. 2012; Downey et al. 2013; Hartman et al. 2016a; Veldstra et al. 2015).

The cannabis influence factor was proposed as a measure of driving impairment from cannabis use and calculated as the molar ratio between the sum of THC and THCOH in plasma and THCCOOH in plasma. The large roadside case/control studies that led to the development of blood alcohol concentrations (BAC) corresponding to legal impairment showed a clear relationship between increasing BAC and the odds ratio of crash risk (Blomberg et al. 2005; Blomberg et al. 2009; Borkenstein

1964; Hurst et al. 1994). A similar effort with cannabis would likely fail because no easily measured biomarker yet exists. Work to develop a THC breathalyzer is still developing and not yet ready for deployment as a forensic tool (Mirzaei et al. 2020).

Tracking performance in both driving simulators and actual driving tests was poorer in volunteers after smoking cannabis containing 20 mg THC (Micallef et al., 2018). In volunteers smoking cannabis to achieve a dose of 300 μg per kg body-weight, driving simulator performance was poorer immediately after cannabis consumption and no performance decrement was observed three hours after smoking. In a medical examination similar to the standardized field sobriety test (SFST) and in the driving simulator, poorer performance was observed at THC serum concentrations greater than 15 ng/ml and CIF values greater than 30 (Tank et al. 2019).

In summary, the effect of THC and THCOH binding to CB1 in brain regions associated with attentional salience has demonstrable effects on performance measures associated with driving.

10.5.2 ASSOCIATION OF THC AND HEART ATTACKS

CB1 receptors are found in the myocardium and coronary endothelial cells and on presynaptic terminals of sympathetic neurons and in postsynaptic membranes on blood vessels. Activation of the CB1 receptors produces modulate coronary vasodilation and reduced myocardial contractility (Weis et al. 2010). CB2 receptors are also found in the myocardium and endothelial cells; their role in heart pathologies is less clear. Immune modulation by CB may act in both protective and deleterious effects on heart function. Activation of the transient receptor potential vanilloid 1 channel (TRPV1) may produce a pro-inflammatory state, and the receptor may also be involved in vasorelaxation. PPARs may be involved in maintaining contractility and blood pressure regulations. Also, PPARγ interferes with the activation of transcription factor NF-κB and thus may reduce inflammation (Sierra et al. 2018).

Since the 1970s, many case reports have appeared in the scientific literature of the adverse and sometimes fatal cardiac effects of cannabis (Charles et al. 1979; Lindsay et al. 2005; MacInnes and Miller 1984). Table 2 in Drummer et al. (2019) provides a summary of 13 deaths with evidence of cannabis use within hours with pathological changes in the heart present in all (Drummer, 2019).

Mittleman and co-workers provide the most relevant examination of the association between very recent cannabis use and heart attack. This study was part of the Determinants of Myocardial Infarction Onset Study (MIOS) conducted on a population of 2624 men and 1258 women aged 20–92 who entered treatment after suffering a myocardial infarction (MI). The study was designed as a case-crossover study in which each individual patient serves as his/her own control by examining a hypothesized event trigger, i.e., cannabis use leading to MI, occurring during different time periods prior to the event (Maclure, 2000).

This study revealed that compared with non-users, the risk of MI onset within one hour of cannabis use increased 4.8-fold (95% confidence interval [CI], 2.9–9.5, $P < 0.001$). From one to two hours after use, the risk was 1.7-fold greater than at other times (95% CI, 0.6–5.1, P=0.34) (Mittleman et al. 2001).

Also, as part of the Myocardial Infarct Onset Study (MIOS), a prospective cohort study of 1913 adults who had suffered an MI were followed for a median duration of 3.8 years, weekly cannabis use resulted in a hazard ratio of 4.2 (95% CI, 1.2–14.3) and less than weekly use resulted in a hazard ratio of 1.9 (95% CI, 0.6–6.3). The authors note that cannabis "may pose a particular risk for susceptible individuals with coronary heart disease" (Mukamal et al. 2008).

Drummer et al. reviewed case reports of deaths in 13 individual cannabis users. In all 13, evidence of ongoing cardiac damage was present. In addition, 31 case reports of non-fatal medical presentations of cardiovascular dysfunction following cannabis use also documented ongoing heart damage (Drummer et al. 2019).

Two messages are evident from these studies:

- The risk of heart attack increases significantly immediately after cannabis use
- In individuals who have already suffered a heart attack, cannabis use increases the risk of a second heart attack

In summary, the cardiovascular effects of THC result from activation of the sympathetic nervous system and inhibition of the parasympathetic nervous system. These effects include an immediate increase in heart rate lasting for an hour or longer. This increase is accompanied by increased cardiac output, cardiac work, and oxygen demand (Franz and Frishman 2016; Goyal et al. 2017; Singh et al. 2018). The increased heart rate is known clinically as ventricular tachycardia and is associated with reduced flow through the coronary arteries that supply blood to the heart muscle (Rezkalla et al. 2016; Khouzam et al. 2013).

10.5.3 Anxiolytic Effects of CBD

CBD does not appear to bind to either CB1 or CB2 and has antagonist effects *in vitro* (McPartland et al. 2007; Morales et al. 2017). CBD may act as a negative allosteric modulator of THC and 2-AG; CBD does not, however, mobilize Ca2+ or recruit β-arrestin (Morales et al. 2017), instead of acting as an antagonist at both CB1 and CB2 (Izzo et al. 2009).

The anxiolytic effects of CBD are likely due to its interactions with serotonin receptors. In rat studies, CBD appears to act as a full agonist at the 5HT1A receptor. CBD also has effects on opioid receptors, glycine receptors, and PPARγ (Izzo et al. 2009; Bian et al. 2019; Bih et al. 2015; Morales and Reggio 2017; Oberbarnscheidt and Miller 2020; Premoli et al. 2019).

In a clinical trial of patients with social anxiety disorder, a 600 mg dose of CBD reduced anxiety in a simulated public speaking test compared with a placebo dose. This conclusion was based on both subjective ratings and physiological measures including blood pressure, heart rate, and skin conductance (Bergamaschi et al. 2011).

In another clinical trial of ten individuals with SAD, a 400 mg dose of CBD increased blood flow in the posterior cingulate gyrus and reduced flow in the parahippocampal gyrus compared with a placebo dose measured with single-photon emission computed tomography (SPECT) and MRI imaging. In addition, subjective measures of anxiety were significantly reduced (Crippa et al. 2011).

Currently, an ongoing clinical trial seeks to observe the effects of flexibly dosed CBD in adults over an eight-week period on generalized anxiety disorder, social anxiety disorder, panic disorder, and agoraphobia compared with a placebo. The participants will be assessed during treatment with blood testing, computer testing for focus, attention, and memory as well as self-reported details on mood, anxiety, sleep, alcohol, and/or drug use (ClinicalTrials.gov 2018).

10.6   CONCLUSIONS

At this time in history, both the potential and perils of cannabis use are being discovered. The prevailing view in the 20th century was that cannabis was an evil substance to be avoided. This unfortunate attitude very likely stifled research that could have hastened a greater understanding of the risks and benefits of this plant used by humans since antiquity. Continuing legalization for medical and recreational use in states has likely spurred the increased research interest observed in the 20th century.

This review is necessarily incomplete because of the increasing research interest. Perhaps the overall message is that the state of play is changing quickly. The hope for this review is to provide a brief but informative overview of the extant knowledge of cannabis pharmacokinetics and pharmacodynamics in the early 21st century.

REFERENCES

Alsherbiny MA, Li CG. 2019. Medicinal cannabis—potential drug interactions. *Medicines* 6:3.

Anderson GD, Chan L-N. 2016. Pharmacokinetic drug interactions with tobacco, cannabinoids and smoking cessation products. *Clinical Pharmacokinetics* 55:1353–1368.

Andersson M, Scheidweiler KB, Sempio C, Barnes AJ, Huestis MA. 2016. Simultaneous quantification of 11 cannabinoids and metabolites in human urine by liquid chromatography tandem mass spectrometry using WAX-S tips. *Analytical and Bioanalytical Chemistry* 408:6461–6471.

Asbridge M, Hayden JA, Cartwright JL. 2012. Acute cannabis consumption and motor vehicle collision risk: systematic review of observational studies and meta-analysis. *BMJ* 344:e536.

Asbridge M, Poulin C, Donato A. 2005. Motor vehicle collision risk and driving under the influence of cannabis: evidence from adolescents in Atlantic Canada. *Accident Analysis & Prevention* 37:1025–1034.

Awasthi R, An G, Donovan MD, Boles Ponto, LL. 2017. Relating observed psychoactive effects to the plasma concentrations of delta-9-tetrahydrocannabinol (THC) and its active metabolite: an effect-compartment modeling approach. *J Pharm Sci* https://doi.org/10.1016/j.xphs.2017.09.009

Awasthi R, An G, Donovan MD, Ponto LLB. 2018. Relating observed psychoactive effects to the plasma concentrations of delta-9-tetrahydrocannabinol and its active metabolite: an effect-compartment modeling approach. *Journal of Pharmaceutical Sciences* 107:745–755.

Aylward LL, Hays SM, Zidek A. 2017. Variation in urinary spot sample, 24 h samples, and longer-term average urinary concentrations of short-lived environmental chemicals:

implications for exposure assessment and reverse dosimetry. *Journal of Exposure Science & Environmental Epidemiology* 27:582–590.

Barter ZE, Bayliss MK, Beaune PH, Boobis AR, Carlile DJ, Edwards RJ, Brian Houston J, Lake BG, Lipscomb JC, Pelkonen OR. 2007. Scaling factors for the extrapolation of in vivo metabolic drug clearance from in vitro data: reaching a consensus on values of human micro-somal protein and hepatocellularity per gram of liver. *Current Drug Metabolism* 8:33–45.

Battistella G, Fornari E, Thomas A, Mall J-F, Chtioui H, Appenzeller M, Annoni J-M, Favrat B, Maeder P, Giroud C. 2013. Weed or wheel! FMRI, behavioural, and toxicological investigations of how cannabis smoking affects skills necessary for driving. *PloS One* 8:e52545.

Beckmann CF, DeLuca M, Devlin JT, Smith SM. 2005. Investigations into resting-state connectivity using independent component analysis. *Philosophical Transactions of the Royal Society B: Biological Sciences* 360:1001–1013.

Bergamaschi MM, Karschner EL, Goodwin RS, Scheidweiler KB, Hirvonen J, Queiroz RH, Huestis MA. 2013. Impact of prolonged cannabinoid excretion in chronic daily cannabis smokers' blood on per se drugged driving laws. *Clinical Chemistry* 59:519–526.

Bergamaschi MM, Queiroz RHC, Chagas MHN, De Oliveira DCG, De Martinis BS, Kapczinski F, Quevedo J, Roesler R, Schröder N, Nardi AE. 2011. Cannabidiol reduces the anxiety induced by simulated public speaking in treatment-naive social phobia patients. *Neuropsychopharmacology* 36:1219–1226.

Bian Y-m, He X-b, Jing Y-k, Wang L-r, Wang J-m, Xie X-Q. 2019. Computational systems pharmacology analysis of cannabidiol: a combination of chemogenomics-knowledgebase network analysis and integrated in silico modeling and simulation. *Acta Pharmacologica Sinica* 40:374–386.

Bih CI, Chen T, Nunn AV, Bazelot M, Dallas M, Whalley BJ. 2015. Molecular targets of cannabidiol in neurological disorders. *Neurotherapeutics* 12:699–730.

Bland TM, Haining RL, Tracy TS, Callery PS. 2005. CYP2C-catalyzed delta (9)-tetrahydrocannabinol metabolism: kinetics, pharmacogenetics and interaction with phenytoin. *Biochemical Pharmacology* 70:1096–1103.

Bleeker C, Vree T, Lagerwerf A, Willems-van Bree E. 2008. Recovery and long-term renal excretion of propofol, its glucuronide, and two di-isopropylquinol glucuronides after propofol infusion during surgery. *British Journal of Anaesthesia* 101:207–212.

Blomberg RD, Peck RC, Moskowitz H, Burns M, Fiorentino D. 2005. *Crash risk of alcohol involved driving: a case-control study*. Dunlap & Associates, Inc. Funded by contract DTNH22-94-C-05001 from USDOT and NHTSA; https://trid.trb.org/view/804190

Blomberg RD, Peck RC, Moskowitz H, Burns M, Fiorentino D. 2009. The Long Beach/Fort Lauderdale relative risk study. *Journal of Safety Research* 40:285–292.

Böcker K, Gerritsen J, Hunault C, Kruidenier M, Mensinga TT, Kenemans J. 2010. Cannabis with high Δ^9-THC contents affects perception and visual selective attention acutely: an event-related potential study. *Pharmacology Biochemistry and Behavior* 96:67–74.

Böhnke E, Dietz L, Heinrich T, Aderjan R, Skopp G, Mikus G. 2013. Disposition and enterohepatic circulation of intravenously administered 11-nor-9-carboxy-Δ^9-tetrahydrocannabinol in serum and urine in healthy human subjects. *Journal of Forensic Toxicology & Pharmacology.* 2(2):1–6. doi:10:417212325-417219841.411000107.

Bondallaz P, Favrat B, Chtioui H, Fornari E, Maeder P, Giroud C. 2016. Cannabis and its effects on driving skills. *Forensic Science International* 268:92–102.

Borkenstein RF. 1964. The role of the drinking driver in traffic accidents. Indiana Univ., Department of Police Administration Bloomington, IN.

Bornheim LM, Lasker JM, Raucy JL. 1992. Human hepatic microsomal metabolism of delta 1-tetrahydrocannabinol. *Drug Metabolism and Disposition* 20:241–246.

Bosker WM, Kuypers KP, Theunissen EL, Surinx A, Blankespoor RJ, Skopp G, Jeffery WK, Walls HC, van Leeuwen CJ, Ramaekers JG. 2012. Medicinal Δ^9-tetrahydrocannabinol (dronabinol) impairs on-the-road driving performance of occasional and heavy cannabis users but is not detected in Standard Field Sobriety Tests. *Addiction* 107:1837–1844.

Brown JD, Winterstein AG. 2019. Potential adverse drug events and drug–drug interactions with medical and consumer cannabidiol (CBD) use. *Journal of Clinical Medicine* 8:989.

Burstein SH. 2019. Eicosanoid mediation of cannabinoid actions. *Bioorganic & Medicinal Chemistry* 27:2718–2728.

Busardò FP, Pellegrini M, Klein J, di Luca NM. 2017. Neurocognitive correlates in driving under the influence of cannabis. *CNS & Neurological Disorders-Drug Targets (Formerly Current Drug Targets-CNS & Neurological Disorders)* 16:534–540.

Calhoun VD, Pekar JJ, McGinty VB, Adali T, Watson TD, Pearlson GD. 2002. Different activation dynamics in multiple neural systems during simulated driving. *Human Brain Mapping* 16:158–167.

Chan R, De Bruyn T, Wright M, Broccatelli F. 2018. Comparing mechanistic and preclinical predictions of volume of distribution on a large set of drugs. *Pharmaceutical Research* 35:1–11.

Charles R, Holt S, Kirkham N. 1979. Myocardial infarction and marijuana. *Clinical Toxicology* 14:433–438.

Citti C, Pacchetti B, Vandelli MA, Forni F, Cannazza G. 2018. Analysis of cannabinoids in commercial hemp seed oil and decarboxylation kinetics studies of cannabidiolic acid (CBDA). *Journal of Pharmaceutical and Biomedical Analysis* 149:532–540.

Compton RP. 2017. Marijuana-impaired driving-a report to congress. United States. National Highway Traffic Safety Administration. Report no. DOT HS 812 XXX, June 2017. At https://www.nhtsa.gov/sites/nhtsa.dot.gov/files/documents/812440-marijuana-impaired-driving-report-to-congress.pdf

Crippa JAS, Derenusson GN, Ferrari TB, Wichert-Ana L, Duran FL, Martin-Santos R, Simões MV, Bhattacharyya S, Fusar-Poli P, Atakan Z. 2011. Neural basis of anxiolytic effects of cannabidiol (CBD) in generalized social anxiety disorder: a preliminary report. *Journal of Psychopharmacology* 25:121–130.

Cristino L, Bisogno T, Di Marzo V. 2020. Cannabinoids and the expanded endocannabinoid system in neurological disorders. *Nature Reviews Neurology* 16:9–29.

Del Balzo G, Gottardo R, Mengozzi S, Dorizzi RM, Bortolotti F, Appolonova S, Tagliaro F. 2018. "Positive" urine testing for cannabis is associated with increased risk of traffic crashes. *Journal of Pharmaceutical and Biomedical Analysis* 151:71–74.

del Caño GG, Montaña M, Aretxabala X, González-Burguera I, de Jesús ML, Barrondo S, Sallés J. 2014. Nuclear phospholipase C-β1 and diacylglycerol LIPASE-α in brain cortical neurons. *Advances in Biological Regulation* 54:12–23.

Demuth DG, Molleman A. 2006. Cannabinoid signalling. *Life Sciences* 78:549–563.

Desrosiers NA, Himes SK, Scheidweiler KB, Concheiro-Guisan M, Gorelick DA, Huestis MA. 2014a. Phase I and II cannabinoid disposition in blood and plasma of occasional and frequent smokers following controlled smoked cannabis. *Clinical Chemistry* 60:631–643.

Desrosiers NA, Lee D, Concheiro-Guisan M, Scheidweiler KB, Gorelick DA, Huestis MA. 2014b. Urinary cannabinoid disposition in occasional and frequent smokers: is THC-glucuronide in sequential urine samples a marker of recent use in frequent smokers? *Clinical Chemistry* 60:361–372.

Desrosiers NA, Ramaekers JG, Chauchard E, Gorelick DA, Huestis MA. 2015. Smoked cannabis' psychomotor and neurocognitive effects in occasional and frequent smokers. *Journal of Analytical Toxicology* 39:251–261.

Devinsky O, Cilio MR, Cross H, Fernandez-Ruiz J, French J, Hill C, Katz R, Di Marzo V, Jutras-Aswad D, Notcutt WG. 2014. Cannabidiol: pharmacology and potential therapeutic role in epilepsy and other neuropsychiatric disorders. *Epilepsia* 55:791–802.

Dietz L, Glaz-Sandberg A, Nguyen H, Skopp G, Mikus G, Aderjan R. 2007. The urinary disposition of intravenously administered 11-nor-9-carboxy-delta-9-tetrahydrocannabinol in humans. *Therapeutic Drug Monitoring* 29:368–372.

Downey LA, King R, Papafotiou K, Swann P, Ogden E, Boorman M, Stough C. 2013. The effects of cannabis and alcohol on simulated driving: influences of dose and experience. *Accident Analysis & Prevention* 50:879–886.

Drummer OH, Gerostamoulos D, Woodford NW. 2019. Cannabis as a cause of death: a review. *Forensic Science International* 298:298–306.

Drummer OH, Gerostamoulos J, Batziris H, Chu M, Caplehorn J, Robertson MD, Swann P. 2004. The involvement of drugs in drivers of motor vehicles killed in Australian road traffic crashes. *Accident Analysis & Prevention* 36:239–248.

Dussy FE, Hamberg C, Luginbühl M, Schwerzmann T, Briellmann TA. 2005. Isolation of Δ^9-THCA-A from hemp and analytical aspects concerning the determination of Δ^9-THC in cannabis products. *Forensic Science International* 149:3–10.

Elvik R. 2013. Risk of road accident associated with the use of drugs: a systematic review and meta-analysis of evidence from epidemiological studies. *Accident Analysis & Prevention* 60:254–267.

Elzinga S, Ortiz O, Raber JC. 2015. The conversion and transfer of cannabinoids from cannabis to smoke stream in cigarettes. *Natural Products Chemistry & Research* 3(1):1–5.

Fabritius M, Chtioui H, Battistella G, Annoni J-M, Dao K, Favrat B, Fornari E, Lauer E, Maeder P, Giroud C. 2013. Comparison of cannabinoid concentrations in oral fluid and whole blood between occasional and regular cannabis smokers prior to and after smoking a cannabis joint. *Analytical and Bioanalytical Chemistry* 405:9791–9803.

Fanali G, Cao Y, Ascenzi P, Trezza V, Rubino T, Parolaro D, Fasano M. 2011. Binding of Δ^9-tetrahydrocannabinol and diazepam to human serum albumin. *IUBMB Life* 63:446–451.

Franz CA, Frishman WH. 2016. Marijuana use and cardiovascular disease. *Cardiology in Review* 24:158–162.

Gadegbeku B, Amoros E, Laumon B. 2011. Responsibility study: main illicit psychoactive substances among car drivers involved in fatal road crashes. Pages 293. Annals of Advances in Automotive Medicine/Annual Scientific Conference: Association for the Advancement of Automotive Medicine 55:293–300.

Gibson CR, Lu P, Maciolek C, Wudarski C, Barter Z, Rowland-Yeo K, Stroh M, Lai E, Nicoll-Griffith DA. 2013. Using human recombinant UDP-glucuronosyltransferase isoforms and a relative activity factor approach to model total body clearance of laropiprant (MK-0524) in humans. *Xenobiotica* 43:1027–1036.

Gill KL, Houston JB, Galetin A. 2012. Characterization of in vitro glucuronidation clearance of a range of drugs in human kidney microsomes: comparison with liver and intestinal glucuronidation and impact of albumin. *Drug Metabolism and Disposition* 40:825–835.

Gjerde H, Mørland J. 2016. Risk for involvement in road traffic crash during acute cannabis intoxication. *Addiction* 111:1492–1495.

Glaz-Sandberg A, Dietz L, Nguyen H, Oberwittler H, Aderjan R, Mikus G. 2007. Pharmacokinetics of 11-nor-9-carboxy-Δ^9-tetrahydrocannabinol (CTHC) after intravenous administration of CTHC in healthy human subjects. *Clinical Pharmacology & Therapeutics* 82:63–69.

Goyal H, Awad HH, Ghali JK. 2017. Role of cannabis in cardiovascular disorders. *Journal of Thoracic Disease* 9:2079.

Gronewold A, Skopp G. 2011. A preliminary investigation on the distribution of cannabinoids in man. *Forensic Science International* 210:e7–e11.

Grotenhermen F. 2003. Pharmacokinetics and pharmacodynamics of cannabinoids. *Clinical Pharmacokinetics* 42:327–360.

Grotenhermen F, Leson G, Berghaus G, Drummer OH, Kruger HP, Longo M, Moskowitz H, Perrine B, Ramaekers JG, Smiley A, Tunbridge R. 2007. Developing limits for driving under cannabis. *Addiction* 102(12):1910–1917. https://doi.org/10.1111/j.1360-0443.2007.02009.x

Hartley S, Simon N, Larabi A, Vaugier I, Barbot F, Quera-Salva M-A, Alvarez JC. 2019. Effect of smoked cannabis on vigilance and accident risk using simulated driving in occasional and chronic users and the pharmacokinetic–pharmacodynamic relationship. *Clinical Chemistry* 65:684–693.

Hartman RL, Brown TL, Milavetz G, Spurgin A, Gorelick DA, Gaffney G, Huestis MA. 2016a. Controlled vaporized cannabis, with and without alcohol: subjective effects and oral fluid-blood cannabinoid relationships. *Drug Testing and Analysis* 8:690–701.

Hartman RL, Brown TL, Milavetz G, Spurgin A, Pierce RS, Gorelick DA, Gaffney G, Huestis MA. 2015. Cannabis effects on driving lateral control with and without alcohol. *Drug and Alcohol Dependence* 154:25–37.

———. 2016b. Cannabis effects on driving longitudinal control with and without alcohol. *Journal of Applied Toxicology* 36:1418–1429.

Hartman RL, Huestis MA. 2013. Cannabis effects on driving skills. *Clinical Chemistry* 59:478–492.

Harvey D, Mechoulam R. 1990. Metabolites of cannabidiol identified in human urine. *Xenobiotica* 20:303–320.

Hasin DS. 2018. US epidemiology of cannabis use and associated problems. *Neuropsychopharmacology* 43:195–212.

Hays SM, Aylward LL, Blount BC. 2015. Variation in urinary flow rates according to demographic characteristics and body mass index in NHANES: potential confounding of associations between health outcomes and urinary biomarker concentrations. *Environmental Health Perspectives* 123:293–300.

Heuberger JA, Guan Z, Oyetayo O-O, Klumpers L, Morrison PD, Beumer TL, van Gerven JM, Cohen AF, Freijer J. 2015. Population pharmacokinetic model of THC integrates oral, intravenous, and pulmonary dosing and characterizes short-and long-term pharmacokinetics. *Clinical Pharmacokinetics* 54:209–219.

Hollister L, Gillespie H, Ohlsson A, Lindgren JE, Wahlen A, Agurell S. 1981. Do plasma concentrations of Δ^9-tetrahydrocannabinol reflect the degree of intoxication? *The Journal of Clinical Pharmacology* 21:171S–177S.

Hu DG, Nair PC, Haines AZ, McKinnon RA, Mackenzie PI, Meech R. 2019. The UGTome: the expanding diversity of UDP glycosyltransferases and its impact on small molecule metabolism. *Pharmacology & Therapeutics* 204:107414.

Huestis MA. 2015. Deterring driving under the influence of cannabis. *Addiction* 110:1697–1698.

Huestis MA, Henningfield JE, Cone EJ. 1992a. Blood cannabinoids. I. Absorption of THC and formation of 11-OH-THC and THCCOOH during and after smoking marijuana. *Journal of Analytical Toxicology* 16:276–282.

Huestis MA, Sampson AH, Holicky BJ, Henningfield JE, Cone EJ. 1992b. Characterization of the absorption phase of marijuana smoking. *Clinical Pharmacology & Therapeutics* 52:31–41.

Hunault CC, Mensinga TT, de Vries I, Kelholt-Dijkman HH, Hoek J, Kruidenier M, Leenders ME, Meulenbelt J. 2008. Delta-9-tetrahydrocannabinol (THC) serum concentrations and pharmacological effects in males after smoking a combination of tobacco and cannabis containing up to 69 mg THC. *Psychopharmacology* 201:171–181.

Hurst PM, Harte D, Frith WJ. 1994. The grand rapids dip revisited. *Accident Analysis & Prevention* 26:647–654.

Hwang E-K, Lupica CR. 2020. Altered corticolimbic control of the nucleus accumbens by long-term Δ⁹-tetrahydrocannabinol exposure. *Biological Psychiatry* 87:619–631.

Izzo AA, Borrelli F, Capasso R, Di Marzo V, Mechoulam R. 2009. Non-psychotropic plant cannabinoids: new therapeutic opportunities from an ancient herb. *Trends in Pharmacological Sciences* 30:515–527.

Jiang R, Yamaori S, Takeda S, Yamamoto I, Watanabe K. 2011. Identification of cytochrome P450 enzymes responsible for metabolism of cannabidiol by human liver microsomes. *Life Sciences* 89:165–170.

Jones AW, Holmgren A, Kugelberg FC. 2008. Driving under the influence of cannabis: a 10-year study of age and gender differences in the concentrations of tetrahydrocannabinol in blood. *Addiction* 103:452–461.

Joshi N, Onaivi ES. 2019. Endocannabinoid system components: overview and tissue distribution. In: Bukiya A (eds) *Recent Advances in Cannabinoid Physiology and Pathology: Advances in Experimental Medicine and Biology* vol 1162. Springer, Cham https:.doi .org/10.1007/978-3-030-21737-2_1

Kano M. 2014. Control of synaptic function by endocannabinoid-mediated retrograde signaling. *Proceedings of the Japan Academy, Series B* 90:235–250.

Kasteel E, Darney K, Kramer N, Dorne J, Lautz L. 2020. Human variability in isoform-specific UDP-glucuronosyltransferases: markers of acute and chronic exposure, polymorphisms and uncertainty factors. *Archives of Toxicology* 94:2637–2661.

Kelly P, Jones RT. 1992. Metabolism of tetrahydrocannabinol in frequent and infrequent marijuana users. *Journal of Analytical Toxicology* 16:228–235.

Khiabani HZ, Bramness JRG, Bjørneboe A, Mørland JR. 2006. Relationship between THC concentration in blood and impairment in apprehended drivers. *Traffic Injury Prevention* 7:111–116.

Khouzam RN, Kabra R, Soufi MK. 2013. Marijuana, bigeminal premature ventricular contractions and sluggish coronary flow: are they related? *Journal of Cardiology Cases* 8:121–124.

Klausner H, Wilcox H, Dingell J. 1975. The use of zonal ultracentrifugation in the investigation of the binding of Δ⁹-tetrahydrocannabinol by plasma lipoproteins. *Drug Metabolism and Disposition* 3:314–319.

Klumpers LE, Cole DM, Khalili-Mahani N, Soeter RP, Te Beek ET, Rombouts SA, van Gerven JM. 2012. Manipulating brain connectivity with Δ⁹-tetrahydrocannabinol: a pharmacological resting state FMRI study. *Neuroimage* 63:1701–1711.

Knights KM, Miners JO. 2010. Renal UDP-glucuronosyltransferases and the glucuronidation of xenobiotics and endogenous mediators. *Drug Metabolism Reviews* 42:63–73.

Knights KM, Spencer SM, Fallon JK, Chau N, Smith PC, Miners JO. 2016. Scaling factors for the in vitro–in vivo extrapolation (IV–IVE) of renal drug and xenobiotic glucuronidation clearance. *British Journal of Clinical Pharmacology* 81:1153–1164.

Korzekwa K, Nagar S. 2017. Drug distribution part 2. Predicting volume of distribution from plasma protein binding and membrane partitioning. *Pharmaceutical Research* 34:544–551.

Laumon B, Gadegbeku B, Martin J-L, Biecheler M-B. 2005. Cannabis intoxication and fatal road crashes in France: population based case-control study. *BMJ* 331:1371.

Law B, Mason P, Moffat A, Gleadle R, King L. 1984. Forensic aspects of the metabolism and excretion of cannabinoids following oral ingestion of cannabis resin. *Journal of Pharmacy and Pharmacology* 36:289–294.

Li M-C, Brady JE, DiMaggio CJ, Lusardi AR, Tzong KY, Li G. 2012. Marijuana use and motor vehicle crashes. *Epidemiologic Reviews* 34:65–72.

Lim SY, Sharan S, Woo S. 2020. Model-based analysis of cannabidiol dose-exposure relationship and bioavailability. *Pharmacotherapy: The Journal of Human Pharmacology and Drug Therapy* 40:291–300.

Lindsay AC, Foale RA, Warren O, Henry JA. 2005. Cannabis as a precipitant of cardiovascular emergencies. *International Journal of Cardiology* 104:230–232.

Lipscomb JC, Kedderis GL. 2002. Incorporating human interindividual biotransformation variance in health risk assessment. *Science of the Total Environment* 288:13–21.

Lipscomb JC, Teuschler LK, Swartout JC, Striley CA, Snawder JE. 2003. Variance of microsomal protein and cytochrome P450 2E1 and 3A forms in adult human liver. *Toxicology Mechanisms and Methods* 13:45–51.

Liu Z, Galettis P, Broyd SJ, van Hell H, Greenwood LM, de Krey P, Steigler A, Zhu X, Schneider J, Solowij N. 2020. Model-based analysis on systemic availability of co-administered cannabinoids after controlled vaporised administration. *Internal Medicine Journal* 50:846–853.

Lowe RH, Abraham TT, Darwin WD, Herning R, Cadet JL, Huestis MA. 2009. Extended urinary Δ^9-tetrahydrocannabinol excretion in chronic cannabis users precludes use as a biomarker of new drug exposure. *Drug and Alcohol Dependence* 105:24–32.

Lozovaya N, Min R, Tsintsadze V, Burnashev N. 2009. Dual modulation of CNS voltage-gated calcium channels by cannabinoids: focus on CB1 receptor-independent effects. *Cell Calcium* 46:154–162.

Lu H-C, Mackie K. 2016. An introduction to the endogenous cannabinoid system. *Biological Psychiatry* 79:516–525.

Lucas CJ, Galettis P, Schneider J. 2018. The pharmacokinetics and the pharmacodynamics of cannabinoids. *British Journal of Clinical Pharmacology* 84:2477–2482.

Lupica CR, Hu Y, Devinsky O, Hoffman AF. 2017. Cannabinoids as hippocampal network administrators. *Neuropharmacology* 124:25–37.

MacCallum CA, Russo EB. 2018. Practical considerations in medical cannabis administration and dosing. *European Journal of Internal Medicine* 49:12–19.

MacInnes D, Miller K. 1984. Fatal coronary artery thrombosis associated with cannabis smoking. *The Journal of the Royal College of General Practitioners* 34:575.

Mandema JW, Verotta D, Sheiner LB. 1992. Building population pharmacokineticpharmacodynamic models. I. Models for covariate effects. *Journal of Pharmacokinetics and Biopharmaceutics* 20:511–528.

Margaillan G, Rouleau M, Fallon JK, Caron P, Villeneuve L, Turcotte V, Smith PC, Joy MS, Guillemette C. 2015. Quantitative profiling of human renal UDP-glucuronosyltransferases and glucuronidation activity: a comparison of normal and tumoral kidney tissues. *Drug Metabolism and Disposition* 43:611–619.

Marsot A, Audebert C, Attolini L, Lacarelle B, Micallef J, Blin O. 2017. Population pharmacokinetics model of THC used by pulmonary route in occasional cannabis smokers. *Journal of Pharmacological and Toxicological Methods* 85:49–54.

Martin J-L, Gadegbeku B, Wu D, Viallon V, Laumon B. 2017. Cannabis, alcohol and fatal road accidents. *PloS One* 12:e0187320.

Mazur A, Lichti CF, Prather PL, Zielinska AK, Bratton SM, Gallus-Zawada A, Finel M, Miller GP, Radomińska-Pandya A, Moran JH. 2009. Characterization of human hepatic and extrahepatic UDP-glucuronosyltransferase enzymes involved in the metabolism of classic cannabinoids. *Drug Metabolism and Disposition* 37:1496–1504.

Maclure M, Mittleman MA. 2000. Should we use a case-crossover design. *Annu Rev Public Health* 21:193–221. https://doi.org/10.1146/annurev.publhealth.21.1.193

McPartland J, Glass M, Pertwee R. 2007. Meta-analysis of cannabinoid ligand binding affinity and receptor distribution: interspecies differences. *British Journal of Pharmacology* 152:583–593.

McPartland JM, Matias I, Di Marzo V, Glass M. 2006. Evolutionary origins of the endocannabinoid system. *Gene* 370:64–74.

Meech R, Hu DG, McKinnon RA, Mubarokah SN, Haines AZ, Nair PC, Rowland A, Mackenzie PI. 2019. The UDP-glycosyltransferase (UGT) superfamily: new members, new functions, and novel paradigms. *Physiological Reviews* 99:1153–1222.

Ménétrey A, Augsburger M, Favrat B, Pin MA, Rothuizen LE, Appenzeller M, Buclin T, Mangin P, Giroud C. 2005. Assessment of driving capability through the use of clinical and psychomotor tests in relation to blood cannabinoids levels following oral administration of 20 mg dronabinol or of a cannabis decoction made with 20 or 60 mg Δ^9-THC. *Journal of Analytical Toxicology* 29:327–338.

Methaneethorn J, Naosang K, Kaewworasut P, Poomsaidorn C, Lohitnavy M. 2020a. Development of a physiologically-based pharmacokinetic model of Δ^9-tetrahydrocannabinol in mice, rats, and pigs. *European Journal of Drug Metabolism and Pharmacokinetics* 45:487–494.

Methaneethorn J, Poomsaidorn C, Naosang K, Kaewworasut P, Lohitnavy M. 2020b. A Δ^9-tetrahydrocannabinol physiologically-based pharmacokinetic model development in humans. *European Journal of Drug Metabolism and Pharmacokinetics* 45:495–511.

Micallef J, Dupouey J, Jouve E, Truillet R, Lacarelle B, Taillard J, Daurat A, Authié C, Blin O, Rascol O. 2018. Cannabis smoking impairs driving performance on the simulator and real driving: a randomized, double-blind, placebo-controlled, crossover trial. *Fundamental & Clinical Pharmacology* 32:558–570.

Middleton DR, Watts MJ, Lark RM, Milne CJ, Polya DA. 2016. Assessing urinary flow rate, creatinine, osmolality and other hydration adjustment methods for urinary biomonitoring using NHANES arsenic, iodine, lead and cadmium data. *Environmental Health* 15:1–13.

Mirzaei H, O'Brien A, Tasnim N, Ravishankara A, Tahmooressi H, Hoorfar M. 2020. Topical review on monitoring tetrahydrocannabinol in breath. *Journal of Breath Research* 14:034002.

Mittleman MA, Lewis RA, Maclure M, Sherwood JB, Muller JE. 2001. Triggering myocardial infarction by marijuana. *Circulation* 103:2805–2809.

Morales P, Hurst DP, Reggio PH. 2017. Molecular targets of the phytocannabinoids: a complex picture. *Prog Chem Nat Prod* 103:103–131. doi:10.1007/978-3-319-45541-9_4

Morales P, Reggio PH. 2017. An update on non-CB1, non-CB2 cannabinoid related G-protein-coupled receptors. *Cannabis and Cannabinoid Research* 2:265–273.

Mukamal KJ, Maclure M, Muller JE, Mittleman MA. 2008. An exploratory prospective study of marijuana use and mortality following acute myocardial infarction. *American Heart Journal* 155:465–470.

Naef M, Russmann S, Petersen-Felix S, Brenneisen R. 2004. Development and pharmacokinetic characterization of pulmonal and intravenous delta-9-tetrahydrocannabinol (THC) in humans. *Journal of Pharmaceutical Sciences* 93:1176–1184.

Newmeyer MN, Swortwood MJ, Barnes AJ, Abulseoud OA, Scheidweiler KB, Huestis MA. 2016. Free and glucuronide whole blood cannabinoids' pharmacokinetics after controlled smoked, vaporized, and oral cannabis administration in frequent and occasional cannabis users: identification of recent cannabis intake. *Clinical Chemistry* 62:1579–1592.

Newmeyer MN, Swortwood MJ, Taylor ME, Abulseoud OA, Woodward TH, Huestis MA. 2017. Evaluation of divided attention psychophysical task performance and effects on pupil sizes following smoked, vaporized and oral cannabis administration. *Journal of Applied Toxicology* 37:922–932.

O'Sullivan SE. 2016. An update on PPAR activation by cannabinoids. *British Journal of Pharmacology* 173:1899–1910.

Oberbarnscheidt T, Miller NS. 2020. The impact of cannabidiol on psychiatric and medical conditions. *Journal of Clinical Medicine Research* 12:393.

Odell MS, Frei MY, Gerostamoulos D, Chu M, Lubman DI. 2015. Residual cannabis levels in blood, urine and oral fluid following heavy cannabis use. *Forensic Science International* 249:173–180.

Ohlsson A, Lindgren J, Wahlen A, Agurell S, Hollister L, Gillespie H. 1981. Plasma levels of delta 9-tetrahydrocannabinol after intravenous, oral, and smoke administration. *NIDA Research Monograph* 34:250–256.

Ohlsson A, Lindgren JE, Wahlén A, Agurell S, Hollister LE, Gillespie HK. 1982. Single dose kinetics of deuterium labelled Δ^1-tetrahydrocannabinol in heavy and light cannabis users. *Biomedical Mass Spectrometry* 9:6–10.

Oshida K, Vasani N, Thomas RS, Applegate D, Rosen M, Abbott B, Lau C, Guo G, Aleksunes LM, Klaassen C. 2015. Identification of modulators of the nuclear receptor peroxisome proliferator-activated receptor α (PPARα) in a mouse liver gene expression compendium. *PloS One* 10:e0112655.

Patilea-Vrana GI, Anoshchenko O, Unadkat JD. 2019. Hepatic enzymes relevant to the disposition of (-)-Δ^9-tetrahydrocannabinol (THC) and its psychoactive metabolite, 11-OH-THC. *Drug Metab Dispos* 47(3):249–256. https://doi.org/10.1124/dmd.118.085548

Peters SK, Dunlop K, Downar J. 2016. Cortico-striatal-thalamic loop circuits of the salience network: a central pathway in psychiatric disease and treatment. *Frontiers in Systems Neuroscience* 10:104.

Pistis M, O'Sullivan SE. 2017. The role of nuclear hormone receptors in cannabinoid function. *Advances in Pharmacology* 80:291–328.

Poulin P, Burczynski FJ, Haddad S. 2016. The role of extracellular binding proteins in the cellular uptake of drugs: impact on quantitative in vitro-to-in vivo extrapolations of toxicity and efficacy in physiologically based pharmacokinetic-pharmacodynamic research. *Journal of Pharmaceutical Sciences* 105:497–508.

Poulin P, Haddad S. 2015. Albumin and uptake of drugs in cells: additional validation exercises of a recently published equation that quantifies the albumin-facilitated uptake mechanism (s) in physiologically based pharmacokinetic and pharmacodynamic modeling research. *Journal of Pharmaceutical Sciences* 104:4448–4458.

Premoli M, Aria F, Bonini SA, Maccarinelli G, Gianoncelli A, Della Pina S, Tambaro S, Memo M, Mastinu A. 2019. Cannabidiol: recent advances and new insights for neuropsychiatric disorders treatment. *Life Sciences* 224:120–127.

Ramaekers JG, Berghaus G, van Laar M, Drummer OH. 2004. Dose related risk of motor vehicle crashes after cannabis use. *Drug and Alcohol Dependence* 73:109–119.

Ramaekers JG, Kauert G, Theunissen E, Toennes SW, Moeller M. 2009. Neurocognitive performance during acute THC intoxication in heavy and occasional cannabis users. *Journal of Psychopharmacology* 23:266–277.

Ramaekers JG, Kauert G, van Ruitenbeek P, Theunissen EL, Schneider E, Moeller MR. 2006a. High-potency marijuana impairs executive function and inhibitory motor control. *Neuropsychopharmacology* 31:2296–2303.

Ramaekers JG, Moeller M, van Ruitenbeek P, Theunissen EL, Schneider E, Kauert G. 2006b. Cognition and motor control as a function of Δ^9-THC concentration in serum and oral fluid: limits of impairment. *Drug and Alcohol Dependence* 85:114–122.

Ramaekers JG, Robbe H, O'Hanlon J. 2000. Marijuana, alcohol and actual driving performance. *Human Psychopharmacology: Clinical and Experimental* 15:551–558.

Rezkalla S, Stankowski R, Kloner RA. 2016. *Cardiovascular effects of marijuana.* SAGE Publications, Los Angeles, CA.

Rogeberg O, Elvik R. 2016. The effects of cannabis intoxication on motor vehicle collision revisited and revised. *Addiction* 111:1348–1359.

Romano E, Torres-Saavedra P, Voas RB, Lacey JH. 2017. Marijuana and the risk of fatal car crashes: what can we learn from FARS and NRS data? *The Journal of Primary Prevention* 38:315–328.

Ronen A, Gershon P, Drobiner H, Rabinovich A, Bar-Hamburger R, Mechoulam R, Cassuto Y, Shinar D. 2008. Effects of THC on driving performance, physiological state and subjective feelings relative to alcohol. *Accident Analysis & Prevention* 40:926–934.

Sachse-Seeboth C, Pfeil J, Sehrt D, Meineke I, Tzvetkov M, Bruns E, Poser W, Vormfelde S, Brockmöller J. 2009. Interindividual variation in the pharmacokinetics of Δ^9-tetrahydrocannabinol as related to genetic polymorphisms in CYP2C9. *Clinical Pharmacology & Therapeutics* 85:273–276.

Scheidweiler KB, Desrosiers NA, Huestis MA. 2012. Simultaneous quantification of free and glucuronidated cannabinoids in human urine by liquid chromatography tandem mass spectrometry. *Clinica Chimica Acta* 413:1839–1847.

Scherer M, Harrell P, Romano E. 2015. Marijuana and other substance use among motor vehicle operators: a latent class analysis. *Journal of Studies on Alcohol and Drugs* 76:916–923.

Schurman LD, Lu D, Kendall DA, Howlett AC, Lichtman AH. 2020. Molecular mechanism and cannabinoid pharmacology. In Nader M, Hurd Y (eds) *Substance Use Disorders: Handbook of Experimental Pharmacology*. 258. Springer, Cham. https://doi.org/10 .1007/164_2019_298.

Schwilke EW, Karschner EL, Lowe RH, Gordon AM, Cadet JL, Herning RI, Huestis MA. 2009. Intra-and intersubject whole blood/plasma cannabinoid ratios determined by 2-dimensional, electron impact GC-MS with cryofocusing. *Clinical Chemistry* 55:1188–1195.

Schwope DM, Bosker WM, Ramaekers JG, Gorelick DA, Huestis MA. 2012. Psychomotor performance, subjective and physiological effects and whole blood Δ^9-tetrahydrocannabinol concentrations in heavy, chronic cannabis smokers following acute smoked cannabis. *Journal of Analytical Toxicology* 36:405–412.

Schwope DM, Karschner EL, Gorelick DA, Huestis MA. 2011. Identification of recent cannabis use: whole-blood and plasma free and glucuronidated cannabinoid pharmacokinetics following controlled smoked cannabis administration. *Clinical Chemistry* 57:1406–1414.

Sempio C, Huestis MA, Mikulich-Gilbertson SK, Klawitter J, Christians U, Henthorn TK. 2019. Population pharmacokinetic modeling of plasma Δ^9-tetrahydrocannabinol and an active and inactive metabolite following controlled smoked cannabis administration. *British Journal of Clinical Pharmacology* 86:611–619.

Sewell RA, Poling J, Sofuoglu M. 2009. The effect of cannabis compared with alcohol on driving. *American Journal on Addictions* 18:185–193.

Sierra S, Luquin N, Navarro-Otano J. 2018. The endocannabinoid system in cardiovascular function: novel insights and clinical implications. *Clinical Autonomic Research* 28:35–52.

Singh A, Saluja S, Kumar A, Agrawal S, Thind M, Nanda S, Shirani J. 2018. Cardiovascular complications of marijuana and related substances: a review. *Cardiology and Therapy* 7:45–59.

Skopp G, Pötsch L, Mauden M, Richter B. 2002. Partition coefficient, blood to plasma ratio, protein binding and short-term stability of 11-nor-Δ^9-carboxy tetrahydrocannabinol glucuronide. *Forensic Science International* 126:17–23.

Slivicki RA, Xu Z, Kulkarni PM, Pertwee RG, Mackie K, Thakur GA, Hohmann AG. 2018. Positive allosteric modulation of cannabinoid receptor type 1 suppresses pathological pain without producing tolerance or dependence. *Biological Psychiatry* 84:722–733.

Strougo A, Zuurman L, Roy C, Pinquier J, Van Gerven J, Cohen A, Schoemaker R. 2008. Modelling of the concentration—effect relationship of THC on central nervous system parameters and heart rate—insight into its mechanisms of action and a tool for clinical research and development of cannabinoids. *Journal of Psychopharmacology* 22:717–726.

Tank A, Tietz T, Daldrup T, Schwender H, Hellen F, Ritz-Timme S, Hartung B. 2019. On the impact of cannabis consumption on traffic safety: a driving simulator study with habitual cannabis consumers. *International Journal of Legal Medicine* 133:1411–1420.

Teixeira H, Proença P, Castanheira A, Santos S, López-Rivadulla M, Corte-Real F, Marques EP, Vieira DN. 2004. Cannabis and driving: the use of LC–MS to detect Δ^9-tetrahydrocannabinol (Δ^9-THC) in oral fluid samples. *Forensic Science International* 146 Supplement:S61–S63.

Tsuboi K, Uyama T, Okamoto Y, Ueda N. 2018. Endocannabinoids and related N-acylethanolamines: biological activities and metabolism. *Inflammation and Regeneration* 38:1–10.

Ujváry I, Hanuš L. 2016. Human metabolites of cannabidiol: a review on their formation, biological activity, and relevance in therapy. *Cannabis Cannabinoid Res* 1:90–101.

van der Stelt M, Di Marzo V. 2005. Anandamide as an intracellular messenger regulating ion channel activity. *Prostaglandins & Other Lipid Mediators* 77:111–122.

Vandrey R, Herrmann ES, Mitchell JM, Bigelow GE, Flegel R, LoDico C, Cone EJ. 2017. Pharmacokinetic profile of oral cannabis in humans: blood and oral fluid disposition and relation to pharmacodynamic outcomes. *Journal of Analytical Toxicology* 41:83–99.

Veldstra J, Bosker W, De Waard D, Ramaekers JG, Brookhuis K. 2015. Comparing treatment effects of oral THC on simulated and on-the-road driving performance: testing the validity of driving simulator drug research. *Psychopharmacology* 232:2911–2919.

Verster JC, Roth T. 2011. Standard operation procedures for conducting the on-the-road driving test, and measurement of the standard deviation of lateral position (SDLP). *International Journal of General Medicine* 4:359.

———. 2014. Excursions out-of-lane versus standard deviation of lateral position as outcome measure of the on-the-road driving test. *Human Psychopharmacology: Clinical and Experimental* 29:322–329.

Wall ME, Perez-Reyes M. 1981. The metabolism of Δ^9-tetrahydrocannabinol and related cannabinoids in man. *The Journal of Clinical Pharmacology* 21:178S–189S.

Wall ME, Sadler BM, Brine D, Taylor H, Perez-Reyes M. 1983. Metabolism, disposition, and kinetics of delta-9-tetrahydrocannabinol in men and women. *Clinical Pharmacology & Therapeutics* 34:352–363.

Weis F, Beiras-Fernandez A, Sodian R, Kaczmarek I, Reichart B, Beiras A, Schelling G, Kreth S. 2010. Substantially altered expression pattern of cannabinoid receptor 2 and activated endocannabinoid system in patients with severe heart failure. *Journal of Molecular and Cellular Cardiology* 48:1187–1193.

Widman M, Agurell S, Ehrnebo M, Jones G. 1974. Binding of (+)-and (-)-Δ^1-tetrahydrocannabinols and (-)-7-hydroxy-Δ^1-tetrahydrocannabinol to blood cells and plasma proteins in man. *Journal of Pharmacy and Pharmacology* 26:914–916.

Widman M, Nilsson I, Nilsson J, Agurell S, Borg H, Granstrand B. 1973. Plasma protein binding of 7-hydroxy-Δ^1-tetrahydrocannabinol: an active Δ^1-tetrahydrocannabinol metabolite. *Journal of Pharmacy and Pharmacology* 25:453–457.

Wiley JL, Marusich JA, Huffman JW. 2014. Moving around the molecule: relationship between chemical structure and in vivo activity of synthetic cannabinoids. *Life Sciences* 97:55–63.

Wolowich WR, Greif R, Kleine-Brueggeney M, Bernhard W, Theiler L. 2019. Minimal physiologically based pharmacokinetic model of intravenously and orally administered delta-9-tetrahydrocannabinol in healthy volunteers. *European Journal of Drug Metabolism and Pharmacokinetics* 44:691–711.

Ye M, Nagar S, Korzekwa K. 2016. A physiologically based pharmacokinetic model to predict the pharmacokinetics of highly protein-bound drugs and the impact of errors in plasma protein binding. *Biopharmaceutics & Drug Disposition* 37:123–141.

Yeh H-C, Lin Y-S, Kuo C-C, Weidemann D, Weaver V, Fadrowski J, Neu A, Navas-Acien A. 2015. Urine osmolality in the US population: implications for environmental biomonitoring. *Environmental Research* 136:482–490.

Zhang L, Beal SL, Sheiner LB. 2003. Simultaneous vs. sequential analysis for population PK/PD data I: best-case performance. *Journal of Pharmacokinetics and Pharmacodynamics* 30:387–404.

Zhou H. 2003. Pharmacokinetic strategies in deciphering atypical drug absorption profiles. *The Journal of Clinical Pharmacology* 43:211–227.

Zhu H-J, Wang J-S, Markowitz JS, Donovan JL, Gibson BB, Gefroh HA, DeVane CL. 2006. Characterization of P-glycoprotein inhibition by major cannabinoids from marijuana. *Journal of Pharmacology and Experimental Therapeutics* 317:850–857.

Index

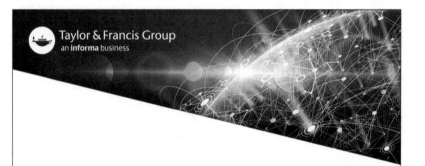